Mathematics  FOR THE
Clinical Laboratory

FOURTH
EDITION

Mathematics FOR THE Clinical Laboratory

Lorraine J. Doucette, MS, MLS(ASCP)CM

MLS Program Director

Department of Medical and Research Technology

University of Maryland School of Medicine

Baltimore, Maryland

Former Academic Chair, MLT, MLA and Phlebotomy Programs

Anne Arundel Community College

Arnold, Maryland

ELSEVIER

Elsevier
3251 Riverport Lane
St. Louis, Missouri 63043

Notice

Practitioners and researchers must always rely on their own experience and knowledge in evaluating and using any information, methods, compounds or experiments described herein. Because of rapid advances in the medical sciences, in particular, independent verification of diagnoses and drug dosages should be made. To the fullest extent of the law, no responsibility is assumed by Elsevier, authors, editors or contributors for any injury and/or damage to persons or property as a matter of products liability, negligence or otherwise, or from any use or operation of any methods, products, instructions, or ideas contained in the material herein.

Previous editions copyrighted 2016, 2011, and 1997.

Library of Congress Control Number: 2020936800

Executive Content Strategists: Jamie L. Blum
Content Development Specialist: Sara Watkins
Publishing Services Manager: Shereen Jameel
Senior Project Manager: Karthikeyan Murthy
Book Designer: Margaret Reid

Printed in India

Last digit is the print number: 9 8 7 6 5 4

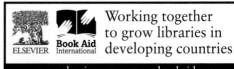

Reviewers

Mary Ruth Beckham, MEd, MT(ASCP)
Director, Program in Clinical Laboratory
  Science
Baylor, Scott & White Health
Temple, Texas

**Mary Coleman, MS, MLS(ASCP)^{CM},
SH(ASCP)^{CM}, CG(ASCP)^{CM}**
Assistant Professor
Department of Medical Laboratory Science
University of North Dakota
Grand Forks, North Dakota

Katherine Davis, MS, MT(ASCP), CLS
CLS Program Director, Assistant Professor
Loma Linda University—School of Allied
  Health Professions
Loma Linda, California

Angelique Decatur, BS, BA, CPhT
Senior Technician Instructor
Everest Colleges—School of Allied Health
Denver, Colorado

Marcella Fickbohm, MS, MT(ASCP)
Medical Laboratory Technology Program
  Coordinator
Manhattan Area Technical College
Manhattan, Kansas

Shawn Marie Froelich, MS, MLS(ASCP)^{CM}
Clinical Coordinator, Assistant Professor
Medical Laboratory Science
Allen College — UnityPoint Health
Waterloo, Iowa

Virginia Haynes, MS, MLS(ASCP)
MLT Program Director
Lake Superior College
Duluth, Minnesota

Debbie Heinritz, MS, MLS(ASCP)^{CM}
MLT Program Director
Health Sciences and Education
Northeast Wisconsin Technical College
Green Bay, Wisconsin

Susan A.K. Higgins, MS, MT(ASCP)SC
Program Director, Clinical Laboratory
  Sciences
Indian Hills Community College
Ottumwa, Iowa

Rory Huschka, MEd, MT(ASCP)
Associate Professor
DeVry University
Phoenix, Arizona

Amy Kapanka, MS, MT(ASCP)SC
MLT Program Director, Professor
MLT Program
Hawkeye Community College
Waterloo, Iowa

Patricia Kelly, MBA, MT(AMT)(ASCP)BB
Dean of Health Sciences
Mississippi Delta Community College
Moorhead, Mississippi

Preface

Mathematics has a reputation as a subject that is difficult to understand and utilize. This perception may lead students to avoid careers that rely on mathematics even if they enjoy science in general. That is unfortunate, because solving mathematical problems should not be a barrier to a career choice.

Students who do not feel comfortable with math may struggle with the math that is associated with the clinical laboratory. This book is written with those students in mind. It will also benefit the student who is comfortable with math, the laboratory professional who may need some review of math concepts, and staff in the physician office laboratory (POL) or clinic who may not have been formally taught any laboratory math.

ORGANIZATION

Content is divided into three sections, beginning with a review of math and calculation basics, followed by coverage of particular areas of the clinical laboratory (including immunohematology and microbiology), and ending with statistical calculations. There is a new section that contains calculations that are not commonly performed in a typical clinical laboratory but may be still taught to students.

Readers who are already proficient in basic mathematics may want to review the introductory chapters quickly and then proceed to the chapters focusing on clinical laboratory skills.

DISTINCTIVE FEATURES OF THIS BOOK

Readers will find recurring margin notes indicating WHAT and HOW of important information. These margin notes guide the reader through the process of identifying in which situation each formula should be used and how to correctly analyze the outcome.

Readers will also notice that the answer for each problem is marked in **boldface** to aid in following the steps used in calculating the unknown. When appropriate, the unknown value to be determined will be noted as a bold-faced green X. As the calculation proceeds step by step, the green boldface will be used to highlight the progress of the calculation.

Examples of calculations for each type of math concept are worked out in a step-by-step manner. A substantial set of practice problems is included in each chapter.

NEW FEATURES INCLUDE:

- A full-color design with a more accessible look and feel.
- Topical margin notes that indicate WHAT and HOW, linking each math concept with its implementation.
- The topics of molarity and normality, and calculations associated with solutions combined into one chapter for a more cohesive presentation.

- A new chapter that includes calculations performed by students but not frequently found in the clinical laboratory.
- A glossary with definitions of important mathematical terms.
- A Greek symbol appendix for quick reference.

EVOLVE RESOURCES

http://evolve.elsevier.com/Doucette/math/

For Students:
- Glossary
- Practice Problems plus Answers

For Instructors:
- Image Collection
- PPT Slides
- Test Bank (not in ExamView)

NOTE TO THE STUDENT

Congratulations on deciding to become a valuable member of the healthcare team as a clinical laboratory professional! Enjoy the sense of accomplishment that will come with learning and performing the math that is essential for accurate and precise laboratory results. Remember, this book will be a valuable resource and companion well into your career.

Welcome to the profession of clinical laboratory science!

Acknowledgements

I would like to thank my family and friends, especially my sons, Steven and Kenneth, who provided love and support to me, as well as my mother who is my inspiration for how to live life to its fullest. It has been a journey for me through the years from when I wrote my first edition in 1997 when my sons were still in grade school to now as they have grown into fine, young men. I lost my husband in 2007 and worked on the second book in the months following his death of complications from kidney failure that began with strep throat at age 9 and ended with peritonitis by *C. difficile* at age 52. I wrote the third edition in a very different emotional place, but I have grown from that experience while I wrote my fourth edition.

I would like to thank laboratory professionals in general for their hard work and dedication to their profession as well as students of clinical laboratory science who use this book to help them learn laboratory mathematics concepts. And last, I would like to thank the staff at Elsevier for helping to make this fourth edition a reality.

Lorraine J. Doucette, MS, MLS(ASCP)^{CM}
MLS Program Director
Department of Medical and Research Technology
University of Maryland School of Medicine
Baltimore, Maryland
Former Academic Chair, MLT, MLA and Phlebotomy Programs
Anne Arundel Community College
Arnold, Maryland

Contents

CHAPTER 1

Basic Arithmetic, Rounding Numbers, and Significant Figures

OBJECTIVES

At the end of this chapter, the reader should be able to do the following:

1. Perform basic arithmetic calculations, including addition, subtraction, multiplication, and division with positive and negative numbers.
2. Perform calculations that require multiple steps in the correct order.
3. Convert fractions to their lowest equivalent form.
4. Perform calculations involving fractions using ratio and proportion.
5. Convert numbers between their percentage and decimal forms.
6. State the rules for rounding numbers in the following situations:

    a. The number to be rounded ends in a number less than 5.
    b. The number to be rounded ends in a number greater than 5.
    c. The number to be rounded ends in 5.
7. State the rules for addition, subtraction, multiplication, and division using significant figures.
8. Perform calculations (incorporating rounding numbers), including addition, subtraction, multiplication, and division to achieve the correct result.
9. Determine the number of significant figures that are in a number.

BASIC ARITHMETIC

This chapter as well as Chapters 2 and 3 are designed as a review of basic mathematical concepts. Students already proficient in these concepts may wish to briefly review them and begin at Chapter 4. Note: Significant figures are not used in Examples 1-1 through 1-16g.

WHAT   **Positive and Negative Numbers**

A positive number is a number that has a value greater than zero; a negative number is a number with a value less than zero. Figure 1-1 is a number line that demonstrates this concept. A plus sign $(+)$ is used to identify a positive number, and a negative, or minus, sign $(-)$ is used to identify a negative number. If only positive numbers are used in an equation, the $(+)$ sign is usually omitted.

WHAT   **Addition of Positive Numbers**

The sum of two or more positive numbers will also be a positive number:

$$(+13) + (+16) + (+22) = +51$$
$$(+12) + (+4) = +16$$
$$(+6) + (+5) + (+28) + (+32) = +71$$
$$(+4) + (+3) + (+3) + (+2) = +12$$

HOW   *Example 1-1*

What is the sum of $+64$ and $+45$?
    Because both numbers are a positive number, the sum will also be a positive number. Therefore, the sum of $+64$ and $+45$ is $+109$.

Example 1-1a   What is the sum of $+45$ and $+38$?

          The sum of these numbers is $+83$.

Example 1-1b   What is the sum of $+105$ and $+107$?

          The sum of these numbers is $+212$.

Example 1-1c   What is the sum of $+3$ and $+86$?

          The sum of these numbers is $+89$.

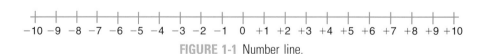

FIGURE 1-1 Number line.

HOW   *Example 1-2*

What is the sum of $+22$, $+37$, $+61$, $+18$, and $+44$?

The sum of this group of numbers will also be a positive number and is determined by simple addition:

$$(+22) + (+37) + (+61) + (+18) + (+44) = +182$$

Therefore, the sum of this group of numbers is $+182$.

Example 1-2a   Using Example 1-2 as a guide, what is the sum of $+2$, $+8$, $+11$, and $+23$?

The sum of this group of numbers is $+44$.

Example 1-2b   Using Example 1-2 as a guide, what is the sum of $+45$, $+83$, $+37$, $+75$, and $+105$?

The sum of this group of numbers is $+345$.

Example 1-2c   Using Example 1-2 as a guide, what is the sum of $+71$, $+16$, $+38$, and $+104$?

The sum of this group of numbers is $+229$.

WHAT   Addition of Negative Numbers

The sum of two or more negative numbers will also be a negative number. That is because when two or more negative numbers are added together, they stay on the left (or negative) side of the number line, and the sum will always be a negative number.

$$(-5) + (-14) + (-2) = -21$$
$$(-7) + (-32) + (-18) = -57$$

HOW   *Example 1-3*

What is the sum of -17 and -38?

Remember: The sum of two negative numbers will be a negative number.

$$(-17) + (-38) = -55$$

Therefore, the sum of these two negative numbers is -55.

Example 1-3a   Using Example 1-3 as a guide, what is the sum of -2 and -7?

The sum of these numbers is -9.

Example 1-3b   Using Example 1-3 as a guide, what is the sum of -15 and -65?

The sum of these numbers is -80.

Example 1-3c   Using Example 1-3 as a guide, what is the sum of -14 and -55?

The sum of these numbers is -69.

Example 1-3d   Using Example 1-3 as a guide, what is the sum of the following group of numbers?

$$-6, -2, -3, -9$$

The sum of this group of numbers is determined by simple addition:

$$(-6) + (-2) + (-3) + (-9) = -20$$

Therefore, the sum of this group of numbers is -20.

Example 1-3e   Using Example 1-3 as a guide, what is the sum of -10, -18, -42, and -11?

The sum of this group of numbers is -81.

Example 1-3f   Using Example 1-3 as a guide, what is the sum of -59, -48, -62, and -12?

The sum of this group of numbers is -181.

Example 1-3g   Using Example 1-3 as a guide, what is the sum of -30, -18, -13, -26, and -84?

The sum of this group of numbers is -171.

WHAT   Addition of Both Positive and Negative Numbers

The sum of an addition of both positive and negative numbers will be the sign of the larger number involved in the addition. If you think of the numbers on the number line as players in a "tug of war" game (Figure 1-2), the larger number will be able to pull the smaller number to the sign direction of the larger number; that is, if the larger number is positive, the smaller number is pulled to the positive direction. When a negative number is added to a positive number, it is actually subtracted from the positive number. For example: What is the sum of -23 and $+12$? Because the larger number is a negative number, the sum will have a negative number. By convention, when placing the numbers in correct order to perform the calculation, the

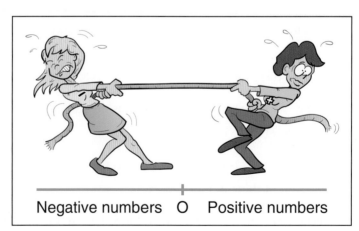

FIGURE 1-2 "Tug of war" between the positive and negative sides of the number line. (This figure was published in Doucette: *Basic Mathematics for the Health-Related Professions*, p. 18, copyright Elsevier, 2000.)

positive number is listed first, followed by the negative number. The negative number is actually subtracted from the positive number to arrive at the sum.

$$+12 - 23 = -11$$

The sum of these two numbers is -11, a negative number.

HOW **Example 1-4**

What is the sum of $+31$ and -65?

When presented with an equation that contains both positive and negative numbers, first list the numbers in the equation so that the positive number(s) are listed first, followed by the negative number(s):

$$(+31) + (-65)$$

Then, solve the equation:

$$(+31) + (-65) = X$$
$$31 - 65 = -34$$

In this equation, the negative number was larger than the positive number, leading to the sum being a negative number. Remember: Think of the numbers as being a "tug of war." The sign of the larger number will determine the sign of the final sum (see Figure 1-2). In this example, since the number -65 is a larger number than $+31$, the final sum of 34 is a negative number (i.e., -34).

Example 1-4a Using Example 1-4 as a guide, what is the sum of -17 and $+41$?

The sum is $+24$ because the equation is set up as $+41 - 17 = X$.

Example 1-4b Using Example 1-4 as a guide, what is the sum of -32 and $+14$?

The sum is -18 because the equation is set up as $+14 - 32 = X$.

Example 1-4c Using Example 1-4 as a guide, what is the sum of -8 and $+3$?

The sum is -5 because the equation is set up as $+3 - 8 = X$.

Example 1-4d Using Example 1-4 as a guide, what is the sum of the following group of numbers?

$$-79, +11, -15, +43$$

When performing a calculation with both positive and negative numbers, always list the positive numbers first, followed by the negative numbers.

$$+11, +43, -79, -15$$

Then, determine the sum of the positive numbers:

$$+11 + 43 = +54$$

Next, determine the sum of the negative numbers:

$$-79 + -15 = -94$$

Last, set up the final equation of the sums of the positive and negative numbers:

$$(+54) + (-94) = X$$

Now solve for X:

$$54 - 94 = X$$
$$X = -40$$

Example 1-4e   Using Example 1-4d as a guide, what is the sum of the following group of numbers: $-66, -92, +83, +12$?

The sum of this group of numbers is -63 because first determine the sum of the positive numbers, or $+83 + 12 = +95$. Next, determine the sum of the negative numbers, or $-66 + -92 = -158$. Then, subtract -158 from $+95$ or $95 - 158 = X$, which equals -63.

Example 1-4f   Using Examples 1-4d and 1-4e as a guide, what is the sum of the following group of numbers: $-21, +5, +8, -4$?

The sum of this group of numbers is -12.

WHAT   ## Subtraction of Two or More Positive Numbers

If the difference is greater than zero, it remains a positive number. However, if a larger positive number is subtracted from a smaller positive number, the difference will have a value less than zero and will be a negative number.

HOW   ***Example 1-5***

What is the answer to the following equation?

$$(+34) - (+5) = X$$

The answer can be found using simple subtraction.

$$(+34) - (+5) = +29$$

The answer, $+29$, is a positive number, since it has a value greater than zero.

Example 1-5a   Using Example 1-5 as a guide, what is the answer to the following equation?

$$(+59) - (+29) = X$$

$59 - 29 = +30$, a positive number, since 29 is less than 59.

Example 1-5b   Using Example 1-5 as a guide, what is the answer to the following equation?

$$(+18) - (+4) = X$$

$(+18) - (+4) = +14$, a positive number, since 18 is a larger number than 4.

Example 1-5c Using Example 1-5 as a guide, what is the answer to the following equation?

$$(+101) - (+82) = X$$

$(+101) - (+82) = +19$, a positive number, since 101 is greater than 82.

Example 1-5d Using Example 1-5 as a guide, what is the answer to this equation?

$$(+56) - (+75) = X$$

Using simple subtraction:

$$56 - 75 = X$$

$X = -19$, a negative number, since 75 is greater than 56.

Example 1-5e Using Example 1-5 as a guide, what is the answer to this equation?

$$(+12) - (+38) = X$$

The answer is -26, since 38 is greater than 12.

Example 1-5f Using Example 1-5 as a guide, what is the answer to this equation?

$$(+55) - (+75) = X$$

The answer is -20, since 75 is greater than 55.

Example 1-5g Using Example 1-5 as a guide, what is the answer to this equation?

$$(+3) - (+7) = X$$

The answer is -4, since 7 is greater than 3.

WHAT Subtraction of Two or More Negative Numbers

When two negative numbers are subtracted from each other, the remainder remains negative as long as it is less than zero. However, as with positive numbers, if a larger negative number is subtracted from a smaller negative number, the difference will have a value greater than zero and be a positive number. Refer to the number line in Figure 1-1. This is because when a negative number is subtracted from a positive or negative number, it is actually added to the positive or negative number because of the following rule:

Two Negatives Rule
Two negatives become a positive (Figure 1-3).
    Whether the final result is a positive or negative number depends on how much "pull" there is on the number line by the numbers in the equation.

HOW Example 1-6

Solve the following equation:

$$(-53) - (-11) = X$$

In this equation, because the negative 11 is being subtracted from the negative 53, the double negatives convert to a positive (+) sign for the number 11.

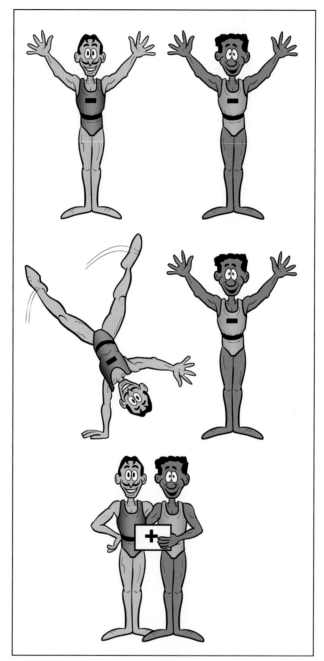

FIGURE 1-3 Two negatives become a positive. (This figure was published in Doucette: *Basic Mathematics for the Health-Related Professions*, p. 24, copyright Elsevier, 2000.)

$$(-53) + 11 = X$$

This equation can be rearranged to have the positive number listed first:

$$11 - 53 = X$$
$$X = -42$$

The final answer is still a negative number because the (-11) did not have enough "pull" to pull the final result into the positive numbers.

Example 1-6a   Using Example 1-6 as guide, solve the following equation:

$$(-21) - (-23) = X$$

Again, because two negatives make a positive, the sign associated with the number 23 is changed to a positive:

$$(-21) + (23) = X$$

The equation can be rearranged so that the positive number is listed first:

$$23 - 21 = X$$
$$X = +2$$

In this case, the final result is a positive number because the number 23 had enough "pull" to pull the final result over the zero value in the number line.

Example 1-6b   Using Example 1-6 as a guide, what is the answer to the following problem?

$$(-9) - (-5) = X$$

The problem is rearranged to be:

$$5 - 9 = X$$
$$X = -4$$

Example 1-6c   Using Example 1-6 as a guide, what is the answer to the following problem?

$$(-32) - (-37) = X$$

Again, by rearranging the problem:

$$37 - 32 = X$$
$$X = +5$$

WHAT **Subtraction of a Positive Number From a Negative Number**

When a positive number is subtracted from a negative number, it is actually ADDED to the negative number.

HOW   ***Example 1-7***

Solve the following equation:

$$(-42) - (+15) = X$$

The number 15 is added to the 42 to have a final answer of -57.

Example 1-7a   Using Example 1-7 as a guide, solve the following equation:

$$-85 - (+42) = X$$
$$X = -127$$

Example 1-7b   Using Example 1-7 as a guide, solve the following equation:

$$(-124) - (+135) = X$$
$$X = -259$$

Example 1-7c   Using Example 1-7 as a guide, solve the following equation:

$$(-38) - (+17) = X$$
$$X = -55$$

WHAT   ## Subtraction of a Negative Number From a Positive Number

When a negative number is subtracted from a positive number, it is actually added to the positive number becase of the Two Negatives Rule (two negatives make a positive).

HOW   ***Example 1-8***

Solve the following equation:

$$(+40) - (-15) = X$$
$$X = +55$$

The result is a positive number, 55.

Example 1-8a   Using Example 1-8 as a guide, solve the following equation:

$$(+15) - (-13) = X$$
$$X = +28$$

Example 1-8b   Using Example 1-8 as a guide, solve the following equation:

$$(+26) - (-16) = X$$
$$X = +42$$

Example 1-8c   Using Example 1-8 as a guide, solve the following equation:

$$(+82) - (-9) = X$$
$$X = +91$$

WHAT   **Multiplication or Division of Two or More Positive Numbers**

When two or more positive numbers are multiplied or divided, the result will be a positive number.

HOW   ***Example 1-9***

Solve the following equation:

$$(+14) \times (+2) = X$$

This equation of two positive numbers can be solved using simple multiplication:

$$14 \times 2 = 28$$

The product, 28, is also a positive number.

Example 1-9a   Using Example 1-9 as a guide, what is the product of $(+47) \times (+5)$?

Using simple multiplication, the product is $+235$.

Example 1-9b   Using Example 1-9 as a guide, what is the product of $(+7) \times (+43)$?

Using simple multiplication, the product is $+301$.

Example 1-9c   Using Example 1-9 as a guide, what is the product of $(+24) \times (+8)$?

Using simple multiplication, the product is $+192$.

Example 1-9d   Using Example 1-9 as a guide, solve the following equation:

$$+20 \div +4 = X \text{ OR } \frac{20}{4} = X$$

This is solved by simple division arithmetic:

$$X = +5$$

Example 1-9e   Using Example 1-9d as a guide, solve the following equation:

$$+72 \div +6 = X$$
$$X = +12$$

Example 1-9f   Using Example 1-9d as a guide, solve the following equation:

$$+50 \div +10 = X$$
$$X = +5$$

Example 1-9g   Using Example 1-9d as a guide, solve the following equation:

$$+24 \div +3 = X$$
$$\mathbf{X} = +8$$

WHAT   ## Multiplication or Division of Two or More Negative Numbers

When two or more negative numbers are multiplied or divided, the result will be a positive number.

HOW   ***Example 1-10***

Solve the following equation:

$$(-15) \times (-3) = X$$

This is solved by simple multiplication arithmetic:

$$\mathbf{X} = +45$$

Example 1-10a   Using Example 1-10 as a guide, solve the following equation:

$$(-55) \times (-6) = X$$
$$\mathbf{X} = +330$$

Example 1-10b   Using Example 1-10 as a guide, solve the following equation:

$$(-130) \times (-17) = X$$
$$\mathbf{X} = +2,210$$

Example 1-10c   Using Example 1-10 as a guide, solve the following equation:

$$(-8) \times (-23) = X$$
$$\mathbf{X} = +184$$

Example 1-10d   Using Example 1-10 as a guide, solve the following equation:

$$-45 \div -5 = \mathbf{X} \quad \text{OR} \quad \frac{-45}{-5} = X$$

This is solved by simple arithmetic:

$$\mathbf{X} = +9$$

Example 1-10e   Using Example 1-10d as a guide, solve the following equation:

$$-68 \div -4 = X$$
$$\mathbf{X} = +17$$

Example 1-10f   Using Example 1-10d as a guide, solve the following equation:

$$-56 \div -8 = X$$
$$\mathbf{X} = +7$$

Example 1-10g   Using Example 1-10d as a guide, solve the following equation:

$$-55 \div -11 = X$$
$$\mathbf{X} = +5$$

WHAT   Multiplication or Division of Negative and Positive Numbers

The result of a mixture of both positive and negative numbers in both multiplication or division calculations will always be a negative number.

HOW   Example 1-11

Solve the following equation:

$$(-45) \times (+4) = X$$

This is a simple multiplication problem. Remember that the final result will be a negative number.

$$X = -180$$

Example 1-11a   Using Example 1-11 as a guide, what is the product of -16 and $+14$?

The product is -224.

Example 1-11b   Using Example 1-11 as a guide, what is the product of $+15$ and -6?

The product is -90.

Example 1-11c   Using Example 1-11 as a guide, what is the product of -34 and $+9$?

The product is -306.

Example 1-11d   Using Example 1-11 as a guide, solve the following equation:

$$(-28) \div (+4) = X$$

This equation can be solved by simple division; however, remember the final result will be a negative number.

$$(-28) \div (+4) = -7$$

Therefore, the result of this equation is -7.

Example 1-11e   Using Example 1-11d as a guide, solve the following equation:

$$(-60) \div (+5) = X$$
$$X = -12$$

Example 1-11f   Using Example 1-11d as a guide, solve the following equation:

$$(-75) \div (+5) = X$$
$$X = -15$$

Example 1-11g   Using Example 1-11d as a guide, solve the following equation:

$$(-192) \div (+12) = X$$
$$X = -16$$

WHAT   ## Order of Calculations

When an equation contains numbers within parentheses, the calculation within the parenthesis is performed first. For example, the equation $23 + (43 \times 3)$ is solved by first performing the calculation within the parenthesis. The equation then becomes $23 + 129$. The sum of this simple addition problem is 152.

HOW   ***Example 1-12***

Solve the following problem:

$$45 + (11 \times 10) = X$$

First solve what is in the parentheses:

$$(11 \times 10) = 110$$

Next add 110 to 45:

$$45 + 110 = 155$$
$$X = 155$$

Example 1-12a   Using Example 1-12 as a guide, solve the following problem:

$$2 + (9 \times 3) = X$$
$$X = 29$$

Example 1-12b   Using Example 1-12 as a guide, solve the following problem:

$$16 - (2 \times 5) = X$$
$$X = 6$$

Example 1-12c   Using Example 1-12 as a guide, solve the following problem:

$$42 \times (2 \times 5) = X$$
$$X = 420$$

Example 1-12d   Now that you have mastered equations within parentheses, solve the following problem:

$$350 \div [4.0 + (275 \div 5.0)] = X$$

In this example, first solve the division calculation within the parentheses:

$$(275 \div 5.0) = 55$$

Next, solve the equation within the brackets:

$$[4.0 + (55)] = 59$$

Now, solve for X:

$$350 \div 59 = X$$
$$X = 5.9$$

Example 1-12e   Using Example 1-12d as a guide, solve the following problem:

$$125 \div [82 - (70 \div 7.0)] = X$$
$$X = 1.7$$

Example 1-12f   Using Example 1-12d as a guide, solve the following problem:

$$40 + [25 + (3 \times 15)] = X$$
$$X = 110$$

WHAT   Fractions

A fraction is a mathematical way to represent the amount of "parts" within a number or substance. The top number, called the numerator, represents the "part"; the bottom number of the fraction, called the denominator, represents the entire amount of parts. For example, a pizza can be cut into four equal slices, or that same pizza can be cut into eight equal slices, each of which would be half as wide as the four slices (Figure 1-4). If the pizza was cut into four equal slices and you ate one of the slices, then you ate one of the four slices of pizza or ¼ of the pizza (Figure 1-5).

HOW   *Example 1-13*

Using the pizza example in Figure 1-4, what fraction would be made if two slices were eaten?
The 2 becomes the numerator, and the 4 becomes the denominator:

$$X = 2/4 \text{ or equivalent fraction } {}^{1}\!/_{2}$$

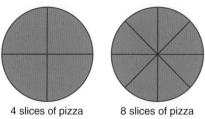

4 slices of pizza   8 slices of pizza

FIGURE 1-4 (A) Four slices of pizza. (B) Eight slices of pizza.

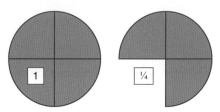

1   ¼

FIGURE 1-5 (A) One whole, (B) ¼.

Example 1-13a   Using Example 1-13 as a guide, if you ate three pieces of the pizza, what fraction would be made?

$$X = {}^3\!/_4$$

Example 1-13b   Using Example 1-13 as a guide, if you ate all four slices of the pizza, what fraction would be made?

$$X = 4/4 \text{ or equivalent of } 1.0$$

WHAT *Equivalent Fractions*

If the pizza discussed in Example 1-13 was cut into 8 equal slices (Figure 1-5; see Figure 1-4), and you ate two of them, then you also ate $^1\!/_4$ of the pizza (or $^2\!/_8$, which can be reduced to $^1\!/_4$). Typically, fractions are written so that the numerator is equal to or as close to 1.0 as possible. Therefore, $^2\!/_8$ becomes $^1\!/_4$, $^2\!/_6$ becomes $^1\!/_3$, $^{10}\!/_{100}$ becomes $^1\!/_{10}$, and so forth. These new fractions are called equivalent fractions because the actual overall concentration is the same. Fractions are reduced to their lowest equivalent fraction by using division and algebra.

HOW *Example 1-14*

Reduce the fraction $^5\!/_{100}$ to its lowest equivalent fraction.

The numerator of a fraction should be as close to 1.0 as possible. A shortcut way is to divide the denominator, 100, by the numerator value 5 to obtain the equivalent fraction $^1\!/_{20}$. To check the accuracy of your calculation, multiply both sides of the new fraction by 5—that is, $^5\!/_5 \times {}^1\!/_{20}$—and the original fraction of $^5\!/_{100}$ can be obtained.

Algebra can also be used, especially when the numerator does not divide easily into the denominator. Using Example 1-14 and algebra, the following equation is constructed:

$$1/X = 5/100$$

Crossmultiplying both sides yields $(1)(100) = (5)X$:

$$100 = 5X$$
$$100/5 = X$$
$$20 = X$$

Therefore, $5/100 = 1/20$.

HOW

Example 1-14a   Using Example 1-14 as a guide, reduce the fraction $4/80$ to its lowest equivalent fraction.

The fraction $4/80$ can be reduced to its equivalent fraction of $1/20$.

Example 1-14b   Using Example 1-14 as a guide, reduce the fraction $2/6$ to its lowest equivalent fraction.

The fraction $2/6$ can be reduced to its equivalent fraction of $1/3$.

Example 1-14c   Using Example 1-14 as a guide, reduce the fraction $4/100$ to its lowest equivalent fraction.

The fraction $4/100$ can be reduced to its equivalent fraction of $1/25$

WHAT   ## Ratio and Proportion With Fractions

From the pizza discussion in Example 1-13 and Figures 1-4 through 1-6, the fractions can also be thought of as ratios of the number of pizza slices to the amount of pizza slices that were cut. For example, eating one slice of pizza out of a pizza cut into four slices is a 1:4 ratio. Ratios are written with a colon separating the part from the whole. This same ratio can be written as the fraction $1/4$.

Many calculations in the laboratory use the concept of ratio and proportion. This concept will also be covered in Chapter 4. Whenever a different quantity, but NOT different concentration of a substance, is required, ratio and proportion calculations are performed. A ratio represents the relationship of one value to another. A 1:1 ratio represents an equal relationship as shown in Example 1-13b, where all four slices were eaten from a pizza cut into four slices. The fraction $4/4$ is equal to a 1:1 ratio whereas a 1:4 ratio means that one value (the pizza cut into four slices) is four times that of the other (an individual slice).

Ratio and proportion are used when a new quantity of a substance is required, and are based on an existing ratio. Examples 1-14 and 1-14a through 1-14c demonstrated how to reduce a fraction to its lowest equivalent form. When performing additions and subtractions of fractions,

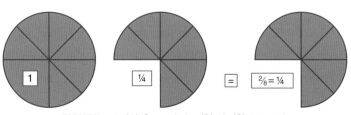

FIGURE 1-6 (A) One whole, (B) ¼, (C) $2/8 = 1/4$.

the denominators of each fraction must be the same value. By using ratio and proportion an equivalent fraction can be determined.

Example 1-15

Calculate the sum of the following fractions:

$$\frac{1}{8} + \frac{2}{8} + \frac{2}{4} = X$$

Because the denominators all need to be of the same value, $2/4$ must be converted to its equivalent with a denominator of 8 by the following equation:

$$(\text{Old fraction})\frac{2}{4} = \frac{X}{8}(\text{New fraction})$$

By crossmultiplying the numerator of $2/4$ with the denominator of $X/8$ and the denominator of $2/4$ with the numerator of $X/8$, the equation can be solved:

$$(2)(8) = (X)(4)$$
$$16 = (4)(X)$$

By multiplying both sides of the equation by $1/4$, the equation becomes:

$$\frac{16}{4} = X$$
$$4 = X$$

Thus, $2/4$ is equivalent to $4/8$.

Another way to solve this equation is to multiply both sides of the initial equation by 8:

$$\frac{8}{1} \times \frac{2}{4} = \frac{X}{8} \times \frac{8}{1}$$

The equation then becomes:

$$\frac{16}{4} = \frac{8X}{8}$$

and, by reducing the fractions, the answer is found:

$$4 = X$$

for the equivalent fraction.

Next, complete the addition of all three fractions. Once a set of fractions to be added has the same denominator, simply add the numerators together:

$$\frac{1}{8} + \frac{2}{8} + \frac{4}{8} = X$$
$$\frac{7}{8} = X$$

HOW   ***Example 1-15a***   Using ratio and proportion and Example 1-15 as a guide, what is the fraction $\frac{1}{5}$ equivalent to with a denominator of 15?

$$\frac{1}{5} = \frac{X}{15}$$

$$(1)(15) = (X)(5)$$

$$15 = (5)(X)$$

$$\frac{15}{5} = X$$

$$X = 3$$

Therefore, the fraction $\frac{1}{5}$ is equivalent to $\frac{3}{15}$.

Example 1-15b   Using Example 1-15 as a guide, what is the fraction $\frac{1}{10}$ equivalent to with a denominator of 1000?

The fraction $\frac{1}{10}$ is equivalent to $\frac{100}{1000}$.

Example 1-15c   Using Example 1-15 as a guide, what is the fraction $\frac{1}{25}$ equivalent to with a denominator of 125?

The fraction $\frac{1}{25}$ is equivalent to $\frac{5}{125}$.

Example 1-15d   Using Example 1-15 as a guide, what is the fraction $\frac{1}{3}$ equivalent to with a denominator of 24?

The fraction $\frac{1}{3}$ is equivalent to $\frac{8}{24}$.

WHAT   ***Multiplication and Division of Fractions***

Multiplication of Fractions. When multiplying two or more fractions, the numerators are multiplied together and the denominators are multiplied together.

Example 1-16

What is the product of $\frac{2}{5} \times \frac{1}{10}$?
   The product is determined by multiplying the numerators of each fraction ($2 \times 1 = 2$) followed by multiplying the denominators of each fraction ($5 \times 10 = 50$) to form the product $\frac{2}{50}$, or its reduced form $\frac{1}{25}$.

Example 1-16a   What is the product of $\frac{1}{3} \times 1\frac{5}{8}$?

To solve this problem, first convert the mixed fraction of $1\frac{5}{8}$ into its fraction form. This is done by multiplying the denominator 8 by the whole number 1 and adding that to the numerator to form the equivalent fraction of $\frac{13}{8}$. Next multiply $\frac{13}{8}$ and $\frac{1}{3}$. The product is $\frac{13}{24}$.

Example 1-16b   Using Example 1-16 as a guide, what is the product of $\frac{7}{8} \times \frac{4}{6}$?

The product is $\frac{28}{48}$, reduced to $\frac{7}{12}$.

Example 1-16c   Using Example 1-16a as a guide, what is the product of $1^{3}/4 \times 1^{1}/4$?

The product is $^{35}/4$, reduced to $8^{3}/4$.

Division of Fractions. Division problems have three terms: the dividend (which is the number that is being divided), the divisor (the number that is being used to divide the dividend), and the answer or quotient. When dividing fractions, the divisor fraction is simply flipped so that the numerator is now the denominator and the denominator is now the numerator. The flipped fraction is then multipled by the dividend fraction to calculate the quotient.

Example 1-17

Divide $^{5}/8$ by $^{1}/4$. The $^{5}/8$ is the dividend and the $^{1}/4$ is the divisor. Therefore, the problem becomes $^{5}/8 \times ^{4}/1 = X$.

$$X = 20/8 \text{ or } 2\,^{4}/8 \text{ or } 2\,^{1}/2$$

Example 1-17a   Using Example 1-17 as a guide, divide $^{6}/32$ by $^{4}/8$.

$$X = 48/128 = 3/8$$

Example 1-17b   Using Example 1-17 as a guide, divide $^{1}/5$ by $^{3}/4$.

$$X = 4/15$$

Example 1-17c   Using Example 1-17 as a guide, divide $^{2}/5$ by $^{1}/4$.

$$X = 1\,^{3}/5 \text{ or } 2\,^{3}/5$$

WHAT **Percents**

The use of percents and percentages in the laboratory is very common. A percent is a fraction with a constant denominator of 100 and is the ratio of the quantity of a substance "per 100" total parts.

Numbers may be written three different ways that all mean the same "per 100" relationship. One way is with the percentage (%) sign. For example, bleach used for decontamination is at a concentration of 10%, or ethanol (EtOH) may be at a concentration of 75%. The 10% bleach is a ratio of 10 parts bleach in 100 total parts. A 70% EtOH solution may be prepared by adding 70 mL absolute (100%) EtOH in a 100-mL volumetric flask and then adding 30 mL of water for the remaining volume. Chapter 5 also has more information on percent calculations.

In the second way, percents can be written as a fraction: 10% bleach could be written as $^{10}/100$.

Some common fractions and their percent forms are:

$$\frac{1}{2} = 50\%$$

$$\frac{1}{4} = 25\%$$

$$\frac{1}{10} = 10\%$$

$$\frac{3}{4} = 75\%$$

The third way is in decimal form: 10% can be written as 0.10, 50% can be written as 0.50, and so forth.

WHAT   # ROUNDING NUMBERS

In the laboratory, the preciseness of a measurement is determined by the rules that guide the use of significant figures and rounding numbers. Significant figures will be discussed in detail later in this chapter. "Rounding off" is the process of removing excess digits from a number so that number has its correct quantity of significant figures. For example, when using a calculator, a result shown on the display may contain many digits, far more than necessary for the equation that was solved. By using the rules for rounding numbers, the digits can be reduced to the correct number of significant figures based on the accuracy of a measurement.

WHAT   ## Rules for Rounding Numbers

1. If the First Digit to Be Dropped Is Less Than 5
If the first digit to be dropped is less than 5, then the last remaining digit stays the same.

HOW   ### Example 1-18

The number 15.683 needs to be rounded from five significant figures to four significant figures. Because the digit to be dropped (3) is less than 5, the last remaining digit, 8, stays the same and the number becomes 15.68.

Example 1-18a   Using Example 1-18 as a guide, round the number 3.654 to three significant figures.

Because the number 4 is less than 5, the last remaining digit stays the same, and the number becomes 3.65.

Example 1-18b   Using Example 1-18 as a guide, round the number 6.43 to two significant figures.

The number becomes 6.4.

Example 1-18c   Using Example 1-18 as a guide, round the number 1.421 to three significant figures.

The number becomes 1.42.

WHAT   **2. If the First Digit to Be Dropped Is Greater Than 5**

If the first digit to be dropped is greater than 5, then the last remaining digit is rounded to the next highest number.

HOW   *Example 1-19*

The number 9.68 needs to be rounded from three significant figures to two significant figures. The number 8 is dropped, and because it is higher than 5, the number 6 is rounded to 7. Thus the final number becomes 9.7.

Example 1-19a   Using Example 1-19 as a guide, round the number 3.469 to three significant figures.

The number becomes 3.47.

Example 1-19b   Using Example 1-19 as a guide, round the number 5.37 to two significant figures.

The number becomes 5.4.

Example 1-19c   Using Example 1-19 as a guide, round the number 13.369 to four significant figures.

The number becomes 13.37.

WHAT   **3. If the First Digit to Be Dropped Is the Number 5**

If the first digit to be dropped is the number 5, the last remaining digit is rounded to the next higher number if it is an ODD number. If the last remaining digit is an EVEN number, it is unchanged because statistically, to do so reduces positive bias in rounding. For this rule, remember the last remaining digit always is or becomes an even number.

HOW   *Example 1-20*

The number 6.35 needs to be rounded from three significant figures to two significant figures. As the last digit is 5, and the preceding digit is an odd number (3), the odd number is rounded to the next even number. Thus the final number becomes 6.4.

Example 1-20a   Using Example 1-20 as a guide, round the number 41.675 to four significant figures.

The number 5 is dropped and the 7, an odd number, becomes an 8. The new number is 41.68.

Example 1-20b   Using Example 1-20 as a guide, round the number 7.435 to three significant figures.

The new number is 7.44.

Example 1-20c   Using Example 1-20 as a guide, round the number 5.35 to two significant figures.

The new number is 5.4.

Example 1-20d   The number 8916.5 has to be rounded from five significant figures to four significant figures. The 5 is dropped, but because the preceding digit, 6, is an even number, it is unchanged. Thus the number becomes 8916, not 8917.

Example 1-20e   Using Example 1-20d as a guide, round the number 12.45 to three significant figures.

The new number becomes 12.4.

Example 1-20f   Using Example 1-20d as a guide, round the number 75.865 to four significant figures.

The new number becomes 75.86.

Example 1-20g   Using Example 1-20d as a guide, round the number 7.125 to three significant figures.

The new number becomes 7.12.

WHAT SIGNIFICANT FIGURES

You've just seen how significant figures impact rounding numbers. But what are significant figures? Significant figures are used in the laboratory to determine the precision of measurements. If your supervisor told you to measure out 30 grams of sodium chloride, you would have to know if you needed to measure 30.0 grams or 30.1 grams or 29.9 grams. With any measurement there is an implied degree of uncertainty to the precision of the measurement. If the length of an instrument was measured to be 23.4 inches long by using a ruler that was only precise to the tenths, then the actual measurement could be anywhere between 23.35 and 23.45 inches long. This concept is called implied uncertainty. By using significant figures, the degree of implied uncertainty of measurements can be established.

In general, the exactness of a group of measurements is dependent on the least exact measurement. For example, if you were given the following volumes of 10.0 mL, 15.85 mL, and 7.775 mL for three different solutions that needed to be added together, the *sum* of these three solutions would not be 33.625 but 33.6. This is because of the three measurements taken, 10.0 mL has the least number of significant figures. You do not know if 10.05 mL instead of 10.0 mL was actually measured. The 10.0 mL measurement is precise only to the first decimal place. Because this measurement is limited in its precision, all other measurements must be limited in their precision as well.

However, in other measurements taken, the measurements may need to be much more precise. In many areas of the laboratory, measurements of solids, such as salts, are commonly taken to the second or third decimal place. Liquids may be measured by use of a graduated cylinder or by weighing. In either case, it is common to have the precision of the measurement determined by use of a decimal point and digits to the right of the decimal point. For example, if 5.75 grams of calcium carbonate ($CaCO_3$) has to be weighed, then the medical laboratory scientist (MLS; also referred to as a medical technologist) or medical laboratory technician (MLT) would know to measure to the hundredth gram.

Another common way to express the precision of a particular number is to use scientific notation. For example, 1000 could be written as 1.0×10^3, or 154,388 could be written as

1.54388×10^5. A number less than 1, such as 0.00465, could be written as 4.65×10^{-3}. In most scientific measurements, scientific notation is used most often because it is the most error-free method to denote precision. You will learn more information about scientific notation in Chapter 2.

WHAT **Working With Significant Figures**

WHAT *Significant Figures and Zeroes*

There are three rules to remember that apply to numbers that contain zeroes when working with significant figures.

WHAT **1. Numbers That Contain Zeroes Within Them.** When a number contains a zero or zeroes as part of that number, the zero or zeroes are considered to be significant to that number and are never dropped out of the number.

HOW *Example 1-21*

The number 1350723 has seven significant figures. The zero within the number is a significant number because it designates the thousands position. The decimal point after the last 3 (1350723) signifies that the 3 in the ones position is the least significant number and that the precision of this number is to the nearest whole number.

Example 1-21a   Using Example 1-21 as a guide, how many significant figures are in the number 857.0042?

The number 857.0042 has seven significant figures. The two zeroes to the right of the decimal point are significant because they are within the entire number.

Example 1-21b   Using Example 1-21 as a guide, how many significant figures are in the number 501.03?

The number 501.03 contains five significant figures.

Example 1-21c   Using Example 1-21 as a guide, how many significant figures are in the number 1.006?

The number 1.006 contains four significant figures.

WHAT **2. Numbers That Contain Zeroes at the End of the Number.** When a number greater than 1 contains a zero or zeroes at the end of the number, or to the right of the decimal place, the zero or zeroes are considered to be significant.

HOW *Example 1-22*

The number 6300.0 has five significant figures.

Example 1-22a   Using Example 1-22 as a guide, how many significant figures are in the number 310.00?

The number 310.00 contains five significant figures.

Example 1-22b   Using Example 1-22 as a guide, how many significant figures are in the number 47.00?

The number 47.00 contains four significant figures.

Example 1-22c   Using Example 1-22 as a guide, how many significant figures are in the number 34.00?

The number 34.00 contains four significant figures.

WHAT **3. Numbers Less Than 1 That Contain Zeroes to the Right of the Decimal Point.** When a number is less than 1, any zeros that are before or after a decimal point but before the first nonzero number within the number are NOT considered to be significant.

HOW *Example 1-23*

The number 0.00663 has three, not five, significant figures. The two zeroes to the right of the decimal point are not considered significant.

Example 1-23a   Using Example 1-19 as a guide, how many significant figures are in the number 0.037?

The number 0.037 has two significant figures, the 3 and 7.

Example 1-23b   Using Example 1-19 as a guide, how many significant figures are in the number 0.006?

The number 0.006 has one significant figure.

Example 1-23c   Using Example 1-19 as a guide, how many significant figures are in the number 0.0333?

The number 0.0333 has three significant figures.

WHAT *Significant Figures in Addition and Subtraction*
There are rules to use when working with significant figures and performing calculations. For calculations involving addition or subtraction, the sum or difference of a group of numbers cannot be any more precise than the least precise number in the group of numbers that were added or subtracted. The final result of an addition or subtraction problem can only have as many digits to the right of the decimal point as the least precise number involved in the problem.

HOW *Example 1-24*

Solve the following equation with the correct amount of significant figures:

$$
\begin{array}{r}
11.5 \\
14.411 \\
+13.65 \\
\hline
39.561 = 39.6
\end{array}
$$

The answer, 39.6, can only be precise to one digit to the right of the decimal point, which is what is found in the least precise number 11.5.

Example 1-24a   Using Example 1-24 as a guide, solve the following equation with the correct amount of significant figures:

$$
\begin{array}{r}
4.05 \\
+\,4.8 \\
\hline
8.85 = 8.8
\end{array}
$$

The sum is 8.8. The 5 of 8.85 is dropped and the 8 stays the same as it is an even number.

Example 1-24b   Using Example 1-24 as a guide, solve the following equation with the correct amount of significant figures:

$$
\begin{array}{r}
2.77 \\
4.489 \\
+\,15.44 \\
\hline
22.699 = 22.70
\end{array}
$$

The sum is 22.70.

Example 1-24c   Using Example 1-24 as a guide, solve the following equation with the correct amount of significant figures:

$$
\begin{array}{r}
34.654 \\
12.895 \\
+\,4.66 \\
\hline
52.209 = 52.21
\end{array}
$$

The sum is 52.21.

Example 1-24d   Using Example 1-24 as a guide, solve the following equation with the correct amount of significant figures:

$$
\begin{array}{r}
10.233 \\
-\,3.45 \\
\hline
6.783 = 6.78
\end{array}
$$

The result of this equation becomes 6.78, not 6.783, because the least precise number, 3.45, has two digits to the right of the decimal point.

Example 1-24e   Using Example 1-24 as a guide, solve the following equation with the correct amount of significant figures:

$$
\begin{array}{r}
168.314 \\
-\,104.4 \\
\hline
63.914 = 63.9
\end{array}
$$

The result is 63.9.

Example 1-24f   Using Example 1-24 as a guide, solve the following equation with the correct amount of significant figures:

$$\begin{array}{r} 71.27 \\ -\ \ 3.4 \\ \hline 67.87 = 67.9 \end{array}$$

The result is 67.9.

Example 1-24g   Using Example 1-24 as a guide, solve the following equation with the correct amount of significant figures.

$$\begin{array}{r} 450.48 \\ -\ \ 10.4 \\ \hline 440.08 = 440.1 \end{array}$$

The result is 440.1.

WHAT   *Significant Figures in Multiplication and Division*

When performing multiplication and division calculations, the final result cannot contain more significant figures than the number in the calculation with the least number of significant figures.

HOW   **Example 1-25**

$$\begin{array}{r} 4.977 \\ \times 1.83 \\ \hline 9.10791 = 9.11 \end{array}$$

The final answer is 9.11 because 1.83, with three significant figures, is the limiting number.

Example 1-25a   Using Example 1-25 as a guide, determine the product of the following equation:

$$\begin{array}{r} 61.45 \\ \times\ \ \ 2.70 \\ \hline 165.915 = 166 \end{array}$$

The product is 166, with three significant figures.

Example 1-25b   Using Example 1-25 as a guide, determine the product of the following equation:

$$\begin{array}{r} 15.1 \\ \times\ \ 11.5 \\ \hline 173.65 = 174 \end{array}$$

The product is 174, with three significant figures.

Example 1-25c   Using Example 1-25 as a guide, determine the product of the following equation:

$$\begin{array}{r} 245.981 \\ \times\ \ \ 3.456 \\ \hline 850.11033 = 850.1 \end{array}$$

The product is 850.1, with four significant figures.

Example 1-25d   Determine the correct amount of significant figures for this division problem:

$$45.14 \div 8.6 = 5.2488 = 5.2$$

The answer becomes 5.2 because 8.6 has the least number of significant figures.

Example 1-25e   Using Example 1-25d as a guide, solve the following equation:

$$6.28 \div 1.1 = 5.709 = 5.7$$

5.709 becomes 5.7 because 1.1 has two significant figures.

Example 1-25f   Using Example 1-25d as a guide, solve the following equation:

$$8.96 \div 2.1 = 4.267$$

4.267 becomes 4.3 because 2.1 has two significant figures.

Example 1-25g   Using Example 1-25d as a guide, solve the following equation:

$$935.44 \div 15.7 = 59.582$$

59.582 becomes 59.6 because 15.7 has three significant figures.

HOW   EXAMPLE PROBLEMS

This section is designed to be useful to both the student and the laboratory professional. Students can use the additional problems to master the material. The laboratory professional can use the examples as templates for solving laboratory calculations. By finding an example similar to the problem that you need to solve, you can substitute into the equation the numbers appropriate to your calculation.

1. **Q.** What is the sum of +2, +9, and +7?
   A. The sum is +18. The problem is solved using simple addition.

2. **Q.** What is the sum of +14, +32, +53, and +47?
   A. The sum is +146. The problem is solved using simple addition.

3. **Q.** What is the sum of −3, −7, and −4?
   A. The sum is −14. The problem is solved using simple addition. The sum of two or more negative numbers will also be a negative number.

4. **Q.** What is the sum of −61, −25, −35, −83, and −98?
   A. The sum is −302. This calculation is solved similar to Example Problem 3.

5. **Q.** What is the sum of −71 and +14?
   A. The sum is −57. Remember to place the positive number first in the equation, followed by the negative number. Remember also that in an addition equation with a positive and a negative number, the final result will be the sign of the larger number as it "pulls" the smaller number across the number line.

6. **Q.** What is the sum of −11 and +34?
   A. The sum is +23. Refer to Example Problem 5 for details.

7. **Q.** What is the sum of −5, +16, −11, and +13?
   A. The sum is 13. Remember to group all of the positive numbers together first, and then group the negative numbers together. Add the positive numbers, then add the negative numbers together, and finally add the sum of the positive numbers with the sum of the negative numbers to give you the final sum.

$$(+16) + (+13) = +29$$
$$(-5) + (-11) = (-16)$$
$$29 - 16 = 13$$

8. **Q.** What is the difference of $(+6) - (+4)$?
   A. The difference is +2. This is a simple subtraction calculation with positive numbers. $6 - 4 = 2$.

9. **Q.** What is the difference of $(-9) - (+4)$?
   A. The difference is −13. When a positive number is subtracted from a negative number, it is actually added to the negative number.

10. **Q.** What is the difference of $(+6) - (+2)$?
    A. The difference is +4. This is a simple subtraction problem of two positive numbers.

11. **Q.** What is the answer if −20 is subtracted from −45?
    A. The answer is −25. The −20 is actually added to the −45 using the Two Negatives Rule where the negative sign becomes a positive sign.

12. **Q.** What is the answer to the following problem?

$$(65.0) \times (5.00) = X$$

   A. The answer is 325.This is solved as a simple multiplication calculation.

13. **Q.** Solve for X.

$$55 \div 5.0 = X$$

   A. The answer is 11. This is a simple division calculation.

14. **Q.** Solve for X.

$$(-60) \div (-5.0) = X$$

   A. The answer is +12. Remember that when two or more negative numbers are multiplied or divided, the result will be a positive number.

15. Q. Solve for X.

$$7.0 \times (15 \div 3.0) = X$$

   A. When peforming a calculation that includes an internal calculation, always peform the calculation within the parentheses first, followed by the rest of the equation. The answer is 35.

16. Q. Solve for X.

$$316 \div (50 + 9.0) = X$$

   A. The answer is 5.4. This calculation is solved similar to Example Problem 15.

17. Q. What is the name of the number that is in the top part of a fraction?
   A. The numerator is the top number in a fraction.

18. Q. What is the name of the number that is in the bottom part of a fraction?
   A. The denomionator is the bottom number in a fraction.

19. Q. Calculate the lowest equivalent fraction for $^5/15$.
   A. The lowest equivalent fraction is $^1/3$.

20. Q. Calculate the lowest equivalent fraction for $^{10}/70$.
   A. The lowest equivalent fraction is $^1/7$.

21. Q. Solve for X.

$$\frac{4}{5} + \frac{1}{2} = X$$

   A. Remember that the denominators for addition and subtraction calculations must be the same value. The equivalent fractions become $^8/10 + {}^5/10 = {}^{13}/10$ or $1\,^3/10$.

22. Q. Solve for X. Use Example Problem 21 as a guide.

$$\frac{2}{3} + \frac{1}{4} = X$$

   A. $X = {}^{11}/12$.

23. Q. Solve for X. Use Example Problem 21 as a guide.

$$\frac{3}{4} - \frac{4}{8} = X$$

   A. $X = {}^2/8$ or $^1/4$.

24. Q. Solve for X.

$$\frac{4}{5} \times \frac{1}{3} = X$$

   A. The answer is $^4/15$. Remember that when multiplying fractions, the numerators are multiplied together and the denominators are multiplied together.

25. **Q.** Solve for X. Use Example Problem 24 as a guide.

$$\frac{2}{5} \times \frac{3}{4} = X$$

A. X = $^3/_{10}$.

26. **Q.** Solve for X.

$$\frac{6}{7} \div \frac{1}{2} = X$$

A. Remember that in division calculations, the divisor fraction is inverted and the calculation becomes a multiplication problem.

$$\frac{6}{7} \times \frac{2}{1} = X$$

$$X = \frac{12}{7} \text{ or } 1\frac{5}{7}$$

27. **Q.** If 4.863 is to be rounded to only two significant figures, what would the final number become?
    A. The final number would be 4.9. The 3 would be dropped and the 6 would round the number 8 up to 9.

28. **Q.** If 0.95482 is to be rounded to three significant figures, what would the final number become?
    A. The final number would be 0.955. The 2 and 8 would be dropped, and because 8 is more than 5, the 4 is rounded up to 5.

29. **Q.** Given that 7.36 is to be rounded to two significant figures, what would the final number become?
    A. 7.36 would be rounded to 7.4. The 6 is dropped, and as 6 is more than 5, the 3 is changed to the number 4.

30. **Q.** The number 0.928 must be changed to contain only two significant figures. What would the final number become?
    A. The final number would become 0.93. The 8 is dropped, and the 2 rounded to the number 3.

31. **Q.** Given that the number 6.97 is to be rounded to two significant figures, what would that number be?
    A. 6.97 would be rounded to 7.0. The 7 would be dropped, and the 9 rounded to 10. This moves the 6 to become 7.

32. **Q.** If the number 7.35 is to be rounded to two significant figures, what would the final number become?
    A. 7.35 would be rounded to 7.4. Remember that when the digit to be dropped is 5, the preceding digit is rounded up if it is an odd number, but unchanged if it is an even number.

33. **Q.** If the number 0.4845 needs to be rounded to three significant figures, what would the number become?

    A. 0.4845 would become 0.484. The 5 is dropped because only three, not four, significant numbers are needed. However, as the preceding digit is an even number, it remains unchanged.

34. **Q.** The number 3.57 has how many significant figures?

    A. This number has three significant figures and is precise to the $1/100$ place.

35. **Q.** The number 14.067 has how many significant figures?

    A. This number has five significant figures and is precise to the $1/1000$ place.

36. **Q.** How many significant figures are contained in the number 0.00352?

    A. This number has three significant figures. Remember that zeroes that are before or after a decimal point but precede any nonzero numbers are not significant.

37. **Q.** How many significant figures are contained in the number 0.05092?

    A. This number has four significant figures. The zeroes on either side of the decimal point are *not* significant, whereas the zero contained within the number is significant.

38. **Q.** How many significant figures are found in the number 5370.00?

    A. 5370.00 contains six significant figures. The zeroes before and after the decimal point are considered to be significant because they describe the preciseness of this number.

39. **Q.** How many significant figures are in the sum of $15.7 + 12.9$?

    A. The sum, 28.6, has three significant figures. Remember: For calculations involving addition or subtraction, the sum or difference of a group of numbers cannot be any more precise than the least precise number in the group of numbers that were added or subtracted. The final result of an addition or subtraction problem can have as many **digits** to the right of the decimal point as the least precise number involved in the problem.

40. **Q.** The sum of $45.29 + 8.4$ has how many significant figures?

    A. The sum, 53.7, has three significant figures. Remember that the sum of a group of numbers must have the number of digits to the right of the decimal point of the least precise number and cannot be more precise than the least precise number (8.4) in the problem.

41. **Q.** $45.2 - 3.6$ results in an answer with how many significant figures?

    A. The answer, 41.6, contains three significant figures.

42. **Q.** The product of 4.55×8.77 contains how many significant figures?

    A. The product, 39.9, contains three significant figures. Remember that in multiplication, the final product cannot contain more significant figures than the least precise number in the problem.

43. **Q.** How many significant figures does the product of 0.382×0.415 contain?

    A. The product, 0.158, contains three significant figures.

44. **Q.** $592.1 \div 8.7$ results in an answer with how many significant figures?

    A. The answer, 68, contains two significant figures. You may have calculated the answer to be 68.06. Remember that, in division, the final answer cannot contain more significant figures than the least significant number in the problem. Because 8.7 contains two significant figures, the final answer is limited to two significant figures.

PRACTICE PROBLEMS

Solve the following practice problems to further master the material. Answers and explanations to some problems can be found in the Answer Key.

Round the following list of numbers to three significant figures.

1. 0.743

2. 17.33

3. 5.687

4. 5.889

5. 5.558

6. 7.735

7. 2.325

Given the following list of numbers, determine the quantity of significant figures in each number.

8. 751.50

9. 5080

10. 987.441

11. 0.91

12. 0.98260

13. 294.00

Solve the following equations. Correct answers must contain the required quantity of significant figures.

14. $18.2 + 19.8 + 15.97 + 14.1 = ?$

15. $42.5 + 15.99 = ?$

16. $(-5) + (-7) = ?$

17. $(-21.0) + (-32.1) + (-15.0) =$

18. $(-32) + (+25) = ?$

19. $(-14) + (+5) = ?$

20. $(-6) + (+12) = ?$

21. $(-5) + (+14) = ?$

22. $(+32) + (-8) + (+15) + (-7) = ?$

23. $215.947 - 32.22 = ?$

24. $0.066 - 0.003 = ?$

25. $(+47) - (+22) = ?$

26. $(+2) - (+9) = ?$

27. $(-16) - (-12) = ?$

28. $(-5) - (+1) = ?$

29. $(-19) - (+14) = ?$

30. $(-8) - (-5) = ?$

31. $8.555 \times 0.11 = ?$

32. $2.824 \times 8.44 = ?$

33. $(-41) \times (-2.0) = ?$

34. $(-4.20) \times (-11.1) = ?$

35. $(-3) \times (+5) = ?$

36. $(-2.3) \times (+1.1) = ?$

37. $(-3.93) \div (-1.44) = ?$

38. $(-25) \div (-5) = ?$

39. $4.77 \div 0.63 = ?$

40. $5.2 \div 4.1 = ?$

41. $4.1 \times (12.0 \div 8.0) = ?$

42. $15.2 + (41.0 - 23.5) = ?$

Reduce the following fractions to their lowest equivalent forms.

43. $\dfrac{15}{20}$

44. $\dfrac{12}{60}$

45. $\dfrac{4}{8}$

46. $\dfrac{3}{9}$

Solve the following calculations.

47. $\dfrac{2}{9} \times \dfrac{1}{4} = X$

48. $1\dfrac{1}{7} \times \dfrac{1}{2} = X$

49. $\dfrac{3}{8} + \dfrac{3}{5} = X$

50. $\dfrac{5}{8} + \dfrac{1}{4} = X$

51. $\dfrac{3}{8} - \dfrac{1}{5} = X$

52. $\dfrac{5}{7} - \dfrac{1}{2} = X$

53. $\dfrac{1}{2} \div \dfrac{1}{3} = X$

54. $\dfrac{5}{8} \div \dfrac{1}{4} = X$

QUICK NOTES

- The sum of two or more positive numbers will be a **positive number.**
- The sum of two or more negative numbers will be a **negative number.**
- The sum of an addition of both positive and negative numbers will be the sign of the **larger number** involved in the addition. When a negative number is added to a positive number, it is actually **subtracted** from the positive number.
- When subtracting two or more positive numbers, if the difference is greater than zero, it remains a positive number. However, if a larger positive number is subtracted from a smaller positive number, the difference will have a value less than zero and will be a negative number.
- When two negative numbers are subtracted from each other, the remainder remains negative as long as it is less than zero. However, as with positive numbers, if a larger negative number is subtracted from a smaller negative number, the **difference** will have a value greater than zero and be a positive number. Remember the Two Negatives Rule: Two negatives make a positive.
- When a positive number is subtracted from a negative number, it is actually **ADDED** to the negative number.
- When a negative number is subtracted from a positive number, it is actually **ADDED** to the positive number because of the Two Negatives Rule.
- When two or more positive numbers are multiplied or divided, the result will be a **positive number.**
- When two or more negative numbers are multiplied or divided, the result will be a **positive number.**
- When there is a mixture of positive and negative numbers in both multiplication and/or division calculations, the results will always be a **negative number.**
- When a calculation contains numbers within parentheses, always perform the calculation within the parentheses first.
- When rounding numbers, the final number cannot be more precise than the least precise number within the calculation.
- When rounding numbers, if the first digit to be dropped is less than 5, then the last remaining digit stays the same.
- When rounding numbers, if the first digit to be dropped is greater than 5, then the last remaining digit is rounded up to the next highest number.
- When rounding numbers, if the first digit to be dropped is equal to 5, then the last remaining digit is rounded up to the next highest number if it is an ODD number but left the same if it is an EVEN number.
- A fraction is a mathematical way to represent the amount of "parts" within a number or substance. The top number, called the numerator, represents the "part"; the bottom number of the fraction, called the denominator, represents the entire amount of parts.

- When performing additions and subtractions of fractions, the denominators of each fraction must be the same value. By using ratio and proportion, an equivalent fraction can be determined.
- When multiplying two or more fractions, the numerators are multiplied together and the denominators are multiplied together.
- Division problems with fractions have three terms: the dividend (which is the number that is being divided), the divisor (the number that is being used to divide the dividend), and the answer or quotient. When dividing fractions, the divisor fraction is simply flipped so that the numerator is now the denominator and the denominator is now the numerator. The flipped fraction is then multipled by the dividend fraction to calculate the quotient.
- To determine significant figures, when a number has zeroes within the number, those zeroes are considered significant and are not removed from the number.
- To determine significant figures, when a number has zeroes at the end of the number, those zeroes are considered significant to the number and not removed.
- To determine significant figures, when a number is less than 1.0, any zeroes that are before or after the decimal point but before the first nonzero number within the number are not considered significant.
- When performing addition or subtraction calculations, the final result can only have as many digits to the right of the decimal point as the least precise number involved in the problem.
- When performing multiplication or division calculations, the final result cannot contain more significant figures than the number in the calculation with the least number of significant figures.

Scientific Notation and Logarithms

OBJECTIVES

At the end of this chapter, the reader should be able to do the following:

1. State the rules for multiplication, division, subtraction, and addition using scientific notation.
2. Convert scientific notation numbers to whole numbers and vice versa.
3. Perform multiplication, division, subtraction, and addition calculations involving scientific notation.
4. State the rules for multiplication, division, subtraction, and addition using logarithms.

5. Perform multiplication, division, subtraction, and addition calculations using logarithms.
6. Define the terms *mantissa* and *characteristic* and explain how they relate to logarithms.
7. Define the terms *mantissa, base,* and *exponents* for scientific notation.

WHAT EXPONENTS AND SCIENTIFIC NOTATION

In mathematics, multiplication is used as a faster method than simple addition when performing multiple addition problems. For example, $6 \times 7 = 42$. The same answer could be found by adding 6 seven times: $6 + 6 + 6 + 6 + 6 + 6 + 6 = 42$.

Exponents are a way to simplify complex multiplication problems.

Exponents are written as x^a, where x is called the base and a is the exponent. The base is the number that is to be multiplied by itself, and the exponent determines how many times it will be multiplied.

For example, 2^4 is equal to $2 \times 2 \times 2 \times 2$ or 16 and 3^3 is equal to $3 \times 3 \times 3$ or 27. In complicated calculations involving many exponents, it is easy to see how the use of exponents can reduce the chance of errors in performing the arithmetic of the calculation.

In the clinical laboratory, scientific notation is often used in calculations to simplify the calculation and is used when expressing standard concentrations of some analytes. For example, a white blood cell count is expressed in units of number of cells counted per

10^9/L (e.g., 4.00 × 10^9/L). Scientific notation is also sometimes used when performing calculations with logarithms, which will be covered later in this chapter. In scientific notation, a number is written in such a way that it is larger than 1 but less than 10 and an integral power of 10. For example, the number 2820000.0 can be expressed as 2.82 × 10^6 because the decimal point can be moved six places to the left. The 2.82 is referred to as the **mantissa number** by some mathematicians. This book will also refer to it as the mantissa number.

$$2\underset{6}{8}\underset{5}{2}\underset{4}{0}\underset{3}{0}\underset{2}{0}\underset{1}{0}.0 = 2.82 \times 10^6$$

There are seven rules (Rules 1–7) for using scientific notation and three rules (Rules 8–10) for determining logarithms or performing calculations with logarithms. If these rules are understood and followed, errors in calculations using scientific notation will be reduced.

WHAT **Rules 1 to 7 for Using Scientific Notation**

Rule 1

Exponents used in scientific notation can be positive or negative numbers. Exponents that are negative usually indicate a number that is less than 1. A negative sign is placed to the left of the exponent to indicate that it is a negative exponent. Exponents that are positive generally do not have any sign associated with them. It is assumed that if a negative sign is not present, then the exponent is positive.

Positive Exponents. Remember that in scientific notation, the mantissa number is written to be between 1 and 10 with a power of 10. Sometimes in the clinical laboratory there will be exceptions in keeping the mantissa number between 1 and 10. You may see some examples of this in the clinical hematology and the clinical chemistry chapters later in this text.

HOW   ***Example 2-1*** $6 \times 10^2 = (6) \times (10) \times (10) = 6 \times 100 = 600$

Example 2-1a $5 \times 10^4 = (5) \times (10) \times (10) \times (10) \times (10) = 5 \times 10000 = 50,000$

Example 2-1b $6 \times 10^1 = (6) \times (10) = 6 \times 10 = 60$

Example 2-1c $7 \times 10^5 = (7) \times (10) \times (10) \times (10) \times (10) \times (10) = 7 \times 100000 = 700,000$

WHAT   **Negative Exponents.** Numbers with negative exponents are expressed with the following formula:

$$b^{-a} = \frac{1}{b^a}$$

HOW *Example 2-2*

In this example, from the equation for negative exponents, b = 10 and a = −5.

$$3 \times 10^{-5} = 3 \times \frac{1}{10^5}$$

$$3 \times \frac{1}{10^5} = 3 \times \frac{1}{100000} = 0.00003$$

Example 2-2a

$$3 \times 10^{-2} = 3 \times \frac{1}{10^2}$$

$$3 \times \frac{1}{10^2} = 3 \times \frac{1}{100} = 0.03$$

Example 2-2b

$$4 \times 10^{-3} = 4 \times \frac{1}{10^3} = 4 \times \frac{1}{1000} = 0.004$$

Example 2-2c

$$8 \times 10^{-2} = 8 \times \frac{1}{100} = 0.08$$

Notice that with scientific notation, the final product could be easily obtained by simply moving the decimal point to the left for a negative exponent and to the right for a positive exponent the number of times indicated by the exponent number itself. In Example 2-1, 6×10^2 was shown to be equal to 600. Instead of multiplying 10 by itself two times, simply use 6.0 as the starting point and move the decimal to the right three places.

$$\underset{\text{base}}{6.0} \qquad \underset{\text{one decimal place}}{60.0} \qquad \underset{\text{two decimal places}}{600.0} \qquad \underset{\text{three decimal places}}{6000.0}$$

For a negative exponent, the decimal place is moved to the left. Using 3×10^{-5} from Example 2-2, the decimal point is moved five places to the left.

$$\underset{\text{base}}{3.0} \quad \underset{\text{one decimal place}}{0.3} \quad \underset{\text{two decimal places}}{0.03} \quad \underset{\text{three decimal places}}{0.003} \quad \underset{\text{four decimal places}}{0.0003} \quad \underset{\text{five decimal places}}{0.00003}$$

WHAT *Rule 2*

If a mantissa number greater than zero has an exponent raised to the zero power, the exponent has a value of 1. This is expressed mathematically as follows:

$$b \times 10^0 = b \times 1 = b$$

A good understanding of how exponents function in scientific notation may help the reader see why the power of 10 raised to the zero power has a value of 1. The exponent tells the reader how many times 10 must be multiplied by itself. The zero exponent simply means that the power of 10 in scientific notation is to be used zero times (i.e., not to be used at all). The mantissa number associated with the power of 10 remains the same (i.e., multiplied by 1). Table 2-1 demonstrates powers of 10 commonly used in the clinical laboratory and their values.

TABLE 2-1 Powers of 10 and Their Associated Values

Exponent	Mantissa Number (a) and Exponent	Value	Example
$10^0 = 1$	$a \times 10^0$	a	$5 \times 10^0 = 5$
$10^1 = 10$	$a \times 10^1$	$a \times 10$	$5 \times 10^1 = 50$
$10^2 = 100$	$a \times 10^2$	$a \times 100$	$5 \times 10^2 = 500$
$10^3 = 1000$	$a \times 10^3$	$a \times 1000$	$5 \times 10^3 = 5000$
$10^6 = 1{,}000{,}000$	$a \times 10^6$	$a \times 1{,}000{,}000$	$5 \times 10^6 = 5{,}000{,}000$
$10^9 = 1{,}000{,}000{,}000$	$a \times 10^9$	$a \times 1{,}000{,}000{,}000$	$5 \times 10^9 = 5{,}000{,}000{,}000$
$10^{-1} = 0.1$	$a \times 10^{-1}$	$a \times 0.1$	$5 \times 10^{-1} = 0.5$
$10^{-2} = 0.01$	$a \times 10^{-2}$	$a \times 0.01$	$5 \times 10^{-2} = 0.05$
$10^{-3} = 0.001$	$a \times 10^{-3}$	$a \times 0.001$	$5 \times 10^{-3} = 0.005$
$10^{-6} = 0.000001$	$a \times 10^{-6}$	$a \times 0.000001$	$5 \times 10^{-6} = 0.000005$
$10^{-9} = 0.000000001$	$a \times 10^{-9}$	$a \times 0.000000001$	$5 \times 10^{-9} = 0.000000005$

HOW   *Example 2-3*

$$3.8 \times 10^0 = ?$$

This problem can be solved two different ways: From Table 2-1, $10^0 = 1$. Substituting this equivalent value into the equation yields 3.8×1, which equals 3.8. From Table 2-1, $a \times 10^0 = a$, or using the example, $5 \times 10^0 = 5$. By substituting the numbers in the problem into the equation, $3.8 \times 10^0 = 3.8$.

Example 2-3a   What is 5.9×10^0 in its nonexponent form?

Using Table 2-1 or the previous example, then $5.9 \times 10^0 = 5.9$.

Example 2-3b   What is 7.4×10^0 in its nonexponent form?

Using Table 2-1 or the previous example, then $7.4 \times 10^0 = 7.4$.

Example 2-3c   What is 5.3×10^0 in its nonexponsent form?

Using Table 2-1 or the previous example, then $5.3 \times 10^0 = 5.3$.

WHAT   *Rule 3*

When multiplying two mantissa numbers using scientific notation, the mantissa numbers themselves are multiplied but the exponents are added. This rule can be expressed as follows:

$$[(b \times 10^a)(c \times 10^d)] = (bc) \times 10^{a+d}$$

HOW   *Example 2-4*

Multiply 3.6×10^2 by 4.8×10^3. Using Rule 3, the following equation is derived:

$$(3.6 \times 10^2) \times (4.8 \times 10^3) = (3.6 \times 4.8) \times (10^5) = 17 \times 10^5 \text{ or } 1.7 \times 10^6$$

This equation can be verified by using simple arithmetic:

$$3.6 \times 10^2 = 360$$
$$4.8 \times 10^3 = 4800$$
$$360 \times 4800 = 1728000 = 1.7 \times 10^6.$$

The difference between 1728000 and 1.7×10^6 is because of significant figure rules of calculations. The number 1728000 is rounded to two significant figures.

Example 2-4a   Multiply 2.25×10^2 by 6.72×10^2.

Using Rule 3, the answer is 1.51×10^5.

Example 2-4b   Multiply 9.3×10^3 by 4.6×10^2.

Using Rule 3, the answer is 4.3×10^6.

Example 2-4c   Multiply 3.6×10^4 by 1.3×10^2.

Using Rule 3, the answer is 4.7×10^6.

WHAT **Rule 4**

When a mantissa (a) number in scientific notation is multiplied by an exponent, the mantissa (a^c) number is multiplied by itself the number of times expressed by the exponent. The power of 10 exponent is multiplied by the exponent. This is expressed mathematically as follows:

$$(a \times 10^b)^c = a^c \times 10^{bc}$$

a^c is equal to "a" multiplied by itself "c" times. This is expressed mathematically as $a^c = a \times a \times a \dots (c \text{ times})$.

HOW **Example 2-5**

$$(2.5 \times 10^2)^2 = 2.5^2 \times 10^{2 \times 2} = (2.5 \times 2.5) \times (10 \times 10 \times 10 \times 10) = 6.2 \times 10^4$$

Example 2-5a $(8.7 \times 10^3)^2 = 8.7^2 \times 10^{3 \times 2} = 75.7 \times 10^6 = 7.57 \times 10^7 = 7.6 \times 10^7$

Example 2-5b $(1.4 \times 10^2)^2 = 1.4^2 \times 10^{2 \times 2} = 1.96 \times 10^4 = 2.0 \times 10^4$

Example 2-5c $(3.2 \times 10^2)^2 = 3.2^2 \times 10^{2 \times 2} = 10.24 \times 10^4 = 1.0 \times 10^5$

WHAT **Rule 5**

In a division calculation involving mantissa (a + c) numbers in scientific notation, the exponent in the denominator (d) is subtracted from the exponent in the numerator of the equation (b). This rule is expressed mathematically as follows:

$$\frac{a \times 10^b}{c \times 10^d} = \frac{a}{c} \times 10^{b-d}$$

HOW   **Example 2-6**

Divide 5.45×10^3 by 2.5×10^2. Using the formula from Rule 5:

$$\frac{5.45 \times 10^3}{2.5 \times 10^2} = \frac{5.45}{2.5} \times 10^{3-2} = 2.2 \times 10^1$$

This answer can be confirmed by simple arithmetic:

$$5.45 \times 10^3 = 5450$$

$$2.5 \times 10^2 = 250$$

$$\frac{5450}{250} = 21.8 = 2.2 \times 10^1$$

Example 2-6a   Divide 5.2×10^3 by $2.7 \times 10^2 = 1.9 \times 10^1$

Example 2-6b   Divide 1.6×10^2 by $4.8 \times 10^1 = 0.33 \times 10^1$ or 3.3×10^0 or 3.3

Example 2-6c   Divide 9.3×10^4 by $8.4 \times 10^3 = 1.1 \times 10^1$

All calculations performed using scientific notation should arrive at the same answer that could be obtained by the slower simple arithmetic method. It is a good idea to check your answers while becoming familiar with scientific notation to make sure that mistakes are not made.

WHAT   **Rule 6**

A different but comparable way of expressing a division problem is the rule that in a division problem the exponent in the numerator can be subtracted from the exponent in the denominator. This is expressed mathematically as follows:

$$\frac{a \times 10^b}{c \times 10^d} = \frac{a}{c} \times \frac{1}{10^{d-b}}$$

HOW   **Example 2-7**

The same calculation from Example 2-6 will be used to demonstrate Rule 6. Using the formula from Rule 6:

$$\frac{5.45 \times 10^3}{2.5 \times 10^2} = \frac{5.45}{2.5} \times \frac{1}{10^{2-3}} = 2.2 \times \frac{1}{10^{-1}}$$

$$2.2 \times \frac{1}{10^{-1}} = 2.2 \times 10^1$$

When a negative exponent is in the denominator of an equation, it becomes a positive exponent when inverted to the numerator. This is why $^1/_{10^{-1}}$ became a positive 10^1.

Example 2-7a $\dfrac{4.8 \times 10^2}{2.7 \times 10^1} = \dfrac{4.8}{2.7} \times \dfrac{1}{10^{1-2}} = 1.8 \times \dfrac{1}{10^{-1}} = 1.8 \times 10^1$

Example 2-7b $\dfrac{8.1 \times 10^4}{1.5 \times 10^2} = \dfrac{8.1}{1.5} \times \dfrac{1}{10^{2-4}} = 5.4 \times \dfrac{1}{10^{-2}} = 5.4 \times 10^2$

Example 2-7c $\dfrac{1.6 \times 10^5}{3.3 \times 10^2} = \dfrac{1.6}{3.3} \times \dfrac{1}{10^{2-5}} = 0.48 \times \dfrac{1}{10^{-3}} = 4.8 \times 10^2$

WHAT   *Rule 7*

When performing addition and subtraction using scientific notation, it is easy to make arithmetic errors. This is because when performing addition and subtraction, the power of 10 exponents used for the scientific notation do not follow the same rules as for multiplication and division. The best way to perform addition and subtraction is to first convert all the numbers in the calculation to their original nonscientific notation form and then perform the addition or subtraction. When using a scientific calculator to perform addition or subtraction involving scientific notation, the EXP (or EE depending on your calculator) function is used. The calculator will convert the numbers to their nonexponent form when performing the calculation. When using a graphing calculator, enter the number followed by pressing the caret key (ˆ), which will then bring the cursor up to the exponent area. Simply type in the exponent value (e.g., −1, 2, 3) and hit ENTER to continue with the calculation. Refer to the instruction manual for your individual calculator for specific instructions.

HOW   *Example 2-8*

Add $5.23 \times 10^4 + 9.2 \times 10^2$.

If we try to manually solve this problem by using the same exponent rule as for multiplication, then the equation that will be derived is as follows:

$$(5.23 + 9.2) \times 10^6$$

Will this equation result in the correct answer? **NO!** Logic tells us that this equation cannot result in the correct answer. If, however, we first convert each number that is in scientific notation back to its simpler form and then perform the addition, we would expect to arrive at the following:

$$52300 + 920 = 53220 \text{ or } 5.3 \times 10^4$$

Example 2-8a $3.81 \times 10^5 + 5.98 \times 10^4 = X$

Solving it manually: $381000 + 59800 = 440800$ or 4.41×10^5.

Example 2-8b $7.7 \times 10^2 + 5.5 \times 10^3 = X$

Solving it manually: $770 + 5500 = 6270$ or 6.3×10^3.

Example 2-8c $6.94 \times 10^2 + 1.80 \times 10^1 = X$

Solving it manually, $694 + 18 = 712$ or 7.12×10^2.

WHAT   **Subtraction Using Scientific Notation**

Subtract 2.3×10^2 from 7.5×10^3.

In subtraction, there is no easy way to perform this calculation without a good chance of error except by first converting all terms into their simpler forms if the subtraction is performed manually or by using a calculator and the EXP (or EE) function.

$$7500 - 230 = 7270 \text{ or } 7.3 \times 10^3$$

Up to this point, all the examples have used positive exponents. The same rules apply when working with negative exponents. A common mistake when performing calculations involving negative exponents is to forget that when a negative number is subtracted from a positive number, it is actually **added** to the positive number because of the following rule that was discussed in Chapter 1:

Two Negatives Rule

Two negatives become a positive.

HOW   ***Example 2-9***

5.0×10^{-2} divided by $6.0 \times 10^{-3} = X$.

Using the rules of division with exponents, the following equation is derived:

$$\frac{5.0 \times 10^{-2}}{6.0 \times 10^{-3}} = \frac{5}{6} \times 10^{-2-(-3)} = 0.8 \times 10^1 = 8.0$$

OR

$$\frac{5.0 \times 10^{-2}}{6.0 \times 10^{-3}} = \frac{5}{6} \times \frac{1}{10^{-3-(-2)}} = 0.8 \times 10^1 = 8.0$$

When -3 is subtracted from -2, it is actually added to -2 and so becomes a positive number $(+1)$ or $[(-2) - (-3) = -2 + 3 = +1]$.

To confirm these answers, convert all numbers to their original nonscientific notation value:

$$5.0 \times 10^{-2} = 0.05$$

$$6.0 \times 10^{-3} = 0.006$$

$$\frac{0.05}{0.006} = 8.0$$

Example 2-9a $\dfrac{9.2 \times 10^{-3}}{4.1 \times 10^{-5}} = \dfrac{9.2}{4.1} \times 10^{-3-(-5)} = 2.2 \times 10^2$

Example 2-9b $\dfrac{8.2 \times 10^{-3}}{1.7 \times 10^{-1}} = 4.8 \times 10^{-3-(-1)} = 4.8 \times 10^{-2}$

Example 2-9c $\dfrac{2.2 \times 10^{-4}}{1.8 \times 10^{-2}} = 1.2 \times 10^{-4-(-2)} = 1.2 \times 10^{-2}$

INTRODUCTION TO LOGARITHMS AND PERFORMING CALCULATIONS WITH LOGARITHMS

WHAT   **Logarithms and Scientific Notation**

The inverse of the exponential function $y = a^x$ is called a logarithmic function, $x = a^y$. The value of the logarithmic function is called the logarithm.

In the laboratory, logarithms are expressed in base 10 and are called common logarithms. Logarithms are used in the calculations of pH for blood gas analysis. In simple terms, a logarithm is the exponent. Table 2-2 demonstrates the multiple of 10 relationship between logarithms and exponents. Logarithms are composed of two parts: a characteristic, which is a whole number; and a mantissa, which is the decimal part. The logarithm can be either positive

TABLE 2-2 Exponents and Their Associated Logarithms

Scientific Notation	Exponent	Logarithm
$1 = 10^0$	0	$\log 1 = 0$
$10 = 10^1$	1	$\log 10 = 1.00$
$100 = 10^2$	2	$\log 100 = 2.000$
$1000 = 10^3$	3	$\log 1000 = 3.0000$
$10000 = 10^4$	4	$\log 10000 = 4.00000$
$100000 = 10^5$	5	$\log 100000 = 5.000000$
$1000000 = 10^6$	6	$\log 1000000 = 6.0000000$
$0.000001 = 10^{-6}$	-6	$\log 0.000001 = -6$
$0.00001 = 10^{-5}$	-5	$\log 0.00001 = -5$
$0.0001 = 10^{-4}$	-4	$\log 0.0001 = -4$
$0.001 = 10^{-3}$	-3	$\log 0.001 = -3$
$0.01 = 10^{-2}$	-2	$\log 0.01 = -2$
$0.1 = 10^{-1}$	-1	$\log 0.1 = -1.0$

or negative. If it is negative, the number it represents has a value between zero and 1. A positive characteristic means that the number the logarithm represents is greater than 1. The log of 1 is equal to zero. Remember that $10^0 = 1$ and that a logarithm is the inverse of the exponent. Table 2-2 is a chart of exponents of 10 and their associated logarithms.

Significant Figures and Logarithms
When working with logarithms, rules of significant figures apply only to the mantissa, not the characteristic of the logarithm.

Determining Logarithms
Logarithms can be determined by use of a calculator or by a logarithm table. Most scientific calculators have a display key to calculate logarithms. The number is entered into the calculator, and the display key "log" is pressed to display the logarithm. Because of the ease of use of the scientific calculator in determining logarithms, use of the logarithm table is becoming less common. The logarithm table at the end of the chapter (Appendix 2-A) contains the logarithms of numbers between 1.0 and 9.9. To use the logarithm table, find the first two digits in column N, and move to the right for the third digit of the number. The four-digit number in the columns is the logarithm of the number, and a decimal is placed to the left of the logarithm.

HOW   *Example 2-10*

Find the logarithm of the number 3.47. To determine the logarithm of 3.47, follow these steps:

1. Find 3.4 in column N.
2. Find the entry to the right of 3.4 under column 7.
3. The four-digit number in column 7 in row 3.4 is .5403.
4. The logarithm of 3.47 is 0.540. The number 0.540 contains three significant figures (540) as does the number 3.47.

Example 2-10a   What is the logarithm of 2.64?

The logarithm of 2.64 is 0.422.

Example 2-10b   What is the logarithm of 7.82?

The logarithm of 7.82 is 0.893.

Example 2-10c   What is the logarithm of 9.63?

The logarithm of 9.63 is 0.984.

When numbers are greater than 9.99, the logarithm table can still be used, but additional steps must be taken.

HOW   ***Example 2-11***

Find the logarithm of **16.4**. To determine the logarithm of 16.4, follow these steps:

1. Express 16.4 as a number less than 10: $16.4 = 1.64 \times 10$.
2. Determine the logarithm of 1.64×10: $\log 1.64 \times 10 = \log 1.64 + \log 10$.
3. Determine the logarithm of **1.64** from the logarithm table.
4. Find **1.6** in column N and find the entry to the right of 1.6 under column 4.
5. The four-digit number in column 4 in row 1.6 is .2148.
6. The logarithm of 1.64 is .2148.
7. Find the logarithm of **10** from Table 2-2.
8. The logarithm of $10 = $ **1**.
9. Since the $\log 1.64 + \log 10 = \log 16.4$, substitute into the equation the appropriate logarithms.
10. $0.2148 + 1.0 = 1.2148$.
11. The number 1.2148 must be reduced to the same number of significant figures as the original number. The number 16.4 contains three significant figures. Because the rules of significant figures apply only to the mantissa, the mantissa must be rounded from four digits to three.
12. The logarithm for $16.4 = 1.215$.

Example 2-11a   What is the logarithm of 26.8?

The logarithm of 26.8 is 1.428.

Example 2-11b   What is the logarithm of 44.7?

The logarithm of 44.7 is 1.650.

Example 2-11c   What is the logarithm of 93.5?

The logarithm of 93.5 is 1.971.

When numbers are less than 1, the logarithm can still be obtained.

HOW   ***Example 2-12***

Find the logarithm of 0.0365. Follow the steps listed to determine the logarithm of 0.0365.

1. The number 0.0365 can be expressed as 3.65×10^{-2}.
2. $\log (3.65 \times 10^{-2}) = \log 3.65 + \log 10^{-2}$.
3. Find the log of 3.65 in the logarithm table.
4. Find 3.6 in column N.
5. Find the entry to the right under column 5.
6. The four-digit entry in column 5, row 3.6 is .5623 rounded to three significant figures, or .562.
7. The logarithm of 3.65 is 0.562.
8. Determine the logarithm of $\mathbf{10^{-2}}$ from Table 2-2.
9. The logarithm of $10^{-2} = -2$.
10. Since the log $0.0365 = \log 3.65 + \log 10^{-2}$, substitute into the equation the appropriate logarithms.
11. $0.562 + -2 = -1.438$.
12. The logarithm of 0.0365 is -1.438.

Example 2-12a   What is the logarithm of 0.413?

The logarithm of 0.413 is -0.384.

Example 2-12b   What is the logarithm of 0.00250?

The logarithm of 0.00250 is -2.602.

Example 2-12c   What is the logarithm of 0.071?

The logarithm of 0.071 is -1.15.

When working with logarithms, Rules 8 through 10 are applied.

Rules 8 to 10 for Determining Logarithms or Performing Calculations With Logarithms

WHAT **Rule 8**
The logarithm of a product of two numbers D and C is the sum of the logarithms of the numbers. This is expressed mathematically as follows:

$$\log(D \times C) = \log D + \log C$$

As shown in Example 2-11, the log of 1.64×10 was equal to the log $1.64 + \log 10$.

HOW **Example 2-13**

$\log (4.58 \times 7.23) = X$. From Rule 8, we know that $\log (4.58 \times 7.23) = \log 4.58 + \log 7.23$.
Using a calculator or the logarithm table, calculate the logarithms of 4.58 and 7.23. The logarithm of $4.58 = 0.661$ and the logarithm of $7.23 = 0.859$. Using the rules of multiplication of logarithms, substitute the logarithms into the formula:

$$\log(D \times C) = \log D + \log C$$
$$\log(4.58 \times 7.23) = 0.661 + 0.859$$
$$0.661 + 0.859 = 1.520$$

The logarithm of $4.58 \times 7.23 = 1.520$.

Example 2-13a   The log of $(3.63 \times 8.51) = X$.

The log of $(3.63 \times 8.51) = \log 3.63 + \log 8.51 = 0.560 + 0.930 = 1.490$.

Example 2-13b   The log of $(2.82 \times 9.34) = X$.

The log of $(2.82 \times 9.34) = 0.450 + 0.970 = 1.420$.

Example 2-13c   The log of $(1.44 \times 8.53) = X$.

The log of $(1.44 \times 8.53) = 0.158 + 0.931 = 1.089$.

WHAT   ***Rule 9***

When performing a division calculation involving logarithms, the log of the denominator is subtracted from the log of the numerator. This is expressed mathematically as follows:

$$\log \frac{E}{F} = \log E - \log F$$

HOW   ***Example 2-14***

$$\text{Find the log of } \frac{7.84}{2.38}.$$

$$\text{Using Rule 9, the } \log \frac{7.84}{2.38} = \log 7.84 - \log 2.28.$$

Determine the logarithms of 7.84 and 2.38 by using a calculator or the logarithm **Appendix 2-A:** The logarithm of $7.84 = 0.894$; the logarithm of $2.38 = 0.377$.

Using the rules of division with logarithms, substitute into the equation the appropriate logarithms:

$$\log \frac{7.84}{2.38} = \log 7.84 - \log 2.38$$

$$\log \frac{7.84}{2.38} = 0.894 - 0.377$$

$$0.894 - 0.377 = 0.517$$

$$\text{The logarithm of } \frac{7.84}{2.38} = 0.517.$$

Example 2-14a   The logarithm of $\dfrac{2.35}{1.67} = X$

The logarithm $= \log 2.35 - \log 1.67 = 0.371 - 0.223 = 0.148$.

Example 2-14b   The logarithm of $\dfrac{1.82}{1.25} = X$

The logarithm $= \log 1.82 - \log 1.25 = 0.260 - 0.097 = 0.163$.

Example 2-14c   The logarithm of $\dfrac{5.25}{3.55} = X$

The logarithm $= \log 5.25 - \log 3.55 = 0.720 - 0.550 = 0.170$.

WHAT   **Rule 10**

The logarithm of a number with a negative exponent is equal to the negative exponent multiplied by the log of the number. This is expressed mathematically as follows:

$$\log g^{-h} = (-h)(\log g)$$

HOW   **Example 2-15**

Find the logarithm of 10^{-4}.

    The logarithm of $10^{-4} = (-4)\,(\log 10)$.

    The log of $10 = 1$. Therefore substituting into the equation: $(-4)\,(1) = -4$.

    Thus the logarithm of $10^{-4} = -4.0$.

    Note: When using a calculator to solve this problem you will get an incorrect result if you enter "10 EXP −4 LOG" to have the logarithm look like 10^{-4} in the calculator. Notice that the result will be −3.0, not −4.0. This is because common logarithms are based on the power of 10. Therefore, in the formula used to illustrate Rule 10, $\log g^{-h} = (-h)\,(\log g)$, it is implied that −h is really 10^{-h}.

    Therefore, when solving the previous problem, "g" would be 1 and "−h" would be 10^{-4}. The format for entering scientific notation into most calculators to determine the logarithm is "(a) EXP (b) LOG," where (a) is ≥ 1.0 and ≤ 9.99 and (b) is the exponent of 10. Therefore the correct entry into the calculator would be "1 EXP −4 LOG." This may not work in all calculators; an alternate method is to enter 10 log × (−4), which will also result in the value of −4.

Example 2-15a   The logarithm of $10^{-6} = X$.

                The logarithm of $10^{-6} = -6$.

Example 2-15b   The logarithm of $10^{-2} = X$.

                The logarithm of $10^{-2} = -2$.

Example 2-15c   The logarithm of $10^{-4} = X$.

                The logarithm of $10^{-4} = -4$.

Example 2-15d   Find the logarithm of 5.40×10^{-3}. To solve this problem, use Rules 8 and 10. Rule 8 states that $\log (D \times C) = \log D + \log C$. Therefore this problem becomes $\log 5.40 + \log 10^{-3}$. Using a calculator, the log of $5.40 = 0.732$. Using Rule 10, the log of $10^{-3} = -3.0$. Therefore the log of $5.40 \times 10^{-3} = \log 5.40 + \log 10^{-3} = 0.732 + -3.00 = -2.268$.

    The result can be confirmed by solving the problem without using scientific notation: $5.40 \times 10^{-3} = 0.00540$. Using a calculator, enter 0.0054, then press LOG. The result, −2.268, is the same.

Example 2-15e   The logarithm of $2.35 \times 10^{-2} = X$.

                The logarithm $= \log 2.35 + \log 10^{-2} = 0.371 + (-2) = -1.629$.

Example 2-15f   The logarithm of $8.92 \times 10^{-3} = \text{X}$.

The logarithm $= \log 8.92 + \log 10^{-3} = 0.950 + (-3) = -2.050$.

Example 2-15g   The logarithm of $4.66 \times 10^{-4} = \text{X}$.

The logarithm $= \log 4.66 + \log 10^{-4} = 0.668 + (-4) = -3.332$.

WHAT Antilogarithms

Sometimes, instead of determining the logarithm of a number, the opposite calculation is required in that the logarithm may be given and the number associated with the logarithm must be determined. The number associated with a logarithm is called the antilogarithm or antilog. The antilog can be determined by a calculator or by the logarithm table. In most calculators, the antilog value is entered into the calculator and the INV function and LOG function are pressed. Some calculators have a second key that must be pressed to access the INV function.

To determine the antilog from the logarithm table, find the number given in the body of the logarithm table, and determine the numbers associated with the row and column in which it is found. The combination of these numbers is the antilog.

HOW *Example 2-16*

Find the antilog of 0.9315. To determine the antilog of 0.9315, follow these steps:

1. Find 0.9315 in the body of the logarithm table.
2. 0.9315 is found in row 8.5, column 4.
3. Combine the values found in the row and column.
4. Row 8.5 + column 4 = 8.540.
5. The antilog of 0.9315 is 8.540.

Prove this by determining the logarithm of 8.540. The logarithm of 8.540 = 0.9315.

Example 2-16a   The antilog of $0.3909 = \text{X}$.

The antilog of $0.3909 = 2.460$.

Example 2-16b   The antilog of $0.2175 = \text{X}$.

The antilog of $0.2175 = 1.650$.

Example 2-16c   The antilog of $0.4713 = \text{X}$.

The antilog of $0.4713 = 2.960$.

HOW **EXAMPLE PROBLEMS**

This section is designed to be useful to both the student and the laboratory professional. Students can use the additional problems to master the material. The laboratory professional can use the examples as templates for solving laboratory calculations. By finding an example similar to the problem that you need to solve, substitute into the equation the numbers appropriate to your calculation.

1. **Q.** Express 140,000,000.00 in exponent form.
   A. 140,000,000.00 is equal to 1.4×10^8.

2. **Q.** Express 3,510,000.00 in exponent form.
   A. 3,510,000.00 is equal to 3.51×10^6.

3. **Q.** Express 6,400.00 in exponent form.
   A. 6,400.00 is equal to 6.4×10^3.

4. **Q.** Express 0.000487 in exponent form.
   A. 0.000487 is equal to 4.87×10^{-4}.

5. **Q.** Express 0.036 in exponent form.
   A. 0.036 is equal to 3.6×10^{-2}.

6. **Q.** Express 0.00255 in exponent form.
   A. 0.00255 is equal to 2.55×10^{-3}.

7. **Q.** What is the value of 4.2×10^0?
   A. 4.2×10^0 is equal to 4.2. This is explained in Rule 2 and shown in Example 2-3. The rule states that any number greater than zero that has an exponent raised to the zero power has a value of 1; therefore 10^0 is equal to 1.0.

8. **Q.** What is the value of 7.1×10^0?
   A. The answer is 7.1. Refer to Example Problem 7 for more information.

9. **Q.** What is the value of 2.87×10^0?
   A. The answer is 2.87. Refer to Example Problem 7 for more information.

10. **Q.** Multiply 3.8×10^4 by 4.2×10^2.
    A. The rule for multiplication with scientific notation states that when multiplying two or more numbers with exponents, the numbers themselves are multiplied, but the exponents are added. Therefore the equation would be:

    $$[(3.8)(4.2)]^{4+2} = 1.6 \times 10^7$$

11. **Q.** Multiply 5.23×10^2 by 2.9×10^3.
    A. $[(5.23) \times (2.9)]^{2+3} = 15.2 \times 10^5$, which becomes 1.5×10^6. Refer to Example Problem 10 for more information.

12. **Q.** Multiply 6.92×10^3 by 2.46×10^6.
    A. $[(6.92) \times (2.46)]^{3+6} = 17.0 \times 10^9 = 1.70 \times 10^{10}$. Refer to Example Problem 10 for more information.

13. **Q.** What is 5.1×10^2 squared?
    A. When multiplying a number in scientific notation by an exponent, the base number is multiplied by itself, the number of times expressed by the exponent's value, whereas the exponent associated with the power of 10 is multiplied by the exponent. Therefore,

    $$[5.1 \times 10^2]^2 = 5.1^2 \times 10^{2 \times 2} = 26 \times 10^4, \text{which becomes } 2.6 \times 10^5.$$

14. **Q.** What is $[3.25 \times 10^2]^3$?

A. $3.25^3 = 3.25 \times 3.25 \times 3.25 = 34.3$

$10^{2\times3} = 10^6$

$[3.25 \times 10^2]^3 = 34.3 \times 10^6 = 3.43 \times 10^7$

Refer to Example Problem 13 for more information.

15. **Q.** What is $[7.812 \times 10^3]^2$?

   A. $[7.812 \times 10^3]^2 = 61.03 \times 10^6 = 6.103 \times 10^7$

Refer to Example Problem 13 for more information.

16. **Q.** Divide 8.1×10^2 by 5.4×10^1.

   A. The rule for division with numbers in scientific notation state that the exponent in the denominator is subtracted from the exponent in the numerator. Therefore,

$$\frac{8.1 \times 10^2}{5.4 \times 10^1} = \frac{8.1}{5.4} \times 10^{2-1} = 1.5 \times 10^1$$

17. **Q.** Divide 4.2×10^{-2} by 9.86×10^{-3}.

   A. $\dfrac{4.2 \times 10^{-2}}{9.86 \times 10^{-3}} = \dfrac{4.2}{9.86} \times 10^{-2-(-3)} = 0.43 \times 10^1 = 4.3$

Refer to Example Problem 13 for more information.

18. **Q.** Divide 5.66×10^3 by 2.15×10^2.

   A. 2.63×10^1. Refer to Example Problem 16 for more information.

19. **Q.** Add 6.2×10^2 to 9.1×10^3.

   A. When performing addition calculations with numbers in scientific notation, convert the numbers back into their nonscientific notation form before proceeding with the addition calculation.

$$6.2 \times 10^2 = 620, \text{ whereas } 9.1 \times 10^3 = 9100.$$

If using a scientific calculator, enter 6.2, press the EXP function key and 2, and then press ENTER or the equal sign. Then save that number (620) in the memory of the calculator, and proceed to enter 9.1×10^3 in the same manner. Perform the addition by recalling 620 to be added to 9100. The sum is 9720 or 9.7×10^3.

20. **Q.** Add 4.5×10^{-2} to 6.1×10^{-1}.

   A. $4.5 \times 10^{-2} = 0.045$

   $6.1 \times 10^{-1} = 0.61$

   $0.045 + 0.61 = 0.655 = 6.6 \times 10^{-1}$

Refer to Example Problem 19 for more information.

21. **Q.** Subtract 8.0×10^2 from 9.3×10^3.

   A. When performing subtraction calculations with numbers in scientific notation, convert the numbers back into their nonscientific notation form before proceeding with the subtraction calculation:

$$8.0 \times 10^2 = 800, \text{ whereas } 9.3 \times 10^3 = 9300$$

If using a scientific calculator, enter 8.0, press the EXP function key and 2, and then press ENTER or the equal sign. Then save that number (800) in the memory of the calculator and proceed to enter 9.3×10^3 in the same manner. Perform the subtraction by recalling 800 to be subtracted from 9300. The difference is 8500 or 8.5×10^3.

22. **Q.** Subtract 4.1×10^{-1} from 3.5×10^{-1}.
    A. Convert both terms into their nonscientific notation form. 4.1×10^{-1} is equal to 0.41, whereas 3.5×10^{-1} is equal to 0.35.

$$0.35 - 0.41 = -0.06 \text{ or } -6.0 \times 10^{-2}$$

23. **Q.** Determine the logarithm of 7.45.
    A. The logarithm can be determined two ways. The first and most common is by the use of a scientific calculator and the LOG function key. Enter 7.45 into the calculator, and press LOG. The logarithm of 7.45 is 0.872. The alternate method is to use a logarithm table. Find 7.4 in the N column and then proceed to column 5 to the right. The four-place number (.8722) is the logarithm. As the number 7.45 has only three significant figures, the mantissa can only contain three significant figures. Therefore the logarithm of 7.45 is 0.872.

24. **Q.** Determine the logarithm of 3.77.
    A. The logarithm of 3.77 is 0.576. Refer to Example Problem 23 for more information.

25. **Q.** Determine the logarithm of 0.0486.
    A. The logarithm can be determined either by the use of a calculator or by using a logarithm table. To use the scientific calculator, enter 0.0486 into the calculator, and press LOG. The alternate is to use a logarithm table. Before using the table, the number 0.0486 must be placed in an appropriate form: $0.0486 = 4.86 \times 10^{-2}$.
    Using the rules of logarithms, the log of $4.86 \times 10^{-2} = \log 4.86 + \log 10^{-2}$. In the logarithm table, find 4.8 in the N column and then proceed to column 6 to the right. The four-place number (.6866) corresponds to 4.86. Next, determine the logarithm of 10^{-2} from Table 2-2. The logarithm of $10^{-2} = -2$. Because the log of $4.86 \times 10^{-2} = \log 4.86 + \log 10^{-2}$, substitute into the equation the values obtained.

$$0.6866 + -2 = \log 0.0486 \text{ or } -1.313$$

26. **Q.** Determine the logarithm of 0.179.
    A. The logarithm of $0.179 = -0.747$. Refer to Example Problem 23 for more information.

27. **Q.** Determine the log of $\dfrac{5.75}{3.87}$.

    A. Using the rules pertaining to division with logarithms,

$$\log \frac{5.75}{3.87} = \log 5.75 - \log 3.87$$

Determine the logarithms of both numbers: $\log 5.75 = 0.760$, $\log 3.87 = 0.588$. Therefore,

$$\log \frac{5.75}{3.87} = 0.760 - 0.588 = 0.172$$

28. **Q.** Determine the logarithm of $\dfrac{0.286}{0.0618}$.

A. The logarithm of $\dfrac{0.286}{0.0618} = 0.665$.

This is determined by first finding the log of 0.286, which is -0.544, and the log of 0.0618, which is -1.209. Using the rules of division (see Rule 9) of logarithms, the log of the denominator is subtracted from the log of the numerator. Thus $-0.544 - (-1.209) = 0.665$.

29. **Q.** Determine the logarithm of $\dfrac{4.75 \times 10^2}{6.82 \times 10^3}$.

    A. The $\log 4.75 \times 10^2 = \log 4.75 + \log 10^2$. The log of $4.75 = 0.677$, and the log of $10^2 = 2$. Using the rules of multiplication of logarithms, the $\log 4.75 \times 10^2 = 0.677 + 2$ or 2.677. The $\log 6.82 \times 10^3 = \log 6.82 + \log 10^3$, which equals $0.834 + 3$ or 3.834. Next, as the equation is a division problem, subtract the log of the denominator from the log of the numerator: $2.677 - 3.834 = -1.157$.
    Therefore the answer is -1.157.

30. **Q.** Determine the logarithm of 3.9×10^{-2}.

    A. To solve the logarithm of a product, the logarithms of both numbers are determined and then added. This is expressed mathematically as $\log (D \times C) = \log D + \log C$. This problem would be expressed as $\log 3.9 + \log 10^{-2}$.
    The log of 3.9 is 0.59, whereas the log of 10^{-2} is -2.0. (Whenever determining the log of 10^a, regardless of whether "a" is a positive number or not, the number 1, not 10, is entered into the calculator along with the appropriate exponent to determine the logarithm. This is because base 10 or scientific logarithms are based on the power of 10, and it is implied that $\log 10^a$ is in actuality log 1 raised to the power of "a.") To solve the problem, add $0.59 + -2$, which results in the sum of -1.41. Therefore the log of $3.9 \times 10^{-2} = -1.410$. This can be verified by calculating the log of 0.039 with a calculator. The result, -1.410, is the same.

31. **Q.** Determine the antilog of 0.4730.

    A. The antilog can be determined by one of two methods. The first is to use the scientific calculator. Most scientific calculators have an INV key or a second key. For calculators with the INV key, simply enter into the calculator the number 0.4730 and press INV and then LOG. If the calculator has a second key or SHIFT key, enter the number and then press SHIFT or second and then LOG. The alternate method is to use the logarithm table. Find .4730 in the body of the table and read across to the N column to find the first two digits of the antilog. The closest number to .4730 in the table is .4728. If the antilog must be precise to four significant figures, interpolate between .4728 and the next antilog .4742 to obtain the fourth digit. Because .4728 is in the seventh column, the third digit is 7. Thus the antilog of 0.4730 is 2.97, or (if you have interpolated) 2.972.

32 **Q.** Determine the antilog of .3856.

    A. The antilog of 0.3856 is 2.430. Refer to Example Problem 31 for more information.

PRACTICE PROBLEMS

Solve the following practice problems to further master the material. Answers and explanations to some problems can be found in the Answer Key.

Express the following numbers in exponent form.

1. 6835.4

2. 814.0

3. 7000.0

4. 0.3519

5. 0.0854

6. 0.000753

7. 0.00000358

Solve the following equations using the rules for working with exponents. Answers must be in correct exponential form.

8. $[(3.26 \times 10^3)(6.44 \times 10^2)]$

9. $[(2.15 \times 10^4)(4.24 \times 10^1)]$

10. $[(7.91 \times 10^{-3})(6.18 \times 10^1)]$

11. $[(3.14 \times 10^{-2})(1.89 \times 10^{-3})]$

12. $[5.7 \times 10^3]^2$

13. $[2.8 \times 10^6]^3$

14. $[3.3 \times 10^{-2}]^2$

15. $[7.8 \times 10^{-3}]^3$

16. $(8.1 \times 10^4) \div (3.5 \times 10^2)$

17. $(2.41 \times 10^2) \div (4.92 \times 10^1)$

18. $(9.135 \times 10^{-3}) \div (2.814 \times 10^{-3})$

19. $(3.6 \times 10^{-4}) \div (8.1 \times 10^{-3})$

20. $(6.65 \times 10^1) + (5.25 \times 10^2)$

21. $(2.8 \times 10^{-2}) + (8.3 \times 10^{-3})$

22. $(4.2 \times 10^3) - (6.8 \times 10^2)$

23. $(3.5 \times 10^{-4}) - (5.6 \times 10^{-2})$

Determine the logarithms of the following numbers.

24. 8.64

25. 4.723

26. 0.341

27. 0.00852

28. 5.21×10^3

29. 4.716×10^{-2}

30. $\log [6.42 \div 4.51]$

31. $\log [(4.8 \times 10^2) \div (2.2 \times 10^1)]$

Determine the antilogs of the following numbers.

32. 0.1818

33. 0.3695

34. 0.2742

35. 0.1430

QUICK NOTES

- Exponents are written as x^a, where x is the base and a is the exponent.
- The whole number associated with the exponent is called the mantissa and has a value between 1.0 and 10.0 with a power of 10.
- If a negative sign is not present in an exponent, the exponent is assumed to be a positive number.
- Numbers with a negative exponent are expressed with the following formula: $b^{-a} = \frac{1}{b^a}$
- If a mantissa number greater than zero has an exponent raised to the zero power, the exponent has a value of 1.

$$b \times 10^0 = b \times 1 = b$$

- When multiplying the mantissa numbers using scientific notation, the mantissa numbers are multiplied but the exponents are added.

$$[(b \times 10^a)(c \times 10^d)] = (bc) \times 10^{a+d}$$

- When a mantissa number in scientific notation is multiplied by an exponent, the mantissa number is multiplied by itself the number of times expressed by the exponent.

$$(a \times 10^b)^c = a^c \times 10^{bc}$$

- In a division calculation involving mantissa numbers in scientific notation, the exponent in the denominator is subtracted from the exponent in the numerator of the equation.

$$\frac{a \times 10^b}{c \times 10^d} = \frac{a}{c} \times 10^{b-d}$$

- In a division problem, the exponent in the numerator can be subtracted from the exponent in the denominator.

$$\frac{a \times 10^b}{c \times 10^d} = \frac{a}{c} \times \frac{1}{10^{d-b}}$$

- If manually performing addition or subtraction using scientific notation, first convert all numbers into their nonscientific notation form.
- The inverse of the exponential function $y = a^x$ is called a logarithmic function, $x = a^y$. The value of this function is called the logarithm.
- Logarithms have two parts: the characteristic, which is the whole number; and a mantissa, which is the decimal part.
- The rules of significant figures only apply to the mantissa of the logarithm.
- The logarithm of a product of two numbers is the sum of the logarithms of the numbers.

$$\log(D \times C) = \log D + \log C$$

- In division of logarithms, the log of the denominator is subtracted from the log of the numerator.

$$\log \frac{E}{F} = \log E - \log F$$

- The logarithm of a number with a negative exponent is equal to the negative exponent multiplied by the log of the number.

$$\log g^{-h} = (-h)(\log g)$$

- To determine the antilogarithm using a calculator, enter the antilog value into the calculator and then the INV function followed by LOG function.

Appendix 2-A Logarithm Table

N	0	1	2	3	4	5	6	7	8	9
1.0	.0000	.0043	.0086	.0128	.0170	.0212	.0253	.0294	.0334	.0374
1.1	.0414	.0453	.0492	.0531	.0569	.0607	.0645	.0682	.0719	.0755
1.2	.0792	.0828	.0864	.0899	.0934	.0969	.1004	.1038	.1072	.1106
1.3	.1139	.1173	.1206	.1239	.1271	.1303	.1335	.1367	.1399	.1430
1.4	.1461	.1492	.1523	.1553	.1584	.1614	.1644	.1673	.1703	.1732
1.5	.1761	.1790	.1818	.1847	.1875	.1903	.1931	.1959	.1987	.2014
1.6	.2041	.2068	.2095	.2122	.2148	.2175	.2201	.2227	.2253	.2279
1.7	.2304	.2330	.2355	.2380	.2405	.2430	.2455	.2480	.2504	.2529
1.8	.2553	.2577	.2601	.2625	.2648	.2672	.2695	.2718	.2742	.2765
1.9	.2788	.2810	.2833	.2856	.2878	.2900	.2923	.2945	.2967	.2989
2.0	.3010	.3032	.3054	.3075	.3096	.3118	.3139	.3160	.3181	.3201
2.1	.3222	.3243	.3263	.3284	.3304	.3324	.3345	.3365	.3385	.3404
2.2	.3424	.3444	.3464	.3483	.3502	.3522	.3541	.3560	.3579	.3598
2.3	.3617	.3636	.3655	.3674	.3692	.3711	.3729	.3747	.3766	.3784
2.4	.3802	.3820	.3838	.3856	.3874	.3892	.3909	.3927	.3945	.3962
2.5	.3979	.3997	.4014	.4031	.4048	.4065	.4082	.4099	.4116	.4133
2.6	.4150	.4166	.4183	.4200	.4216	.4232	.4249	.4265	.4281	.4298
2.7	.4314	.4330	.4346	.4362	.4378	.4393	.4409	.4425	.4440	.4456
2.8	.4472	.4487	.4502	.4518	.4533	.4548	.4564	.4579	.4594	.4609
2.9	.4624	.4639	.4654	.4669	.4683	.4698	.4713	.4728	.4742	.4757
3.0	.4771	.4786	.4800	.4814	.4829	.4843	.4857	.4871	.4886	.4900
3.1	.4914	.4928	.4942	.4955	.4969	.4983	.4997	.5011	.5024	.5038
3.2	.5051	.5065	.5079	.5092	.5105	.5119	.5132	.5145	.5159	.5172
3.3	.5185	.5198	.5211	.5224	.5237	.5250	.5263	.5276	.5289	.5302
3.4	.5315	.5328	.5340	.5353	.5366	.5378	.5391	.5403	.5416	.5428
3.5	.5441	.5453	.5465	.5478	.5490	.5502	.5514	.5527	.5539	.5551
3.6	.5563	.5575	.5587	.5599	.5611	.5623	.5635	.5647	.5658	.5670
3.7	.5682	.5694	.5705	.5717	.5729	.5740	.5752	.5763	.5775	.5786
3.8	.5798	.5809	.5821	.5832	.5843	.5855	.5866	.5877	.5888	.6010
3.9	.5911	.5922	.5933	.5944	.5955	.5966	.5977	.5988	.5999	.6010
4.0	.6021	.6031	.6042	.6053	.6064	.6075	.6085	.6096	.6107	.6117
4.1	.6128	.6138	.6149	.6160	.6170	.6180	.6191	.6201	.6212	.6222
4.2	.6232	.6243	.6253	.6263	.6274	.6284	.6294	.6304	.6314	.6325
4.3	.6335	.6345	.6355	.6365	.6375	.6385	.6395	.6405	.6415	.6425

N	0	1	2	3	4	5	6	7	8	9
4.4	.6435	.6444	.6454	.6464	.6474	.6484	.6493	.6503	.6513	.6522
4.5	.6532	.6542	.6551	.6561	.6571	.6580	.6590	.6599	.6609	.6618
4.6	.6628	.6637	.6646	.6656	.6665	.6675	.6684	.6693	.6702	.6712
4.7	.6721	.6730	.6739	.6749	.6758	.6767	.6776	.6785	.6794	.6803
4.8	.6812	.6821	.6830	.6839	.6848	.6857	.6866	.6875	.6884	.6893
4.9	.6902	.6911	.6920	.6928	.6937	.6946	.6955	.6964	.6972	.6981
5.0	.6990	.6998	.7007	.7016	.7024	.7033	.7042	.7050	.7059	.7067
5.1	.7076	.7084	.7093	.7101	.7110	.7118	.7126	.7135	.7143	.7152
5.2	.7160	.7168	.7177	.7185	.7193	.7202	.7210	.7218	.7226	.7235
5.3	.7243	.7251	.7259	.7267	.7275	.7284	.7292	.7300	.7308	.7316
5.4	.7324	.7332	.7340	.7348	.7356	.7364	.7372	.7380	.7388	.7396
5.5	.7404	.7412	.7419	.7427	.7435	.7443	.7451	.7459	.7466	.7474
5.6	.7482	.7490	.7497	.7505	.7513	.7520	.7528	.7536	.7543	.7551
5.7	.7559	.7566	.7574	.7582	.7589	.7597	.7604	.7612	.7619	.7627
5.8	.7634	.7642	.7649	.7657	.7664	.7672	.7679	.7686	.7694	.7701
5.9	.7709	.7716	.7723	.7731	.7738	.7745	.7752	.7760	.7767	.7774
6.0	.7782	.7789	.7796	.7803	.7810	.7818	.7825	.7832	.7839	.7846
6.1	.7853	.7860	.7868	.7875	.7882	.7889	.7896	.7903	.7910	.7917
6.2	.7924	.7931	.7938	.7945	.7952	.7959	.7966	.7973	.7980	.7987
6.3	.7993	.8000	.8007	.8014	.8021	.8028	.8035	.8041	.8048	.8055
6.4	.8062	.8069	.8075	.8082	.8089	.8096	.8102	.8109	.8116	.8122
6.5	.8129	.8136	.8142	.8149	.8156	.8162	.8169	.8176	.8182	.8189
6.6	.8195	.8202	.8209	.8215	.8222	.8228	.8235	.8241	.8248	.8254
6.7	.8261	.8267	.8274	.8280	.8287	.8293	.8299	.8306	.8312	.8319
6.8	.8325	.8331	.8338	.8344	.8351	.8357	.8363	.8370	.8376	.8382
6.9	.8388	.8395	.8401	.8407	.8414	.8420	.8426	.8432	.8439	.8445
7.0	.8451	.8457	.8463	.8470	.8476	.8482	.8488	.8494	.8500	.8506
7.1	.8513	.8519	.8525	.8531	.8537	.8543	.8549	.8555	.8561	.8567
7.2	.8573	.8579	.8585	.8591	.8597	.8603	.8609	.8615	.8621	.8627
7.3	.8633	.8639	.8645	.8651	.8657	.8663	.8669	.8675	.8681	.8686
7.4	.8692	.8698	.8704	.8710	.8716	.8722	.8727	.8733	.8739	.8745
7.5	.8751	.8756	.8762	.8768	.8774	.8779	.8785	.8791	.8797	.8802
7.6	.8808	.8814	.8820	.8825	.8831	.8837	.8842	.8848	.8854	.8859
7.7	.8865	.8871	.8876	.8882	.8887	.8893	.8899	.8904	.8910	.8915
7.8	.8921	.8927	.8932	.8938	.8943	.8949	.8954	.8960	.8965	.8971

N	0	1	2	3	4	5	6	7	8	9
7.9	.8976	.8982	.8987	.8993	.8998	.9004	.9009	.9015	.9020	.9025
8.0	.9031	.9036	.9042	.9047	.9053	.9058	.9063	.9069	.9074	.9079
8.1	.9085	.9090	.9096	.9101	.9106	.9112	.9117	.9122	.9128	.9133
8.2	.9138	.9143	.9149	.9154	.9159	.9165	.9170	.9175	.9180	.9186
8.3	.9191	.9196	.9201	.9206	.9212	.9217	.9222	.9227	.9232	.9238
8.4	.9243	.9248	.9253	.9258	.9263	.9269	.9274	.9279	.9284	.9289
8.5	.9294	.9299	.9304	.9309	.9315	.9320	.9325	.9330	.9335	.9340
8.6	.9345	.9350	.9355	.9360	.9365	.9370	.9375	.9380	.9385	.9390
8.7	.9395	.9400	.9405	.9410	.9415	.9420	.9425	.9430	.9435	.9440
8.8	.9445	.9450	.9455	.9460	.9465	.9469	.9474	.9479	.9484	.9489
8.9	.9494	.9499	.9504	.9509	.9513	.9518	.9523	.9528	.9533	.9538
9.0	.9542	.9547	.9552	.9557	.9562	.9566	.9571	.9576	.9581	.9586
9.1	.9590	.9595	.9600	.9605	.9609	.9614	.9619	.9624	.9628	.9633
9.2	.9638	.9643	.9647	.9652	.9657	.9661	.9666	.9671	.9675	.9680
9.3	.9685	.9689	.9694	.9699	.9703	.9708	.9713	.9717	.9722	.9727
9.4	.9731	.9736	.9741	.9745	.9750	.9754	.9759	.9763	.9768	.9773
9.5	.9777	.9782	.9786	.9791	.9795	.9800	.9805	.9809	.9814	.9818
9.6	.9823	.9827	.9832	.9836	.9841	.9845	.9850	.9854	.9859	.9863
9.7	.9868	.9872	.9877	.9881	.9886	.9890	.9894	.9899	.9903	.9908
9.8	.9912	.9917	.9921	.9926	.9930	.9934	.9939	.9943	.9948	.9952
9.9	.9956	.9961	.9965	.9969	.9974	.9978	.9983	.9987	.9991	.9996
N	0	1	2	3	4	5	6	7	8	9

Systems of Measurement

OUTLINE

OBJECTIVES

At the end of this chapter, the reader should be able to do the following:

1. State the units of measurement used in the United States Customary System.
2. State the units of measurement used in the metric system.
3. Convert units of measurement within the metric system.
4. Convert units of measurement between the metric system and the United States Customary System.
5. Compare and contrast the freezing and boiling points of water in the Celsius, Fahrenheit, and Kelvin temperature systems.
6. Convert among the Celsius, Fahrenheit, and Kelvin methods of temperature measurement.

WHAT MEASUREMENT OF LENGTH, WEIGHT, AND MASS

United States Customary System

Systems of weights and measures have been in existence since the first trade occurred among prehistoric peoples. The Egyptians used the cubit, which may be the earliest known use of linear measurement. One cubit was the distance between the elbow and the tip of the little finger. Later, the Greeks and Romans adopted many of the measurements used in the Egyptian system. The United States Customary System of measurement is based on the English system of measurement, which draws largely from the Greek and Roman systems. The United States is one of a handful of countries in the world that still use this system. Scientists and most other countries prefer the metric system. However, in the United States, efforts to persuade the American public to adopt the metric system have not succeeded. Americans want their foot-long hot dogs, their gallons of milk, and their miles of road. However, change may come from the business community as international trade agreements mandate the use of the metric system as the standard for measurements.

US Customary System of Measurement of Length and Area

Measurement of length in this system begins with the inch and progresses to the mile and acre.

12 inches	= 1 foot		5280 feet	= 1 mile
3 feet (36 inches)	= 1 yard		1 square foot	= 144 square inches
220 yards	= 1 furlong		1 square yard	= 9 square feet
8 furlongs	= 1 mile		43,560 square feet	= 1 acre
1760 yards	= 1 mile		1 square mile	= 640 acres

US Customary System of Liquid or Dry Measurement

Measurement of liquids begins with the teaspoon and progresses to the gallon.

1 teaspoon	= $\frac{1}{3}$ tablespoon		$5\frac{1}{3}$ fluid ounces	= $\frac{2}{3}$ cup
2 tablespoons	= 1 fluid ounce		6 fluid ounces	= $\frac{3}{4}$ cup
1 fluid ounce	= $\frac{1}{8}$ cup		8 fluid ounces	= 1 cup
2 fluid ounces	= $\frac{1}{4}$ cup		2 cups	= 1 pint
$2\frac{2}{3}$ fluid ounces	= $\frac{1}{3}$ cup		2 liquid pints	= 1 liquid quart
4 fluid ounces	= $\frac{1}{2}$ cup		4 liquid quarts	= 1 gallon

Measurements of dry volumes include the following:

1 dry quart	= 2 dry pints
8 dry quarts	= 1 peck
4 pecks	= 1 bushel

US Systems for Measurement of Mass

At present, there are four different measurement systems used in the United States to measure weight.

1. Troy: used to weigh silver, gold, and other precious metals
2. Apothecaries: used by pharmacists to weigh drugs
3. Avoirdupois: used for general purposes
4. Metric system: used in science

Troy

1 pennyweight	= 24 grains		5760 grains	= 1 pound
20 pennyweights	= 1 ounce		3.2 grains	= 1 carat
12 ounces	= 1 pound			

Apothecaries

1 scruple	= 20 grains		12 ounces	= 1 pound
3 scruples	= 1 dram		5760 grains	= 1 pound
8 drams	= 1 ounce			

Avoirdupois

1 dram	$= 27^{11}/_{32}$ grains
16 drams	= 1 ounce
16 ounces	= 1 pound
7000 grains	= 1 pound

100 pounds	= 1 hundredweight
2000 pounds	= 1 short ton
2240 pounds	= 1 long ton

As you can see, these measurements are not consistent with one another, which leads to confusion among systems. It was because of this inconsistency that another method of measurement that could be standardized was sought. That system is the metric system, which was developed in France in the 1790s.

WHAT ## Metric System

The metric system is based on fixed standards and on a uniform scale of 10. There are three basic units of measurement for length, weight, and volume. The basic units are as follows:

length	= meter (m)
Mass	= gram (g)
Volume	= liter (L)

The meter is defined as the length of the path traveled by light in a vacuum in $\dfrac{1}{299,792,458}$ of a second. The kilogram, or 1000 g, is defined as the mass of water contained by a cube whose sides are one-tenth the length of a meter or one decimeter in length. The liter is defined as the volume of liquid contained within that same cube.

Another measurement is area. This is a derivation of the measurement of length. By multiplying the length times the width of a square surface, the area of the surface can be determined. Area is measured in squared units. Common laboratory metric area measurements are mm^2, cm^2, and m^2.

Prefixes before the basic units of measurement inform the reader if a measurement is larger or smaller than the basic unit. Memorizing the prefixes and their abbreviations in Table 3-1 will be helpful in learning the metric system.

WHAT ### Conversion Among Different Measurements Within the Metric System

Because the metric system is based on a scale of 10, conversion among different measurements within a unit is relatively simple (Table 3-2). A basic ratio and proportion calculation is all that is needed to perform the conversion.

In the clinical laboratory, many analytes—such as glucose—are measured in terms of milligrams per deciliter or the number of milligrams contained in 1 dL of plasma. Other analytes, such as the hormone prolactin, are measured in terms of nanograms per milliliter. In hematology, white blood cells historically are counted in terms of cubic millimeters (mm^3) or currently expressed in units of liters of whole blood. The mean corpuscular volume (MCV) is measured in femtoliters.

In other areas of healthcare, the metric term *micro* (0.000001 or 10^{-6}) tends to be abbreviated as mc, but in the clinical laboratory as the Greek symbol μ. For example, microgram is frequently abbreviated as mcg for drug dosages, but as μg in the clinical laboratory.

TABLE 3-1 Metric System Prefixes and Abbreviations

Prefix	Abbreviation	Comparison to Basic Unit of 1 Gram, Meter, or Liter
Femto	f	10^{-15} smaller
Pico	p	10^{-12} smaller
Nano	n	10^{-9} smaller
Micro	mc	10^{-6} smaller
Milli	m	10^{-3} smaller
Centi	c	10^{-2} smaller
Deci	d	10^{-1} smaller
Deca	Da	10^{1} larger
Hecto	H	10^{2} larger
Kilo	K	10^{3} larger
Mega	M	10^{6} larger

TABLE 3-2 Common Metric System Units

Unit	Abbreviation	Comparable Unit
1 megameter	(Mm) =	1,000,000 or 10^{6} meters
1 kilometer	(Km) =	1000 meters
1 deciliter	(dL) =	0.1 or 10^{-1} liters
10 deciliters	(dL) =	1 liter
1 centimeter	(cm) =	0.01 or 10^{-2} meters
10 centimeters	(cm) =	1 decimeter
1 milliliter	(mL) =	0.001 or 10^{-3} liters
1 millimeter	(mm) =	0.001 or 10^{-3} meters
10 millimeters	(mm) =	1 centimeter
1 microgram	(mcg) =	0.000001 or 10^{-6} grams
1000 micrograms	(mcg) =	1 milligram
1 nanometer	(nm) =	0.000000001 or 10^{-9} meters
1000 nanometers	(nm) =	1 micrometer
1 picogram	(pg) =	0.000000000001 or 10^{-12} grams
1000 picograms	(pg) =	1 nanogram
1 femtoliter	(fL) =	0.000000000000001 or 10^{-15} liters
1000 femtoliters	(fL) =	1 nanoliter
1 cm^2	=	100 mm^2
1 m^2	=	1,000,000 mm^2
1 mm^3	=	1 microliter
1 cm^3	=	1 milliliter

HOW **Example 3-1**

How many milliliters are in a 2.0-L soda bottle?

To convert liters to milliliters, the basic value of each must be known. Table 3-2 shows that 1 mL is 10^{-3} smaller than the base value of 1 L; therefore, there are 1000 mL in 1 L.

As discussed in Chapter 1 and again in Chapter 4, ratio and proportion is a great math tool that can be used for many laboratory calculations provided that there is a proportional relationship between two ratios. A ratio can be expressed as a fraction with a numerator (the top number of the fraction) and a denominator (the lower or bottom number of the fraction). In the following example, both the numerators are in liters and the denominators are in milliliters. The relationship ratio is 1000 mL = 1 L, or 10^3 mL = 1 L. Therefore X mL = 2 liters is also a proportional relationship. To solve a ratio and proportion calculation, the numerator of the first ratio (1 L) is multiplied by the denominator of the second ratio (X mL). The denominator of the first ratio (1000 mL) is then multiplied by the numerator of the second ratio (2 L). This is called crossmultiplication. The liter units will cancel out, leaving the final result in milliliters.

$$\frac{1 \text{ liter}}{1000 \text{ milliliters}} = \frac{2 \text{ liters}}{X \text{ milliliters}}$$

Crossmultiplying the equation derives:

$$(1 \text{ L}) \, X \text{ mL} = (2 \text{ L})(1000 \text{ mL})$$

$$X \text{ mL} = \frac{2 \text{ L}}{1 \text{ L}}(1000 \text{ mL})$$

$$\mathbf{X \text{ mL} = 2000 \text{ mL}}$$

There are 2000 mL (2.0×10^3 mL) in a 2.0-L soda bottle.

Example 3-1a   How many deciliters are in 2.5 L?

$$\frac{X \text{ dL}}{2.5 \text{ L}} = \frac{10 \text{ dL}}{1 \text{ L}}$$

Crossmultiplying the equation and solving for X:

$$(X \text{ dL})(1 \text{ L}) = (2.5 \text{ L})(10 \text{ dL})$$

$$X \text{ dL} = \frac{(2.5 \cancel{\text{L}})(10 \text{ dL})}{1 \cancel{\text{L}}}$$

$$\mathbf{X = 25 \text{ dL}}$$

Using ratio and proportion, the answer is 25 dL or 2.5×10^1 dL.

Example 3-1b   How many milligrams are in 1.0 g?

From Table 3-1, a milligram is 10^{-3} smaller than a gram. Using ratio and proportion:

$$\frac{1 \text{ mg}}{X \text{ g}} = \frac{1 \text{ mg}}{10^{-3}} = 10^3 \text{ mg or } 1000 \text{ mg}$$

Therefore the answer is 1000 mg or 1.0×10^3 mg.

Example 3-1c   How many centimeters are in 1 km?

This problem can be solved in two steps. First, using ratio and proportion or the chart, convert kilometers into meters. There are 1000 m in 1 km. Next, convert the 1000 m into centimeters. Since there are 100 cm in 1 m, then by using ratio and proportion, the final answer is 100,000 cm or 1.0×10^5 cm.

WHAT *String Method*

A shortcut way to perform conversions is called the "string" method. In this method, the number that you want to convert into a different unit is multiplied by an equivalent ratio or ratios equal to 1 (e.g., 10 dL = 1 L or 1 dL = 1×10^{-1} L). The units will cancel out and you will end up with the desired result. A benefit of this method is that although you need to know the relationships between the basic unit and the prefix units, you don't need to know exact equivalents such as how many picograms are in a microgram.

HOW *Example 3-2*

Using the string method to solve Example 3-1a yields the following equation:

$$\left(\frac{2.5\ \cancel{L}}{1}\right) \times \left(\frac{10\,\text{dL}}{1\,\text{L}}\right) = 25\ \cancel{L}$$

Example 3-2a   Example 3-1c can be solved by:

$$\left(\frac{1\ \cancel{Km}}{1}\right)\left(\frac{10^3\ \cancel{m}}{1\ \cancel{Km}}\right)\left(\frac{10^2\ \text{cm}}{1\ \cancel{m}}\right) = 10^5\ \text{cm or } 1.0 \times 10^5\ \text{cm}$$

Example 3-2b   How many picograms are in 4.0 micrograms? A microgram is 1×10^{-6} of a gram or 0.000001 g. A picogram is a million (1 millionth = 1×10^{-6}) times smaller than a microgram, or another way to say it is that a picogram (pg) is 1×10^{-12} of a gram. One picogram can also be expressed as 0.000000000001 g. By using ratio and proportion, the units can be converted from one to the other.

$$\frac{1 \times 10^6\ \text{pg}}{1\ \text{mcg}} = \frac{\text{X pg}}{4.0\ \text{mcg}}$$

Crossmultiplying the equation:

$$(1 \times 10^6)(4.0) = (1)(\text{X})$$
$$4.0 \times 10^6 = \text{X}$$

Therefore, there are 4.0×10^6 pg in 4.0 mcg.

Or use the string method. Using the relationships from Table 3-1:

$$\frac{4\ \cancel{mcg} \times 10^{-6}\ \cancel{g} \times 1\,\text{pg}}{1\ \cancel{mcg} \times 10^{-12}\ \cancel{g}} = 4 \times 10^6\ \text{pg} \quad \text{OR} \quad \left(\frac{4\,\text{mcg}}{1}\right)\left(\frac{10^{-6}\text{g}}{1\text{mcg}}\right)\left(\frac{1\text{pg}}{10^{-12}\text{g}}\right) = 4 \times 10^6\ \text{pg}$$

Example 3-2c   How many nanograms are in 25 pg?

One nanogram is equal to 1000 pg. Using ratio and proportion, there are 2.5×10^{-2} ng in 25 pg.

$$\text{Or: } \left(\frac{25 \text{ pg}}{1}\right)\left(\frac{10^{-12} \text{ g}}{1 \text{ pg}}\right)\left(\frac{10^{+9} \text{ ng}}{1 \text{ g}}\right) = 2.5 \times 10^{-2} \text{ ng}$$

Example 3-2d   How many deciliters are in 75 mL?

There are 10 dL in 1 L and there are 1000 mL in 1 L. Therefore, there are 100 mL in 1 dL. Using the string method, there are 0.75 or 7.5×10^{-1} dL or 0.75 dL in 75 mL.

$$\text{Or: } \left(\frac{75 \text{ mL}}{1}\right)\left(\frac{10^{-3} \text{ L}}{1 \text{ mL}}\right)\left(\frac{10 \text{ dL}}{1 \text{ L}}\right) = 0.75 \text{ dL}$$

Example 3-2e   How many microliters are in 0.5 mL?

There are 1000 mcL in 1 mL. Therefore using the string method there are 500 mcL in 0.5 mL.

$$\text{Or: } \left(\frac{0.5 \text{ mL}}{1}\right)\left(\frac{10^{-3} \text{ L}}{1 \text{ mL}}\right)\left(\frac{10^6 \text{ mcL}}{\text{L}}\right)$$
$$= 500 \text{ mcL or } 5 \times 10^2 \text{ mcL}$$

WHAT   ***Shortcut Method for Conversion Between Metric System Units***

As shown in Example 3-2e, because 1 microliter is 1000 times smaller than 1 mL, a shortcut method of conversion is to move the decimal point of 0.500 mL three spaces to the right to convert it to 500 mcL.

$$0.500 \text{ milliliters} = 0.500 = 500 \text{ microliters}$$

HOW   ***Example 3-3***

Convert 25 pg to nanograms.

Since a picogram is 1000 times smaller than a nanogram, a shortcut method is to move the decimal point of 25 pg three spaces to the left to convert it to nanograms.

$$25 \text{ picograms} = 0.025 = 0.025 \text{ nanograms}$$

In summary, when converting from a larger metric unit to a smaller metric unit, move the decimal point the appropriate amount of spaces to the right, and when converting a smaller metric unit to a larger metric unit, move the decimal point the appropriate amount of spaces to the left. Use Table 3-1 as a guide to determine how many spaces you need to move the decimal point. A way to help you remember which direction to move the decimal point is to use the greater than (>) symbol and place the larger unit to the left of the symbol (the larger end) and the smaller unit to the right of the symbol (the smaller end). The symbol seems to "point" the direction that the decimal point needs to move.

For example: 500 g = X mg. Since there are 1000 milligrams in 1 gram, use the greater than symbol and move the decimal three positions to the right: 500 g > 500,000 mg.

Example 3-3a Convert 2.5 L to milliliters.

A liter is larger than a milliliter, so move the decimal point three spaces to the right: 2.5 L = 2500 mL.

Example 3-3b Convert 17.4 dL to liters.

A deciliter is 10 times smaller than a liter, so move the decimal point one space to the left: 17.4 dL = 1.74 L.

Example 3-3c Convert 300 mg to grams.

A milligram is smaller than a gram, so move the decimal point three spaces to the left: 300 mg = 0.300 g.

WHAT *Conversion Among Units Within the Metric System*

Sometimes a measurement may have to be converted to a different but comparable value to perform a calculation. Molarity is expressed in terms of moles per liter (see Chapter 5 for more information). If a measurement is in milligrams per liter (mg/L) quantities, it must be converted to grams per liter for the molarity equation. The process of "unit conversion" allows units to be converted from one form to another if the correct unit conversion fraction is used in the calculation. Using unit conversion to convert one type of unit to another, a ratio and proportion calculation is performed. The rules of algebra allow the inclusion of a fraction that has a value of 1 to be included in both sides of an equation when performing calculations. Using unit conversion, an equation is formed in which the unit to be changed is multiplied by the unit conversion fraction. This unit conversion fraction has a net value of 1; its purpose is to cancel out of the equation the units that are not desired and convert the original number into the unit that is desired. For example, a number is expressed as a quantity of X mg/dL, and the number needs to be expressed as X mg/L. Using unit conversion, we know that there are 10 dL in 1 L. X mg/dL can be multiplied by 10 dL/1 L (which equals 1). The deciliter units cancel and X mg is multiplied by 10. Thus 10 mg/dL is comparable to 100 mg/L.

HOW *Example 3-4*

Convert 85 mg/dL to milligrams per liter.
85 mg/dL can be written as follows:

$$\frac{85 \text{ mg}}{1 \text{ dL}}$$

There are 10 dL in 1 L. Therefore the fraction $\dfrac{10 \text{ dL}}{1 \text{ L}}$ is equal to 1.

The rules of algebra allow any number to be multiplied by 1 in an equation. Therefore:

$$\left(\frac{85 \text{ mg}}{1 \text{ dL}}\right)\left(\frac{10 \text{ dL}}{1 \text{ L}}\right) = \frac{(85 \text{ mg})(10 \text{ dL})}{(1 \text{ dL})(1 \text{ L})}$$

Cancel the units in the following equation:

$$\frac{(85 \text{ mg})(10 \cancel{\text{ dL}})}{(1 \cancel{\text{ dL}})(1 \text{ L})} = \frac{850 \text{ mg}}{1 \text{ L}}$$

The result is **850 mg/L.**

Example 3-4a   Convert 24 mg/dL to milligrams per liter.

Using Example 3-4 as a guide, and since there are 10 deciliters in 1 liter, multiply 24 by 10 to change 24 mg/dL to 240 mg/L.

Shortcut method to convert mg/dL to mg/L: As long as the numerator stays as mg, since there are 10 dL in 1.0 L, simply add a zero to the numerator number to change between mg/dL and mg/L. For example, 85 mg/dL is equal to 850 mg/L and 24 mg/dL is equal to 240 mg/L.

Example 3-4b   Convert 5.5 g/dL to milligrams per deciliter.

Since the denominator value of deciliter stays the same, this is really about converting grams to milligrams. Since a gram is larger than a milligram, move the decimal three spaces to the right to change 5.5 g/dL to 5500 mg/dL.

Example 3-4c   Convert 322 mg/dL to grams per liter.

This has two problems to solve: converting from milligrams to grams and deciliters to liters. First, convert from deciliters to liters and use Example 3-4a as a guide. The 322 mg/dL becomes 3220 mg/L. (Remember, there are 10 dL in 1.0 L so the amount of mg/L should be 10 times the amount of mg/dL.) Then convert milligrams to grams by moving the decimal three spaces to the left for 3.22 g/L.

WHAT   *Conversion Between United States System and the Metric System*

As the US system is so widely used by Americans, it may become necessary to convert between this system and the metric system. There are a few measurements that are commonly used and are listed in Example 3-5. Table 3-3 compares US system units and metric units. To convert from one unit to another, use the ratio and proportion formula as illustrated in Example 3-4 or multiply the US system measurement by the conversion factor or multiply the metric system measurement by the reciprocal of the conversion factor.

HOW   *Example 3-5*

How many milliliters are there in a 12-ounce soft drink? As seen in Table 3-3, 1 fluid ounce = 29.6 mL. Using ratio and proportion, the following equation is derived:

$$\frac{1 \text{ oz}}{29.6 \text{ mL}} = \frac{12.0 \text{ oz}}{X \text{ mL}}$$

TABLE 3-3 Comparison of US System Units and Metric Units

Convert From US Unit to Metric Unit	Multiply US Unit by Conversion Factor	Metric Unit	To Convert From Metric Unit to US Unit Multiply Metric Unit by Reciprocal of Conversion Unit	US Unit
Inch	25.4	millimeter	1/25.4 = 0.039	inch
Inch	2.54	centimeter	1/2.54 = 0.394	inch
Inch	0.0254	meter	1/0.0254 = 39.37	inch
Yard	0.914	meter	1/0.914 = 1.0914	yard
Mile	1.61	kilometer	1/1.61 = 0.621	mile
Ounce	28.3	gram	1/28.3 = 0.035	ounce
Ounce (fluid)	29.6	milliliter	1/29.6 = 0.034	ounce (fluid)
Pound	0.453	kilogram	1/0.453 = 2.21	pound
Pint	0.474	liter	1/0.474 = 2.11	pint
Gallon	3.79	liter	1/3.79 = 0.264	gallon

Read table from left to right.

Crossmultiplying the equation yields the following:

$$1 X = (12.0)(29.6)$$
$$X = 355 \text{ mL}$$

The result is 355, not 355.2, because the product cannot have more than three significant figures.

Example 3-5a   How many inches are there in a meter?

Using Table 3-3, there are 39.37 inches in a meter.

Example 3-5b   How many pounds are in 65.0 kg?

There are 2.21 pounds in each kilogram, therefore the answer is 2.21 times 65.0 or 144 lb.

Example 3-5c   How many kilograms are in 165 pounds?

The answer is 74.7 kg.

WHAT   Système Internationale

In 1960, the metric system was further revised by the Eleventh General Conference of Weights and Measures in Paris. A new system, the Système Internationale (SI) or International System of Units, was devised to further standardize measurements in the scientific community. This system was again revised in 1971 and is based on seven units: the meter for length, kilogram for mass, mole for concentration, second for time, ampere for electric current, Kelvin for temperature, and candela for light intensity. All other units of measurement can be calculated from one of these seven base units. Within the clinical laboratory, the SI method of measurement is replacing the older metric system.

WHAT ***Conversion Between the Metric System and Système Internationale***

Within the clinical laboratory, the change to SI primarily affects the clinical chemistry laboratory. Because the base unit of concentration in the SI is the mole, the values of many analytes have changed significantly. Enzyme measurements were the first to use the SI system. Before adopting the SI for enzymes, units for enzyme measurements were arbitrary and method based. Some assays, such as the muscle-brain (MB) fraction of the creatinine kinase enzyme used the terms of mass rather than in activity (nanograms/milliliter vs. units/liter).

Urea is a waste product that is excreted in urine and is commonly used to diagnose and treat patients with kidney disease. The urea molecule (NH_2CONH_2) (Figure 3-1) has a molecular weight of 60.07 and in many countries is measured and reported in mmol/L units. However, in the United States, blood urea nitrogen (BUN), not urea, is measured. Only the amount of nitrogen is measured in a BUN assay, and the results are expressed as mg/dL. Because only the nitrogen is measured in the BUN assay, multiplying the BUN value in mg/dL by the factor 2.14 (based on the difference in molecular weights) will result in the urea value in mg/dL.

HOW ***Example 3-6***

Given a BUN result of 12.5 mg/dL, convert it into terms of the urea concentratrion in mg/dL.
Since urea (mg/dL) = BUN (mg/dL) × 2.14, then the urea value in mg/dL = 12.5 × 2.14 or 26.8 mg/dL.

Example 3-6a Convert a BUN value of 25 mg/dL into its urea value in mg/dL.

A 25 mg/dL BUN value is equal to a 53.5 mg/dL urea value.

Example 3-6b Convert a BUN value of 72.5 mg/dL into its urea value in mg/dL.

A 72.5 mg/dL BUN value is equal to a 155.2 mg/dL.

Example 3-6c Given a glucose result of 80.0 mg/dL, what is the result in SI units? SI units are in molar terms (refer to Chapter 5 for additional information); therefore the first step is to determine the molecular weight of glucose. The formula for glucose is $C_6H_{12}O_6$ with a molecular weight of 180.16 g/mol. The next step is to convert 80.0 mg/dL into grams per liter or molar terms:

$$\left(\frac{80.0 \text{ mg}}{1 \text{ dL}}\right)\left(\frac{1 \text{ gram}}{1000 \text{ mg}}\right)\left(\frac{10 \text{ dL}}{1 \text{ L}}\right) = \frac{0.800 \text{ g}}{1 \text{ L}}$$

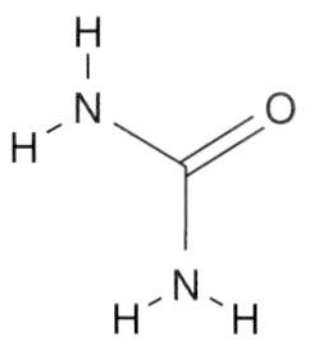

FIGURE 3-1 Urea.

Next, using the formula for molarity (see Chapter 5 for more information), the molarity of glucose can be determined.

$$\text{Molarity or moles/liter} = \frac{\left(\dfrac{\text{gram}}{\text{gram molecular weight}}\right)}{1\ \text{L}}$$

Substituting into the equation the values we have for this problem:

$$\text{M or mol/L} = \frac{\left(\dfrac{0.800\ \text{g}}{180.16\ \text{gmw}}\right)}{1\ \text{L}} = \frac{0.00444\ \text{mol}}{1\ \text{L}}$$

M or mol/L = 0.00444 mol or 4.44 m mol per liter

Therefore the glucose concentration in SI units is 4.44 mmol/L.

A shortcut method is to convert moles to millimoles and grams to milligrams. The formula would be:

$$\text{millimoles/liter} = (\text{milligrams/grams per mole})/1\ \text{L}$$
$$\textbf{millimoles/liter} = (800\ \text{mg}/180.16\ \text{g/mol})/1\ \text{L}$$
$$\textbf{X} = 4.44\ \text{mmol/L}$$

Example 3-6d   Given a urea result of 15 mg/dL, what is the result in terms of millimoles per liter? The molecular weight of urea is 60.07 g/mol.

The urea result of 15 mg/dL is equal to 2.5×10^{-3} mol/L or 2.50 mmol/L.

Example 3-6e   Given a BUN result of 22 mg/dL, what is the result in terms of millimoles per liter? The molecular weight of BUN is 28. By using Example 3-6 as a guide, 22 mg/dL is equal to 220 mg/L and 0.220 g/L. Substituting this value into the molarity formula equals:

$$\text{M or mol/L} = \frac{\left(\dfrac{0.220\ \text{g}}{28\ \text{gmw}}\right)}{1\ \text{L}} = \frac{0.007857\ \text{mol}}{1\ \text{L}}$$

M or mol/L = 0.007857 mol or 7.8 mmol per liter

The BUN result of 22 mg/dL is equal to 7.8 mmol/L.

Example 3-6f   Using Examples 3-6d and 3-6e as a guide, convert a urea result of 164 mg/dL to mmol/L.

Remember to use the molecular weight of urea, which is 60.07 g/mol in this calculation.

A urea result of 164 mg/dL is equal to a 27.3 mmol/L urea value.

Example 3-6g Given a cholesterol result of 245 mg/dL, what is the result in terms of milli-moles per liter? The molecular weight of cholesterol is 386.65 g/mol.

The cholesterol result of 245 mg/dL is equal to 6.34 mmol/L.

Example 3-6h Given a creatinine result of 1.4 mg/dL, what is the result in terms of millimoles per liter? The molecular weight of creatinine is 113.12 g/mol.

The creatinine result of 1.4 mg/dL is equal to 1.2×10^{-1} mmol/L.

WHAT MEASUREMENT OF TEMPERATURE

The thermometers used in the clinical laboratory today trace their origins from discoveries made by Galileo and others in the 15th and 16th centuries. Three types of measurement systems have evolved since that time.

Fahrenheit

Daniel Gabriel Fahrenheit invented the Fahrenheit scale for temperature measurement in 1724. His first attempts used a mercury thermometer and a mixture of water, ice, and sal ammoniac to determine an artificial freezing point, which he labeled as zero, and the boiling point of pure water (212°) as the upper point. In between, he divided his scale into 212 equal parts. His final thermometer used the freezing point of water (32°) as the lower point and the temperature of the human body (96° according to Fahrenheit) as the upper point. Soon after his death, the upper point of the Fahrenheit scale was again changed to 212°, whereas the freezing point remained unchanged, and the scale was divided into 180 equal parts. In 1861, the temperature of the human body was changed to 98.6°F by the work of Dr. Carl Wunderlich.

Celsius

In 1742, the Swedish astronomer Anders Celsius used the same fixed points of freezing and boiling water but set the fixed points to be 0 and 100, respectively. The scale was then divided into 100 equal parts. The Celsius, or centigrade, system of temperature measurement is used almost everywhere in the world and by the scientific community.

Kelvin

In 1852, William Thomson (Lord Kelvin) developed the thermodynamic scale of temperature. This scale, unlike other temperature scales at the time, did not depend on the effect of temperature on any gas or any other substance. Instead, it is based on theories relating to a reversible heat engine. From these theories, he deduced that the temperature of absolute zero would be reached when the engine no longer gave off any heat. There is no upper limit to the Kelvin scale. Kelvin's absolute temperature scale is related to the Celsius scale by the following formula:

$$\text{Kelvin} = t(^{\circ}\text{C}) + 273.15$$

Figure 3-2 shows a comparison between thermometers.

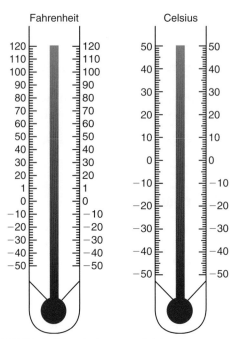

Fahrenheit   Celsius

FIGURE 3-2 Fahrenheit versus Celsius thermometers.

Conversion Between Temperature Scales

Almost all temperatures in the clinical laboratory are taken using the Celsius scale. It is helpful to be able to convert between Celsius and Fahrenheit temperatures. Notice by comparing both scales that the Fahrenheit scale is divided into 180 parts, whereas the Celsius scale is divided into 100 parts. Thus the Fahrenheit degree is $5/9$ of the Celsius degree.

Conversion From Celsius to Fahrenheit

To convert from a Celsius temperature to degrees Fahrenheit, you must remember that the Fahrenheit degree is $5/9$ of a Celsius degree because of the differences of their scales. As the zero of Celsius is equal to 32°F, a constant of 32 must be included in the conversion to make the two scales equal. The following formula describes the relationship between Celsius and Fahrenheit temperatures:

$$°F = \frac{9}{5}°C + 32$$

or

$$°F = [1.8 \times °C] + 32$$

HOW   **Example 3-7**

Convert 4°C to degrees Fahrenheit. Use the conversion formula:

$$°F = \frac{9}{5}°C + 32$$

Substituting into the formula the Celsius temperature of the refrigerator, the following formula is derived:

$$°F = \frac{9}{5}(4\,°C) + 32$$

$$°F = 7.2 + 32$$

$$°F = 39.2$$

Therefore, a 4 °C temperature is equal to a 39.2 °F temperature. By tradition, Fahrenheit temperatures are reported to the nearest $^1/_{10}$ of a degree.

Example 3-7a   Convert 10°C to °F.

Using the conversion formula: $°F = \frac{9}{5}(10) + 32 = 18 + 32 = 50.0\,°F$

10°C is equal to 50.0 °F.

Example 3-7b   Convert 37 °C to °F.

Using the conversion formula: $°F = \frac{9}{5}(37) + 32 = 66.6 + 32 = 98.6\,°F$

37 °C is equal to 98.6 °F.

Example 3-7c   Convert 100 °C to °F.

Using the conversion formula: $°F = \frac{9}{5}(100) + 32 = 180 + 32 = 212.0\,°F$

100 °C is equal to 212.0 °F.

WHAT   *Conversion From Fahrenheit to Celsius*

To convert Fahrenheit to Celsius, the previous formula may be worked backwards. Because the two scales have different freezing temperatures (32 vs. 0), the factor of 32 must first be subtracted from the Fahrenheit temperature. The result of this calculation is then multiplied by $\frac{5}{9}$.

HOW   *Example 3-8*

If a thermometer reads 39 °F, what is that equal to in terms of degrees Celsius? To convert from a Fahrenheit degree to a Celsius degree, first subtract the factor of 32 from the Fahrenheit degree. Next, multiply the result of this calculation by $\frac{5}{9}$. The conversion formula from Fahrenheit to Celsius is as follows:

$$°C = (°F - 32)\frac{5}{9}$$

Substituting the 39 °F temperature into the formula:

$$°C = (39 - 32)\frac{5}{9}$$

$$°C = (7)\frac{5}{9}$$

$$°C = 3.9$$

Therefore a temperature that records 39 °F on a thermometer is equal to a temperature of 3.9 °C.

Example 3-8a   Convert 45.0 °F to °C.

Using the formula: $°C = (°F - 32)\dfrac{5}{9} = 13 \times \dfrac{5}{9} = 7.2°C$

45.0°F is equal to 7.2 °C.

Example 3-8b   Convert 103 °F to °C.

Using the formula: $°C = (°F - 32)\dfrac{5}{9} = 71 \times \dfrac{5}{9} = 39.4°C$

103 °F is equal to 39.4°C.

Example 3-8c   Convert −4 °F to °C.

Using the formula: $°C = (°F - 32)\dfrac{5}{9} = -36 \times \dfrac{5}{9} = -20°C$

−4 °F is equal to −20.0 °C.

HOW **EXAMPLE PROBLEMS**

This section is designed to be useful to both the student and the laboratory professional. Students can use the additional problems to master the material. The laboratory professional can use the examples as templates for solving laboratory calculations. By finding an example similar to the problem that you need to solve, substitute into the equation the numbers appropriate to your calculation.

1. **Q.** Convert 200 pg to grams.
   A. 1 pg is equal to 1×10^{-12} g. Therefore 200 pg is equal to 200×10^{-12} g or 2.00×10^{-10} g.

2. **Q.** Convert 5.0 g to picograms.
   A. One pg is 1×10^{-12} smaller than 1 g. Therefore 5.0×10^{12} pg is equivalent to 5 g.

3. **Q.** Convert 84 mL to microliters.
   A. There are 84,000 mcL or 8.4×10^4 in 84 mL.

4. **Q.** How many milligrams are in 4.82 g?
   A. There are 1000 mg in 1 g. Therefore multiply 4.82 by 1000 to convert milligrams to grams: $4.82 \times 1000 = 4820$ mg.

5. **Q.** How many deciliters are in 1.0 L?
   A. Using the shortcut method of moving the decimal point, 1.0 L would have the decimal point moved one space to the right (since we are going from a larger metric unit to a smaller metric unit) to be 10 dL in 1.0 L.

6. **Q.** How many liters are in 1500 mL?
   A. Using the shortcut method of moving the decimal point, 1500 mL would have the decimal point moved three spaces to the left (since we are going from a smaller metric unit of milliliters to a larger metric unit of liters), resulting in an answer of 1.5 L.

7. **Q.** How many centimeters are in 2 m?
   A. There are 100 cm in 1 m. Therefore, there will be 200 cm in 2 m.

8. **Q.** Express 4.5 mL equivalent to liters.
   A. A milliliter is 1000 times smaller than a liter. To determine how many liters are in 4.5 mL, divide 4.5 by 1000: $^{4.5}/_{1000} = 0.0045$ L or 4.5×10^{-3} L.

9. **Q.** How many meters are in 100 yards?
   A. One meter is slightly longer than 1 yard. The conversion factor used to convert from yards to meters is 0.914. Multiply the amount of yards by 0.914 to convert to meters: 100 yards $\times$ 0.914 = 91.4 m.

10. **Q.** How many kilograms are in 10 pounds of a dry weight?
    A. To convert from pounds to kilograms, multiply the pounds weight by the factor 0.453. $10 \times 0.453 = 4.53$ kg or divide the number of pounds by 2.21.

11. **Q.** A patient weighs 55 kg. How many pounds does the patient weigh?
    A. To convert from kilograms to pounds, multiply the kilogram quantity by 2.21 to convert to pounds:

    $$55 \times 2.21 = 121.6 \text{lb.}$$ By convention report to the nearest pounds.

12. **Q.** Convert 225 pounds to kilograms.
    A. To convert from pounds to kilograms, multiply the pounds by 0.453. There are 102.0 kg in 225 lb.

13. **Q.** Convert 3.5 mg/mL to milligrams per liter.
    A. Use equivalent units to convert milligrams per milliliter to milligrams per liter. There are 1000 mL/L. 1000 mL/L is equivalent to 1. Therefore we can use this fraction to cancel units and convert from milligrams per milliliter to milligrams per liter.

    $$\left(\frac{3.5\,\text{mg}}{1\,\text{mL}}\right)\left(\frac{1000\,\text{mL}}{1\,\text{L}}\right) = \frac{3500\,\text{mg}}{1\,\text{L}}$$

    Therefore 3.5 mg/mL is equivalent to 3.5×10^3 mg/L.

14. **Q.** Convert 258 mg/dL to grams per liter.
    A. This is solved in two parts. First, convert milligrams to grams:

    $$\left(\frac{258\,\text{mg}}{1\,\text{dL}}\right)\left(\frac{1\,\text{g}}{1000\,\text{mg}}\right) = \frac{0.258\,\text{g}}{1\,\text{dL}}$$

    Next, convert deciliters to liters:

    $$\left(\frac{0.258\,\text{g}}{1\,\text{dL}}\right)\left(\frac{10\,\text{dL}}{1\,\text{L}}\right) = \frac{2.58\,\text{g}}{1\,\text{L}}$$

    Therefore 258 mg/dL is equal to 2.58 g/L.

15. **Q.** Convert 0.750 g/L to mg/mL.
    A. This is solved in two parts. First convert grams to milligrams, then convert liters to milliliters.

Therefore the 0.750 g/L becomes 750 mg/L. Then when it is converted to mg/mL, it becomes 0.750 mg/mL. Notice that it is the same number, 0.750. This is because the mg/mL becomes 1000/1000 or 1.0.

16. **Q.** Convert 2.5 g/L to mg/mL.
    A. Using Example 3-15 as a guide, 2.5 g/L becomes 2.5 mg/mL.

17. **Q.** A patient's calcium result is 8.5 mg/dL. Convert this result to SI units.
    A. SI units are in moles per liter. The gram atomic weight, or grams per mole, of calcium is 40.

    First, convert 8.5 mg/dL into grams per liter using the string method:

    $$\left(\frac{8.5 \text{ mg}}{1 \text{ dL}}\right)\left(\frac{1 \text{ g}}{1000 \text{ mg}}\right)\left(\frac{10 \text{ dL}}{1 \text{ L}}\right) = \frac{0.085 \text{ g}}{L}$$

    Next, use the molarity formula to solve for molarity:

    $$M = \frac{\frac{g}{g/mol}}{1 \text{ L}} \text{ or } M = \frac{mol}{1 \text{ L}}$$

    Substitute into the formula the appropriate numbers:

    $$moles/L = \frac{\frac{0.085 \text{ g}}{40 \text{ g/mol}}}{1 \text{ liter}}$$

    $$moles/L = 0.0021 \text{ mol/L or 2.1 mmol/L}$$

18. **Q.** If a patient had a calcium value of 3.2 mmol/L, how many milligrams per deciliter of calcium does the patient have?
    A. 12.8 mg/dL. Refer to Example Problem 17 for additional information. Since the units are milligrams and millimoles, the milligrams do not have to be converted to grams for the molarity calculation.

19. **Q.** Convert a BUN value of 85 mg/dL to a urea value in mg/dL units.
    A. To convert BUN to urea when both are in mg/dL units, multiply the BUN value by 2.14. Therefore a BUN value of 85 mg/dL is the same as a urea value of 182 mg/dL.

20. **Q.** How many degrees Fahrenheit is a 30°C temperature?
    A. The formula to convert °F to °C is as follows:

    $$°F = \frac{9}{5}°C + 32$$

    Substituting into the formula the Celsius temperature:

    $$°F = \frac{9}{5}(30) + 32$$

    $$°F = 86$$

21. **Q.** How many degrees Fahrenheit is a $-10°C$ temperature?
    A. Use the following formula:

$$°F = \frac{9}{5}°C + 32$$

$$°F = \frac{9}{5}(-10°C) + 32$$

$$°F = 14$$

22. **Q.** How many degrees Celsius is a $215°F$ temperature?
    A. The formula to convert $°C$ to $°F$ is as follows:

$$°C = (°F - 32)\frac{5}{9}$$

Substituting into the formula the Fahrenheit temperature:

$$°C = (215°F - 32)\frac{5}{9}$$

$$°C = 101.7$$

23. **Q.** How many degrees Celsius is a $-20°F$ temperature?
    A. The formula to convert $°C$ to $°F$ is as follows:

$$°C = (°F - 32)\frac{5}{9}$$

Substitute into the formula:

$$°C = (-20°F - 32)\frac{5}{9}$$

$$°C = -29$$

HOW **PRACTICE PROBLEMS**

Solve the following practice problems to further master the material. Answers and explanations to some problems can be found in the Answer Key.

Convert the following numbers to their metric equivalents:

1. 55.5 mcg $= ?$ g

2. 3.5 g $= ?$ mg

3. 500 mL $= ?$ dL

4. 500 mL = ? mcL

5. 0.500 mL = ? mcL

6. 0.25 L = ? dL

7. 25 mL = ? L

8. 2.5 L = ? mL

9. 70 mm = ? cm

10. 4.0 km = ? m

11. 2.0 L = ? dL

12. 20 nm = ? mm

13. 2.25 oz = ? g

14. 72 in = ? m

15. 1.5 pints = ? mL

16. 2.0 gal = ? L

Convert the following numbers.

17. 25.0 mg/dL to milligrams per liter

18. 5.0 mg/L to milligrams per deciliter

19. 18.5 g/L to milligrams per deciliter

20. 150.0 mg/dL to grams per liter

21. 180.0 mg/dL to grams per liter

22. 10.0 cm^2 to mm^2

23. Given a magnesium value of 4.0 mg/dL, what is the result in SI units? Gram atomic weight of Mg = 24.

24. Express a glucose value of 130 mg/dL in SI units. Gram molecular weight of glucose = 180.16.

25. Convert a 83.0 mg/dL BUN value to mg/dL urea.

26. Convert a 110.0 mg/dL BUN value to mg/dL urea.

27. Convert a 120.0 mg/dL BUN value to mmol/L urea. The molecular weight of urea = 60.07

28. Convert a 34.0 mg/dL BUN value to mmol/L urea. The molecular weight of urea = 60.07.

Convert the following temperatures.

29. 12°C to °F

30. −5.0°C to °F

31. 205°F to °C

32. −18°F to °C

QUICK NOTES

- The metric system base unit for length is the meter, for mass is the gram, and for volume is the liter.
- A common metric prefix is deci (d), which is 1/10 or 10^{-1} smaller than the base unit. There are 10 dL in 1.0 liter.
- A milli (m) is 1000 times smaller than the base unit, or 10^{-3}. There are 1000 mL in 1.0 liter.
- A micro (mc) is a million times smaller than the base unit, or 10^{-6}. There are 1000 mcL in 1.0 mL and 1×10^{6} mcL in 1.0 liter.
- When converting from a larger metric unit to a smaller metric unit, move the decimal point the appropriate amount of spaces to the right (e.g., 0.750 mg to mcg will equal 750 mcg); when converting a smaller metric unit to a larger metric unit, move the decimal point the appropriate amount of spaces to the left (e.g., 750 mcg to mg will equal 0.750 mg).
- Always check your math conversions by converting a known relationship (e.g., 500 mcL = 0.500 mL) and ensuring you arrive at the correct value.
- When converting Fahrenheit to Celsius, or vice versa, always use the relationship of 98.6°F is equal to 37°C.
- Remember that Fahrenheit temperatures will always be higher than Celsius temperatures unless dealing with very low negative-degree temperatures.
- As a frame of reference, $-12°$ to 0°C is freezer temperature compared to below 32°F, and 4° to 8°C is refrigerator temperature or about 40°F.

BIBLIOGRAPHY

National Center for Biotechnology Information. (n.d.). PubChem Compound Database: Urea. Retrieved from https://pubchem.ncbi.nlm.nih.gov/compound/1176.

Dilutions and Titers

OBJECTIVES

At the end of this chapter, the reader should be able to do the following:

1. State the components and the formula for dilutions.
2. Define the following terms: *sample volume, diluent volume, total volume, dilution factor.*
3. Calculate the sample volume or diluent volume needed for a particular dilution.
4. Calculate the dilution made given the sample volume and diluent volume.
5. Given the dilution and total volume, calculate the sample volume.
6. Given the dilution, sample volume, and total volume, calculate the diluent volume.
7. Calculate the dilution factor, and use it to obtain original concentrations.
8. Explain the difference between dilutions and ratios.
9. Given sufficient information, determine the ratio or dilution.
10. Describe how a serial dilution is performed.
11. Calculate a final concentration when performing serial dilutions.
12. Determine the concentration of any tube in a serial dilution.
13. Determine how a serial dilution should be performed if given the final dilution requested.
14. Compare and contrast dilutions and titers.
15. Compare and contrast ratio and proportion to dilutions.

WHAT **SIMPLE DILUTIONS**

In many areas of the clinical laboratory, a specimen may have to be diluted so that it can be analyzed. In chemistry, the specimen may have a concentration outside of the linear range of the method or instrument used for analysis. Antibiotics are diluted in microbiology to determine the minimal inhibitory concentration for microorganisms. Serial dilutions are performed on serum in immunology to determine titers of antibodies. A poorly performed or interpreted dilution may lead to errors of analysis and subsequently affect patient treatment.

There are two parts to a dilution. The first part is the sample to be diluted; the second is the diluent used to perform the dilution. In Chapter 5 you will learn about solutions. In a solution there are also two parts: the solute (the part that is being placed into the solution) and the solvent (the liquid into which the solute is being diluted). The solute plus the solvent makes a solution. So for a dilution, the sample that is being diluted is the solute and the diluent is the solvent.

Many lyophilized quality control materials have an accompanying liquid called the diluent to be used for reconstitution. This diluent may contain buffers necessary for the correct concentration of the analytes to be tested. If deionized water is used instead of the manufacturer's supplied diluent, the control material will not be correctly buffered, and inaccurate results may occur. Therefore it is essential that the proper diluent be used for reconstitution.

When a dilution is required, often it is referred to as a "1 to 2" dilution or a "1 to 10" dilution. For example, a dilution of equal parts of sample may be written as or 1 to 2, or ½. If written as a 1:2 with a colon separating the numbers, in this textbook that refers to a ratio, which will be covered later in this chapter.

A 1 to 10 dilution means that for every 1 part of sample there is a total of 10 parts of the solution. In a 1 to 10 dilution, 1 part of the sample is used and 9, *not* 10, parts of the diluent are used. If 10 parts of the diluent would be used, then there would be a total of 11 parts to the solution.

A simple dilution uses the following formula:

$$\frac{\text{Sample volume (SV)}}{\text{Sample volume } + \text{ Diluent volume (DV)}}$$

or

$$\frac{\text{Sample volume}}{\text{Total volume (TV)}}$$

NOTE: Throughout this chapter, sample volume may be abbreviated SV, diluent volume abbreviated DV, and total volume abbreviated TV.

Notice that the sample volume is included in the denominator of the equation because it is part of the total volume of the solution. Many dilution errors are made by forgetting this crucial fact.

HOW   **Example 4-1**

What is the sample volume and what is the diluent volume in a 1 to 5 dilution?
Use the dilution formula to solve the problem:

$$\frac{\text{Sample volume}}{\text{Sample volume } + \text{ Diluent volume}} =$$

$$\frac{1 \text{ part sample}}{1 \text{ part sample } + 4 \text{ parts diluent}} = 1 \text{ to } 5 \text{ dilution}$$

A 1 to 5 dilution is made with 1 part sample and 4 parts diluent.

Example 4-1a   What is the sample volume and diluent volume in a 1 to 20 dilution?

Using the dilution formula, there would be **1 part sample and 19 parts diluent** to make a 1 to 20 dilution.

Example 4-1b   What is the sample volume and diluent volume in a 1 to 25 dilution?

Using the dilution formula, there would be **1 part sample and 24 parts diluent** to make a 1 to 25 dilution.

Example 4-1c   What is the sample volume and diluent volume in a 1 to 100 dilution?

Using the dilution formula, there would be 1 part sample to 99 parts diluent to make a 1 to 100 dilution.

Example 4-1d   A 10 mcL sample is added to 90 mcL diluent. What dilution was made?

Using the dilution formula:

$$\frac{10 \text{ parts sample}}{10 \text{ parts sample} + 90 \text{ parts diluent}} = \frac{10}{100} = \frac{1}{10}$$

A 10 mcL sample and 90 mcL of diluent make a 1 to 10 dilution.

Example 4-1e   A 20 mcL sample is added to 80 mcL diluent. What dilution was made?

Using the dilution formula:

$$\frac{20 \text{ parts sample}}{20 \text{ parts sample} + 80 \text{ parts diluent}} = \frac{20}{100} = \frac{1}{5}$$

A 20 mcL sample and 80 mcL of diluent make a 1 to 5 dilution.

WHAT   HOW TO MAKE DILUTIONS WHEN THE TOTAL VOLUME IS DETERMINED

Sometimes the total volume of a dilution is already determined, usually based on the sample size needed for analysis, but how do you decide what the sample and diluent volume should be? You can use ratio and proportion to determine the sample and diluent volume. Allow extra volumes for the sample and diluent so that there is room to pipette the diluted sample if there will be manual pipetting involved. For example, if you need 100 mcL total volume, and you make your dilution so that there is exactly 100 mcL, it will be impossible to accurately pipette all 100 mcg using a manual pipette. An easy way is to make double what you need.

HOW   Example 4-2

A 1 to 4 dilution of serum is to be made on a sample that is too high to measure on the chemistry analyzer for the creatinine method that is used (i.e., "outside of the linear range of the instrument"). The total volume of the dilution is to be 100 mcL. What volumes of serum and diluent (deionized water) are needed?

To solve this problem, use ratio and proportion:

$$\frac{1 \text{ part sample volume}}{4 \text{ parts total volume}} = \frac{X \text{ parts sample volume}}{100 \text{ parts total volume}}$$

Crossmultiplying the equation yields the following:

$$(1)(100 \text{ mcL}) = (4 \text{ mcL})(X)$$

$$100 \text{ mcL} = (4 \text{ mcL})(X)$$

(Divide both sides by 4)25 mcL = X

25.0 mcL is the sample volume and 100.0 − 25.0 or 75.0 mcL is the diluent volume.

Example 4-2a   A 1 to 10 dilution must be prepared to make a total volume of 100.0 mcL. How much serum must be used?

Again, use ratio and proportion to solve this problem.

$$\frac{1 \text{ part sample volume}}{10 \text{ parts total volume}} = \frac{X \text{ parts sample volume}}{100 \text{ parts total volume}}$$

Crossmultiplying the equation yields the following:

$$(1)(100 \text{ mcL}) = (10 \text{ mcL})(X)$$
$$100 \text{ mcL} = (10 \text{ mcL})(X)$$
$$10 \text{ mcL} = X$$

Therefore **10 mcL of serum** will be used for the dilution. To determine the amount of diluent needed, subtract 10 from 100: 100 mcL total volume − 10 mcL sample volume = **90 mcL diluent volume**.

Example 4-2b   A 1 to 3 dilution of serum must be performed. How many parts of the sample must be used, and how many parts of the diluent must be used?

Using the dilution formula, a **1 to 3 dilution** consists of **1 part sample to 2 parts diluent**.

$$\frac{1 \text{ SV}}{1 \text{ SV} + 2 \text{ DV}} = \frac{1}{3 \text{ dilution}}$$

Example 4-2c   Using this 1 to 3 dilution, a total volume of 90 mcL is needed. How is this dilution performed?

Using ratio and proportion, **30 mcL of serum** are used, and **60 mcL of diluent** are used to make a total volume of 90 mcL. This is also 1 part serum to 2 parts diluent (30 × 2 = 60).

Example 4-2d   A 1 to 4 dilution of a sample must be performed, with a total volume of 200 mcL. How much serum would be needed?

Using ratio and proportion, **50 mcL of serum** would be needed and **150 mcL of diluent** would be used.

Example 4-2e   If you had a total volume of 100 mcL and you used 25 mcL of serum to make your dilution, what was the value of the actual dilution you performed?

Now to add a little twist to it: Determine the dilution that is performed given the sample volume and total volume.

Using ratio and proportion:

$$\frac{1 \text{ part sample volume}}{X \text{ parts total volume}} = \frac{25 \text{ parts sample volume}}{100 \text{ parts total volume}}$$

Crossmultiplying the equation yields:

$$(25 \text{ mcL})(X) = (1)(100 \text{ mcL})$$
$$25(\text{mcL})(X) = 100 \text{ mcL}$$
$$X = 4 \text{ mcL}$$

Therefore a dilution made with 25 mcL in a total volume of 100 mcL is a 1 to 4 dilution.

Example 4-2f   If you had a total volume of 250 mcL and you used 50 mcL of serum to make your dilution, what would be the value of the actual dilution you performed?

Using ratio and proportion again, a dilution made with 50 mcL in a total volume of 250 mcL is a 1 to 5 dilution.

Example 4-2g   If you had a total volume of 100 mcL and you used 10 mcL of serum to make your dilution, what would be the value of the actual dilution you performed?

The actual value of the dilution would be a 1 to 10 dilution.

WHAT **DILUTION VARIATIONS**

What is the value of a dilution with 0.5 part sample to 9.5 parts diluent?

The value would be a 1 to 20 dilution. At first, you might have thought that it is a 1 to 10 dilution; however, the dilution fraction's numerator must be a whole number of at least 1.0. Therefore the 0.5 has to be doubled to 1 and the denominator number of 10.0 (0.5 sample volume + 9.5 diluent volume) is doubled to 20.

HOW   *Example 4-3*

What is the dilution that is made with 0.25 sample volume and 2.75 diluent volume?

Because 0.25 is less than 1 by a factor of 4, multiply both sides of the dilution formula by a factor of 4:

$$\frac{0.25 \text{ SV}}{0.25 \text{ SV} + 2.75 \text{ DV}} = \frac{0.25 \text{ SV}}{3.00 \text{ TV}} \times \frac{4}{4} = \frac{1.0}{12.00}$$

The dilution made is a 1 to 12 dilution.

Example 4-3a   What is the dilution that is made with 0.50 sample volume and 1.50 diluent volume?

Because 0.50 is less than 1 by a factor of 2, both 0.50 (SV) and 2.0 (TV) are each multiplied by 2 to yield 1.0 (SV) and 4.0 (TV). Therefore this is a 1 to 4 dilution.

Example 4-3b   What is the dilution made with 0.20 SV and 1.80 DV?

Both the 0.20 SV and the 2.0 TV are multiplied by a factor of 5 to yield a dilution of 1 to 10.

Example 4-3c   What is the dilution made with 0.5 sample volume and 6.0 diluent volume?

Both the 0.5 SV and the 6.5 TV are multiplied by a factor of 2 to yield a dilution of 1 to 13.

WHAT # DILUTED SPECIMEN VALUES

Once the specimen has been diluted and analyzed, the result obtained must be corrected for the dilution. A common preventable laboratory error is the failure to correct a diluted specimen's result properly. An easy way to correct the result is to use a "factor." This factor is the reciprocal of the dilution that was performed. In the first example and in the preceding example, a 1 to 4 dilution was performed. The factor for these dilutions is the reciprocal of 1 to 4, or 4.

$$1 \div \frac{1}{4} \text{ OR } \frac{1}{\frac{1}{4}} = 4$$

The creatinine result obtained from Example 4-2 would be multiplied by 4 to obtain its true value.

HOW ### Example 4-4

Using Example 4-2, suppose that the linear range of the creatinine assay the instrument could measure was from 0.1 mg/dL to 15.0 mg/dL. A patient sample is analyzed, and the result is too high to be measured on the instrument. A 1 to 5 dilution is performed on the serum, and the reanalyzed diluted sample result is 5.0 mg/dL. The diluted sample result must be multiplied by the dilution factor to determine the concentration in the undiluted sample.

$$5.0 \text{ mg/dL} \times 5(\text{dilution factor}) = 25.0 \text{ mg/dL}$$

Therefore the patient's actual creatinine result is 25.0 mg/dL, *not* 5.0 mg/dL. Failure to perform this crucial step would mean the reporting of a creatinine level of 5.0 mg/dL instead of 25.0 mg/dL, which could be harmful to the patient. Remember that the diluted concentration times the dilution factor is equal to the true sample concentration.

Example 4-4a

A patient's glucose result is outside the linear range of the analyzer; 10.0 mcL of serum are added to 90.0 mcL of diluent and the diluted sample reanalyzed. The glucose value of the diluted sample is 75.0 mg/dL. What glucose value is reported to the physician, and what is the dilution factor that will be used to calculate this result?

The first step is to determine the dilution that was performed:

$$\frac{10.0 \text{ mcL}}{10.0 \text{ mcL} + 90.0 \text{ mcL}} = \frac{10.0}{100.0} = \frac{1}{10}$$

Next, the dilution factor is the reciprocal of the dilution that was performed, in this case 1 to 10.

$$\text{Dilution factor} = \frac{1}{\frac{1}{10}} = 10$$

The last step is to multiply the diluted result by the factor:

$$75.0 \text{ mg/dL} \times 10 = 750.0 \text{ mg/dL}$$

The technologist reports a glucose value of 750.0 mg/dL to the physician. This example demonstrates how critical it is to perform the dilution calculations correctly. In this example, a glucose value of 75.0 mg/dL is within the reference intervals, a value of 750.0 mg/dL is life threatening.

Example 4-4b   A patient's aspartate aminotransferase (AST) value is outside of the linear range. The patient's serum sample is diluted by taking 25 mcL of serum and 75 mcL of diluent. It is reanalyzed, and the diluted value that is obtained is 400 IU. What is the actual true AST value?

The dilution was performed by adding 25 mcL of serum to 75 mcL of diluent in a 1 to 4 dilution ($^{25}/_{100}$). The patient's true AST value is 1600 IU (400 × 4).

Example 4-4c   A different patient's glucose sample needed to be diluted. An amount of 30 mcL of serum is added to 150 mcL of diluent. The diluted sample's result was 145 mg/dL. What is the true glucose value?

The dilution that was performed was a 1 to 6 dilution. Therefore the patient's actual glucose result is 145 × 6 or 870 mg/dL.

Example 4-4d   A patient's alanine aminotransferase (ALT) value is outside of the linear range; 50 mcL of serum was added to 200 mcL of diluent. The diluted specimen was reanalyzed and a value of 350 IU was obtained. What is the patient's true ALT value?

The dilution that was performed was a 1 to 5 dilution. Therefore 350 × 5 = 1750, so the true ALT value is 1750 IU.

WHAT DILUTIONS VERSUS RATIOS

Learning about dilutions and ratios can be confusing for students because different textbooks refer to them in different ways. In the laboratory it is best to ask scientists how they interpret ratios and dilutions to avoid mistakes. As mentioned at the beginning of this chapter, in this book, dilutions will be referred to with a slash, as in $^1/_2$, whereas ratios will be referred to with a colon, as in 1:4. In a ratio, the numerator is the part or amount of the sample used, whereas the denominator is the part or amount of diluent used.

Ratio 1:4 = one part sample, four parts diluent

Contrast this with a dilution in which the numerator denotes the parts of the sample used but the denominator is the total parts (diluent plus the sample).

$$\text{A 1 to 4 dilution is}: \frac{1 \text{ part sample volume}}{1 \text{ part sample volume } + \text{ 3 parts diluent volume}} = \frac{1}{4}$$

Dilution $\frac{1}{4}$ = one part sample, three parts diluent

Note that for a 1 to 4 dilution, there were THREE parts diluent. An easy way to turn a dilution into a ratio is to remove the sample volume from the denominator. In a 1 to 4 dilution, by removing the 1 part sample volume from the denominator, the fraction becomes $\frac{1}{3}$, or a 1:3 ratio.

A 1:4 ratio of 1 part sample and 4 parts diluent is a 1 to 5 dilution.

$$\text{Ratio}: \frac{1 \text{ part SV}}{4 \text{ parts DV}} = \frac{1}{4} \qquad \text{Dilution}: \frac{1 \text{ part SV}}{4 \text{ parts DV } + \text{ 1 part SV}} = \frac{1}{5}$$

As shown, another way of stating the difference between ratios and dilutions is that a dilution is formed by the ratio of the sample volume to the total volume. The ratio tells you how much of the sample and diluent are necessary to form the dilution. Using the previous example, the 1:4 ratio tells you that you need 1 part sample to 4 parts diluent to make a 1 to 5 dilution.

Example 4-5

To clarify the difference between a ratio and a dilution, suppose 50 mcL of serum was added to 100 mcL of diluent. Consider the following questions:

What is the ratio of serum to diluent?

The ratio of serum to diluent is 50 parts serum to 100 parts diluent or a 1:2 (1 to 2) ratio.

What is the dilution in this example?

Fifty parts of serum were diluted into 100 parts of diluent. Using the dilution formula:

$$\frac{50 \text{ mcL SV}}{50 \text{ mcL SV} + 100 \text{ mcL DV}} = \frac{50 \text{ mcL SV}}{150 \text{ mcL TV}} = \frac{1}{3}$$

Therefore 50 parts sample to 100 parts diluent is a 1 to 2 ratio, but a 1 to 3 dilution.

This is a critical distinction when calculating the original concentration as Example 4-4 demonstrates.

Example 4-5a   If 15 mcL of sample was added to 90 mcL of diluent, what is the ratio and what is the dilution?

15 mcL added to 90 mcL is a 1 to 6 ratio and a 1 to 7 dilution.

Example 4-5b   If 30 mcL of sample was added to 90 mcL of diluent, what is the ratio and what is the dilution?

30 mcL added to 90 mcL is a 1 to 3 ratio and a 1 to 4 dilution.

Example 4-5c   If 10 mcL of sample was added to 90 mcL of diluent, what is the ratio and what is the dilution?

10 mcL added to 90 mcL is a 1 to 9 ratio and a 1 to 10 dilution.

SERIAL DILUTIONS AND TUBE DILUTIONS

Serial dilutions are performed when large dilutions must be made with small volumes of sample and diluent. For example, suppose that a $\frac{1}{1000}$ dilution of serum was needed for a test. Theoretically 1.0 mL of sample and 999.0 mL of diluent could be used (or 0.5 mL of sample and 499.5 mL of diluent).

However, this is a large volume of diluent and sample. Using serial dilutions, much smaller sample and diluent volumes can be used. A serial dilution is simply a series of sequential dilutions of the sample until the final dilution is reached. By definition, a serial dilution uses the same dilution for each tube in the series. A tube dilution series uses different dilutions for each tube. In both cases, the final dilution is the product of each individual dilution:

Final dilution = (dilution 1)(dilution 2)(dilution 3), etc.

In immunology, serial dilutions are performed using the same dilution over and over again. If a serial dilution was composed of a series of 1 to 10 dilutions, that dilution series can be referred to as a "tenfold" dilution series. Common serial dilution series used in immunology are $\frac{1}{2}$, $\frac{1}{4}$, and $\frac{1}{10}$. If reagents are to be added directly to serially diluted tubes, it is important to discard from the last tube in the series the same sample volume used for all other dilutions in the series. For example, if a tenfold dilution was performed with five tubes with a sample volume of 10 mcL and a diluent volume of 90 mcL, 10 mcL from the fifth tube must be discarded. If the 10 mcL is not removed from the last tube, its total volume would be 100 mcL. However, all the other tubes have a total volume of 90 mcL because 10 mcL is removed from each to be used in the next dilution in the series. By removing the 10 mcL from the last tube, when additional reagents are added to the diluted tubes, all tubes in the reaction sequence will have the same volume.

In chemistry, samples may be serially diluted, or a tube dilution series may be used. In either a serial dilution or tube dilution series, if the original concentration is known, then the concentration of each tube in the series can be calculated in one of two ways.

HOW   ***Example 4-6***

A tube dilution series is performed on a sample to check the pipetting skills of a medical laboratory technician student. Five tubes are used in the dilution. The concentration of the sample is 1650 mg/dL. The sample is diluted ⅕ (tube 1), rediluted ½ (tube 2), diluted again ¼ (tube 3), then diluted ⅕ (tube 4), and then diluted ¹⁄₁₀ (tube 5). After the student performs the dilution, the diluted specimen will be analyzed, and the student will be graded for precision of pipetting. What will be the diluted concentration in each tube? Figure 4-1 is a schematic of the multiple dilution.

HOW   **Method 1 to Determine the Concentration of Each Tube**

1. Divide the first tube in the series by the dilution factor used in its dilution (⅕ dilution was performed; factor = 5).

   The sample concentration in tube 1 is as follows:

   $$\frac{1650 \text{ mg/dL}}{5} \text{ or } 330 \text{ mg/dL}$$

2. Divide the concentration of the first tube by the dilution performed for the second tube (dilution was ½, therefore factor = 2).

   The concentration of tube 2 is as follows:

   $$\frac{330 \text{ mg/dL}}{2} \text{ or } 165 \text{ mg/dL}$$

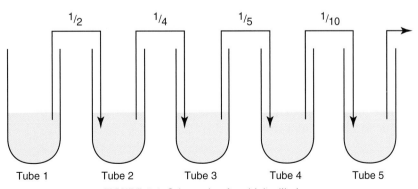

FIGURE 4-1 Schematic of multiple dilutions.

3. Divide the concentration of the second tube by the dilution performed for the third tube (dilution was $^1/_4$; therefore factor = 4).

The concentration of tube 3 is as follows:

$$\frac{165 \text{ mg/dL}}{4} \text{ or } 41.25 \text{ mg/dL}$$

4. Divide the concentration of the third tube by the dilution performed for the fourth tube (dilution was $^1/_5$; therefore the factor = 5).

The concentration of tube 4 is as follows:

$$\frac{41.25}{5} \text{ or } 8.25 \text{ mg/dL}$$

5. Divide the concentration of the fourth tube by the dilution performed for the fifth tube (dilution was $^1/_{10}$; therefore the factor = 10).

Tube 5 has a concentration of the following:

$$\frac{8.25}{10} \text{ or } 0.825 \text{ mg/dL}$$

HOW   **Method 2 to Determine the Concentration of Each Tube**

1. Divide the original concentration by the dilution factor used for tube 1 to determine the concentration of tube 1.

$$\frac{1650}{5} = 330 \text{ mg/dL}$$

2. Determine the dilution, and therefore the dilution factor, for tube 2 by multiplying the dilutions performed on tubes 1 and 2.

$$\underset{\text{Tube 1}}{\left(\frac{1}{5}\right)} \times \underset{\text{Tube 2}}{\left(\frac{1}{2}\right)} = \underset{\substack{\text{Dilution for tube 2} \\ \text{Dilution factor} = 10}}{\frac{1}{10}}$$

Divide the original concentration by the dilution factor for tube 2.

$$\frac{1650}{10} = 165 \text{ mg/dL}$$

3. Determine the dilution, and therefore the dilution factor, for tube 3 by multiplying the dilutions performed on tubes 1, 2, and 3.

$$\underset{\text{Tube 1}}{\left(\frac{1}{5}\right)} \times \underset{\text{Tube 2}}{\left(\frac{1}{2}\right)} \times \underset{\text{Tube 3}}{\left(\frac{1}{4}\right)} = \underset{\substack{\text{Dilution for tube 3} \\ \text{Dilution factor} = 40}}{\frac{1}{40}}$$

Or multiply the dilution of tube 2 by the dilution performed on tube 3.

$$\left(\frac{1}{10}\right)\left(\frac{1}{4}\right)=\frac{1}{40}$$

Divide the original concentration by the dilution factor for tube 3.

$$\frac{1650}{40}=41.25 \text{ mg/dL}$$

4. Determine the dilution, and the dilution factor, for tube 4 by multiplying the dilutions performed on tubes 1, 2, 3, and 4.

$$\underset{\text{Tube 1}}{\left(\frac{1}{5}\right)} \times \underset{\text{Tube 2}}{\left(\frac{1}{2}\right)} \times \underset{\text{Tube 3}}{\left(\frac{1}{4}\right)} \times \underset{\text{Tube 4}}{\left(\frac{1}{5}\right)} = \underset{\substack{\text{Dilution for tube 4} \\ \text{Dilution factor} = 200}}{\frac{1}{200}}$$

Or multiply the dilution of tube 3 by the dilution performed on tube 4.

$$\left(\frac{1}{40}\right)\left(\frac{1}{5}\right)=\frac{1}{200}$$

Divide the original concentration by the dilution factor for tube 4.

$$\frac{1650}{200}=8.25 \text{ mg/dL}$$

5. Determine the dilution, and the dilution factor, for tube 5 by multiplying the dilutions performed on tubes 1, 2, 3, 4, and 5.

$$\underset{\text{Tube 1}}{\left(\frac{1}{5}\right)} \times \underset{\text{Tube 2}}{\left(\frac{1}{2}\right)} \times \underset{\text{Tube 3}}{\left(\frac{1}{4}\right)} \times \underset{\text{Tube 4}}{\left(\frac{1}{5}\right)} \times \underset{\text{Tube 5}}{\left(\frac{1}{10}\right)} = \underset{\substack{\text{Dilution for tube 5} \\ \text{Dilution factor} = 2000}}{\frac{1}{2000}}$$

Or multiply the dilution of tube 4 by the dilution performed on tube 5.

$$\left(\frac{1}{200}\right)\left(\frac{1}{10}\right)=\frac{1}{2000}$$

Divide the original concentration by the dilution factor for tube 5.

$$\frac{1650}{2000}=0.825 \text{ mg/dL}$$

To check this result, multiply 1650 by the product of the individual dilutions:

$$(1650)\left(\tfrac{1}{5}\times\tfrac{1}{2}\times\tfrac{1}{4}\times\tfrac{1}{5}\times\tfrac{1}{10}\right)=(1650)\left(\tfrac{1}{2000}\right)=0.825 \text{ mg/dL}$$

Any of the dilutions performed in a serial or tube dilution series can be rechecked in this manner to verify the accuracy of the calculations that were performed.

Usually, serial dilutions are performed as a method of diluting a sample using the smallest quantities of sample and diluent possible. In the laboratory, often how a dilution is performed is limited by the types of pipettes available. Many dilutions are performed using the volumes of the available pipettes as the base from which the dilutions are calculated. It makes little sense to calculate a dilution in which 5 mcL of sample is required when the smallest volume pipette available is a 10 mcL pipette.

HOW

Example 4-7

A 1 to 1000 dilution of a serum sample must be made. How is this done using small volumes of serum and diluent?

Perform a serial dilution on the serum specimen. Figure 4-2 is a schematic of the dilution.

Step 1: Perform a 1 to 10 dilution of the serum (10 mcL of serum to 90 mcL of diluent): tube 1.

Step 2: Perform a 1 to 10 dilution of tube 1 (10 mcL in tube 1 to 90 mcL of diluent in tube 2): tube 2.

Step 3: Perform a 1 to 10 dilution of tube 2 (10 mcL in tube 2 to 90 mcL of diluent in tube 3): tube 3.

Tube 1 is diluted 1 to 10.
Tube 2 is diluted 1 to 100:

$$\left(\frac{1}{10}\right)\left(\frac{1}{10}\right) = \frac{1}{100}$$

Tube 3 is diluted 1 to 1000:

$$\left(\frac{1}{100}\right)\left(\frac{1}{10}\right) = \frac{1}{1000}$$

In this manner, only 10 mcL of sample and 270 mcL of diluent are required to make the 1 to 1000 dilution.

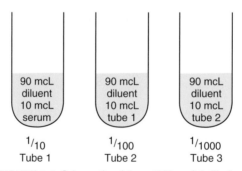

FIGURE 4-2 Schematic of 1 to 1000 serial dilution.

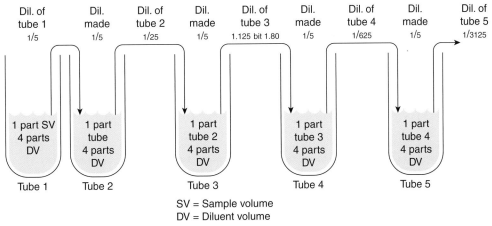

Dil. of tube 1	Dil. made	Dil of tube 2	Dil. made	Dil. of tube 3	Dil. made	Dil. of tube 4	Dil. made	Dil. of tube 5
1/5	1/5	1/25	1/5	1.125 bit 1.80	1/5	1/625	1/5	1/3125

1 part SV
4 parts
DV

1 part
tube
4 parts
DV

1 part
tube 2
4 parts
DV

1 part
tube 3
4 parts
DV

1 part
tube 4
4 parts
DV

Tube 1   Tube 2   Tube 3   Tube 4   Tube 5

SV = Sample volume
DV = Diluent volume

FIGURE 4-3 Schematic of 1 to 5 serial dilution.

Example 4-7a   What is the final dilution on a serial dilution series with five tubes, each a 1 to 5 dilution (also called a fivefold dilution)?

A fivefold dilution is five 1 to 5 dilutions: $\dfrac{1}{5} \times \dfrac{1}{5} \times \dfrac{1}{5} \times \dfrac{1}{5} \times \dfrac{1}{5} = \dfrac{1}{3125}$ (Figure 4-3).

Therefore the final dilution is 1 to 3125.

Example 4-7b   What is the final dilution on a tenfold serial dilution made with six tubes?

A tenfold serial dilution means that each dilution is a 1 to 10 dilution.

$$\frac{1}{10} \times \frac{1}{10} \times \frac{1}{10} \times \frac{1}{10} \times \frac{1}{10} \times \frac{1}{10} = \frac{1}{1000000}$$

The final dilution is 1 to 1,000,000.

Example 4-7c   What is the final dilution on a twofold serial dilution made with four tubes?

A twofold serial dilution means that each dilution is a 1 to 2 dilution.

$$\frac{1}{2} \times \frac{1}{2} \times \frac{1}{2} \times \frac{1}{2} = \frac{1}{16}$$

The final dilution is 1 to 16.

In immunology, serial dilutions are often made of serum samples. How could a final dilution of 1 to 320 be made?

The first step is to determine the serial dilution scheme. Some questions to consider are: What dilutions should be made? How many dilutions are necessary? Common serial dilution schemes use a factor of 2, 4, 5, or 10 to make the serial dilutions. A 1 to 320 dilution could be made a number of ways. A 1 to 2 serial dilution could be made to a final concentration of 1 to 32, followed by a 1 to 10 dilution ($^1/_2 \rightarrow {}^1/_4 \rightarrow {}^1/_8 \rightarrow {}^1/_{16} \rightarrow {}^1/_{32}$, then $^1/_{10}$ of the $^1/_{32}$ dilution). Or the dilution scheme could be increased by the factor of 10 from the start. Figure 4-4 demonstrates this serial dilution scheme. The dilution is made from a starting point of a $^1/_{20}$ dilution followed by a series of $^1/_2$ serial dilutions.

Figures 4-5, 4-6, and 4-7 show common serial dilution protocols used in the clinical laboratory.

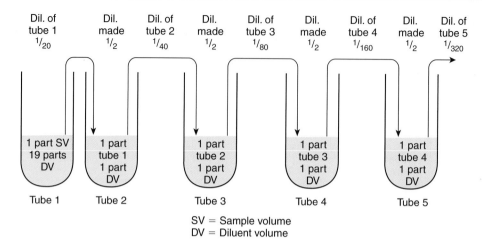

SV = Sample volume
DV = Diluent volume

FIGURE 4-4 Schematic of 1 to 320 serial dilution.

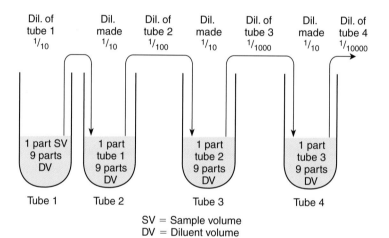

SV = Sample volume
DV = Diluent volume

FIGURE 4-5 Schematic of tenfold serial dilutions.

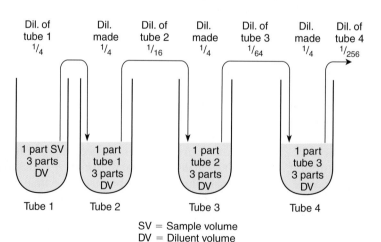

SV = Sample volume
DV = Diluent volume

FIGURE 4-6 Schematic of fourfold serial dilutions.

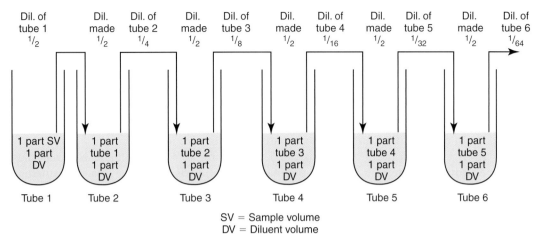

FIGURE 4-7 Schematic of twofold serial dilutions.

NOTE: All tubes must be well mixed before sampling for the subsequent tube.

WHAT **TITERS**

In immunology, titers are measured to determine the quantity of antibody present in a patient's sample. Sometimes this information is used to determine the patient's level of protective antibodies (Ab) against disease, such as in rubella or mumps. Other times, it is used to determine the concentration of antibodies that lead to disease, such as autoantibodies present in the patient's serum. A titer is the inverse of the dilution used in which a reaction occurred when testing antigen-antibody (Ag-Ab) interactions. A low titer of a protective antibody may mean that the patient does not have immunity to the particular disease being tested. When performing a titer analysis, serial dilutions of the patient's serum are made in individual test tubes or wells and antigen is added to each tube or well. The dilution in which the last measurable reaction occurred is the dilution used as the titer.

HOW *Example 4-8*

A rubella titer analysis is performed on an OB-GYN patient. Serial dilutions of the patient's serum are made at $^1/_{20}$, $^1/_{40}$, $^1/_{80}$, $^1/_{160}$, $^1/_{320}$, $^1/_{640}$, and $^1/_{1280}$. Rubella antigen is added to each tube. A positive reaction is found in all but the $^1/_{1280}$ dilution. What is the patient's titer?

The patient's rubella titer is 640, because at the $^1/_{640}$ dilution the last positive reaction occurred.

Example 4-8a   An infectious mononucleosis antibody titer analysis is performed on a 16-year-old boy. A fourfold dilution series is positive at the $^1/_4$, $^1/_{16}$, and $^1/_{64}$ dilutions but negative at $^1/_{256}$.

What is the boy's antibody titer?

As the last positive dilution was $^1/_{64}$, the patient's titer is 64.

EXAMPLE PROBLEMS

This section is designed to be useful to both the student and the laboratory professional. Students can use the additional problems to master the material. The laboratory professional can use the examples as templates for solving laboratory calculations. By finding an example similar to the problem that you need to solve, substitute into the equation the numbers appropriate to your calculation.

1. **Q.** In a 1 to 5 dilution, how many parts of diluent are needed?
   A. A 1 to 5 dilution ($^1/_5$) consists of 1 part sample to 4 parts diluent. This is because the **total** volume is 5 parts (1 part sample + 4 parts diluent). This is mathematically expressed as:

$$\frac{Sample\ volume}{Sample\ volume\ +\ Diluent\ volume}$$

   or

$$\frac{Sample\ volume}{Total\ volume}$$

2. **Q.** In a 1 to 3 dilution, how many parts of diluent are needed?
   A. A 1 to 3 dilution consists of 1 part sample to 2 parts diluent.

3. **Q.** In a 1 to 10 dilution, how many parts of diluent are needed?
   A. A 1 to 10 dilution consists of 1 part sample to 9 parts diluent.

4. **Q.** If 10 mL of sample are added to 190 mL of diluent, what is the dilution factor?
   A. The dilution factor is the reciprocal of the dilution. In this question, 10 mL of sample is added to 190 mL of diluent. The dilution performed can be calculated by using the formula in problem 1. The dilution is a $^1/_{20}$ dilution (10 parts sample to 200 parts total volume). Therefore the dilution factor is the reciprocal of $^1/_{20}$ or 20.

5. **Q.** In a 1 to 10 dilution, what is the dilution factor?
   A. The dilution factor is the reciprocal of the dilution, or 10.

6. **Q.** In a 1 to 5 dilution, what is the dilution factor?
   A. The dilution factor is 5, which is the reciprocal of the dilution that was made.

7. **Q.** If 0.25 part of a sample is diluted into 4.75 parts of diluent, what is the dilution factor?
   A. The numerator in the dilution formula has to be larger than 1. Since 0.25 is less than 1, both sides of the equation [SV/(SV + DV)] are multiplied by 4, resulting in a dilution of 1 to 20. The dilution factor is 20.

8. **Q.** A serum sample is outside of the linear range of the analyzer for an analyte. A 1 to 3 ratio of serum to diluent is performed and the sample reanalyzed. What factor would the technologist need to multiply the result of the diluted sample by to obtain the correct concentration of the analyte?
   A. A 1:3 ratio is 1 part sample to 3 parts diluent. This is exactly the same as a 1 to 4 ($^1/_4$) dilution. The diluted result must be multiplied by 4, not by 3, to obtain a correct result.

9. **Q.** A $^1/_{10}$ dilution is to be performed on a sample; 50 mcL of serum is available and 50 mcL is needed for the test, but the technologist cannot use all the serum for the sample, as a repeat analysis may be necessary. How should the dilution be performed?

A. To determine the sample volume necessary, divide the total volume by the dilution factor of 10. A ¹⁄10 dilution can be performed using 5 mcL of serum to 45.0 mcL of diluent (⁵⁄50 = ¹⁄10). Pipetting 5 mcL of sample may not be practical, so by multiplying all parts by a factor of 2 yields a more easily performed dilution of 10 mcL of serum to 90 mcL of diluent. This leaves 40 mcL of serum available for further testing.

10. **Q.** A serum amylase is diluted ¹⁄100 with a result of 45.0 IU/L. What is the patient's actual amylase result?

   A. Because the sample is diluted ¹⁄100, the diluted result must be multiplied by the dilution factor. This dilution factor is the reciprocal of the dilution performed. In this problem, as a ¹⁄100 dilution is performed, the dilution factor is 100. Therefore the result of 45 IU/L is multiplied by 100 to yield the actual amylase result of 4500 IU/L.

11. **Q.** In a multiple dilution series, 20 mcL of serum and 80 mcL of diluent are added and mixed in tube 1. From tube 1, 10 mcL are taken and placed into 40 mcL of diluent in tube 2. What is the final dilution in tube 2?

   A. The final dilution is the product of the individual dilutions in the multiple dilution series. The first dilution is a ¹⁄5 dilution, as 20 mcL of sample are added to a total volume of 100 mcL (²⁰⁄100 = ¹⁄5). The second dilution is also ¹⁄5 as 10 mcL of serum are added to a total volume of 50 mcL (¹⁰⁄50 = ¹⁄5). Therefore the final dilution is as follows:

$$\text{Final dilution} = \left(\frac{1}{5}\right)\left(\frac{1}{5}\right) = \frac{1}{25}$$

   The sample in tube 2 is diluted ¹⁄25.

12. **Q.** Using the same dilution from question 11, if the original concentration of the sample had been 50 mg/dL, what is the concentration of the sample in tube 1?

   A. To determine the concentration of the first tube in a serial or multiple dilution series, divide the sample concentration in the first tube in the series by the dilution factor used in its dilution. In this case, 50 mg/dL are divided by the factor of 5, as a ¹⁄5 dilution was performed in tube 1. This yields a concentration of 10 mg/dL in tube 1.

13. **Q.** A tenfold serial dilution is performed with a final dilution of ¹⁄10,000. The beginning dilution in the series in tube 1 is a ¹⁄10 dilution. If the original concentration had been 75,000 ng/dL, what would the concentration be in tube 3?

   A. A tenfold serial dilution means that each tube in the series is diluted ¹⁄10. Therefore the first tube is diluted ¹⁄10 and the second is diluted ¹⁄10 with the sample volume coming from tube 1. The third tube is also diluted ¹⁄10 with its sample volume coming from the diluted tube 2. The dilutions and concentrations in each tube can be calculated two different ways. The first method calculates the individual concentrations in each tube by dividing each tube by its dilution factor. For example, tube 1 is diluted ¹⁄10. If the original concentration is 75,000 ng/mL, the concentration in tube 1 is ⁷⁵,⁰⁰⁰⁄10 or 7500. The concentration in tube 2 can be calculated by dividing the concentration of tube 1 by the dilution performed in tube 2. In this case, ⁷⁵⁰⁰⁄10 equals 750. Tube 3 can be calculated by dividing the concentration of tube 2 by the dilution factor of 10 as well: ⁷⁵⁰⁄10 = 75. Therefore the concentration of tube 3 is 75 ng/mL.

   Another method to determine the concentrations of each individual tube in a series is to multiply the individual dilutions performed on the previous tubes and divide the original concentration by the reciprocal of the product of the individual dilutions. For example, tube 1 is a $^1/_{10}$ dilution, tube 2 is a $^1/_{10}$ dilution, and tube 3 is a $^1/_{10}$ dilution. The actual dilution in tube 3 is as follows:

$$\left(\frac{1}{10}\right)\left(\frac{1}{10}\right)\left(\frac{1}{10}\right) = \frac{1}{1000}$$

Therefore, in tube 3, a $^1/_{1000}$ dilution was performed. By dividing the original concentration by 1000, the concentration in tube 3 can be calculated as follows:

$$\frac{75,000}{1000} = 75 \text{ ng/mL}$$

Therefore both methods yield the same result: 75 ng/mL in tube 3.

14. **Q.** If a serial dilution is performed, and the final concentration of the sample is 0.433 mg/dL with a dilution factor of 1500, what is the original concentration?

A. To determine the original concentration, multiply the dilution factor by the final diluted sample. In this case, 1500×0.433 mg/dL $= 649.5$ mg/dL. The original concentration is 649.5 mg/dL.

15. **Q.** A serial dilution was performed, with a final concentration of the sample equal to 0.350 mg/dL. The dilution factor was 2200. What is the original concentration?

A. The original concentration is 770 mg/dL.

16. **Q.** A multiple dilution series is performed to determine the antistreptolysin O titer of a patient. The multiple dilutions consisted of $^1/_{100}$, $^1/_{125}$, $^1/_{166}$, $^1/_{250}$, $^1/_{500}$, $^1/_{625}$, $^1/_{833}$, and $^1/_{1250}$ dilutions of the patient's serum. One milliliter of each dilution is added to test tubes. Streptolysin antigen was added to all tubes, incubated, and streptolysin O cells were then added. The presence of the streptolysin O antibody in the patient's serum binds the streptolysin antigen and prevents hemolysis of the O cells. The $^1/_{250}$ dilution tube is the first tube to exhibit hemolysis. What is the patient's titer?

A. The last dilution tube not to exhibit hemolysis, or to demonstrate a positive reaction, is the tube with the $^1/_{166}$ dilution. Therefore the patient's titer is 166 Todd units.

HOW **PRACTICE PROBLEMS**

Solve the following practice problems to further master the material. Answers and explanations to some problems can be found in the Answer Key.

Calculate the dilution factors for the following problems.

1. 20 mcL sample added to 80 mcL diluent

2. 10 mcL sample added to 190 mcL diluent

3. 50 mcL sample added to 200 mcL diluent

4. 2 mL sample added to 10 mL diluent

5. 10 mcL sample added to 90 mcL diluent

6. 0.20 mL sample added to 3.8 mL diluent

7. 0.250 mL sample added to 0.750 mL diluent

8. If 5 parts sample are added to 95 parts diluent, what is the ratio as defined in this book and what is the dilution?

9. If 2 parts sample are added to 12 parts diluent, what is the ratio as defined in this book and what is the dilution?

10. If 0.5 part sample is added to 19.5 parts diluent, what is the ratio as defined in this book and what is the dilution?

11. A 1 to 6 dilution was performed on a sample. The diluted value was analyzed and determined to be 100 mg/dL. What is the true value of the analyte?

12. A 1 to 2 dilution was performed on a sample. The diluted value was determined to be 280 mg/dL. What is the true value of the analyte?

Use the following information to answer questions 13 to 16.

A multiple dilution series was performed. The sample was diluted $\frac{1}{4}$, $\frac{1}{4}$, $\frac{1}{4}$, and $\frac{1}{4}$.

13. What is the final dilution?

14. What is the final dilution factor?

15. What is the concentration in tube 3 if the original concentration was 100?

16. What is the dilution factor for tube 2?

Use the following information to answer questions 17 to 20.

A series of five $\frac{1}{5}$ dilutions was performed.

17. What is the final dilution?

18. What is the final dilution factor?

19. If the original concentration was 50, what is the concentration in tube 4?

20. What is the dilution factor for tube 3?

21. A measles antibody titer was performed on a 5-year-old girl. The girl's serum was tested with measles antigen in the following sequence: undiluted, diluted $\frac{1}{4}$, $\frac{1}{16}$, $\frac{1}{64}$, $\frac{1}{256}$, and $\frac{1}{1032}$. Positive reactions were noted for the undiluted, $\frac{1}{4}$, $\frac{1}{16}$, and $\frac{1}{64}$ tubes. What is the girl's titer?

22. An antithyroid microsomal antibody test was performed on a 45-year-old woman. The dilution sequence was performed in a microtiter plate by first adding 50 mcL of serum to 100 mcL of diluent in well 1; 50 mcL of the first dilution was added to 100 mcL of diluent in well 2; 50 mcL from well 2 was added to 100 mcL of diluent in well 3; wells 4 through 12 were serially diluted in a fourfold dilution series. What would the dilution be in well 6?

QUICK NOTES

- The basic formula for a dilution is sample volume/total volume.
- The total volume consists of two parts: the sample volume and the diluent volume.
- Another way to write the dilution formula is: Sample volume/Sample volume + Diluent volume.
- A ratio is simply the sample volume/diluent volume.

- A 1:3 ratio is a 1 to 4 dilution.
- The numerator of a sample volume quantity must be a value of 1.0 or higher. If not, both sides of the equation must be multiplied by the value that will allow the sample volume to be at least 1.0 or larger than 1.0. For example, 0.5/3.0 must be multiplied by 2/2 to become 1/6 or a 1 in 6 dilution.
- The actual value of a sample that is diluted is determined by multiplying the dilution factor (the reciprocal of the dilution that was made [e.g., a 1 to 6 dilution has a dilution factor of 6]) by the analyzed result that was obtained using the diluted specimen (e.g., if a 1 to 6 dilution is made on a serum specimen and that diluted serum is analyzed for glucose). The diluted serum result is 100 mg/dL. The actual value is multiplied by the dilution factor of 6 for a glucose result of 600 mg/dL.
- Serial dilutions are a way to make a very large dilution of a serum specimen without using a large quantity of that serum.
- A titer is the dilution in which the last measurable reaction occurred. It is used in immunology to determine the strength of an antigen-antibody reaction and to determine if someone has antibody immunity to certain viruses.

Calculations Associated with Solutions

OBJECTIVES

At the end of this chapter, the reader should be able to do the following:

1. Define the following terms: *molarity, normality, mole, molar, molal, molality, gram, equivalent weight.*
2. Calculate molar concentrations of solutions.
3. Calculate normal concentrations of solutions.
4. Calculate molal concentrations of solutions.
5. Interconvert molar solution concentrations with normal solution concentrations.
6. Define the following abbreviations or terms: $\%^{w/v}$, $\%^{v/v}$, $\%^{w/w}$, anhydrous, hydrated, density.

7. Perform calculations to determine $\%^{w/v}$, $\%^{v/v}$, or $\%^{w/w}$ concentrations of solutions.
8. Perform calculations to interchange between percentage concentrations and molarity or normality concentrations.
9. Calculate the concentration of solutes and solvents by using ratio and proportion.

WHAT **MOLARITY**

In science, it is important that there is a standardized way of quantifying the concentrations of various solutions. A solution is a mixture of solvent and solute.

Solvent = the liquid into which the solute is diluted. In the clinical laboratory, the solvent may be deionized water, saline, ethanol, methanol, or an organic solvent.
Solute may be a solid, such as dry chemicals, or a liquid.

By standardizing the method in which various concentrations of solutions can be made, the concentrations of the solutions can become reproducible.

The basic solid measurement unit used in science is the gram (g). Many solutions made in the laboratory use gram quantities of a solid chemical in the solution. An example is 0.85%

normal saline, which is used often in the immunohematology laboratory. To make this solution, 8.5 g of solid crystals of sodium chloride (NaCl) are dissolved into a small quantity of water in a 1.0 L volumetric flask. Once the sodium chloride is dissolved, additional water is added to the 1.0 L calibration mark. The Latin term *quantum satis* (qs), which means "the quantity is satisfied" or that a sufficient quantity is added, is often used to describe the addition of the solvent to the calibration mark. For example, if you prepared the 0.85% normal saline solution, 8.5 g of NaCl would be weighed, dissolved in a small quantity of water in a 1.0 L volumetric flask, and then qs with water to the calibration mark.

The basic volume measurement unit used in science is the liter (L). In many solutions in the laboratory, gram quantities of a solid are diluted into a solvent to prepare a total of 1.0 L of solution. The quantitation of the concentration of the solution can be standardized by use of molarity (M). The molarity of a solution is comprised of three parts: the gram weight of the solute, the solute's gram molecular weight (gmw), and the solvent quantity.

The gram weight of the solute divided by its gram molecular weight is called a mole. A molar solution refers to a solution with a particular molarity. A 1.0 M solution contains 1.0 mol of solute in 1.0 L of solution. A molar solution can be referred to as M or moles/L.

Often in the laboratory the concentration of the solution that is necessary for a test and the quantity of solution that is needed is known. What is not known and must be computed is the amount of the solute (moles) needed to derive the necessary concentration of the solution. To calculate the amount of moles needed for a solution of a particular molar concentration, the gram atomic weight, or gram molecular weight of the element or compound that is needed, must be found. These weights may be found by using a periodic table or any table that lists the gram atomic weights of the elements. The molecular weight of a compound is the sum of the atomic weights of each element in the compound. A periodic table is found on p. 150. A periodic table lists each element by categorizing the elements according to atomic number, energy level, and electron orbital position. Table 5-1 lists the atomic weights of common elements used in the clinical laboratory. The atomic weights have been rounded to the hundredths. Because they have been rounded, when deciding the quantity of significant figures for a result in a calculation involving atomic weights, the preciseness of the atomic weights is ignored in the decision. For calculations for drugs or complicated molecules, the manufacturer's spec sheet will contain the gmw of the chemical.

HOW   **Example 5-1**

What is the gram molecular weight of KCl?
The gram molecular weight is the sum of the atomic weights of K and Cl. Using **Table 5-1**, the gram atomic weight of potassium is 39.10 and the gram atomic weight of chloride is 35.45. Therefore the gram molecular weight of KCl is as follows:

$$39.10 + 35.45 = 74.55$$

The gram molecular weight of KCl is 74.55.

Example 5-1a   What is the gram molecular weight of HCl?

The gram molecular weight of HCl is the sum of the gram atomic weights of hydrogen and chloride. Therefore the gram molecular weight of HCl is:

$$1.01 + 35.45 = 36.46$$

The gram molecular weight of HCl is 36.46.

TABLE 5-1 Atomic Weights of Common Elements Used in the Clinical Laboratory

Element Name	Element Abbreviation	Atomic Wt (rounded value)
Aluminum	Al	26.98
Calcium	Ca	40.08
Carbon	C	12.01
Chlorine	Cl	35.45
Copper	Cu	63.55
Hydrogen	H	1.01
Iodine	I	126.90
Iron	Fe	55.85
Lead	Pb	207.20
Lithium	Li	6.94
Magnesium	Mg	24.30
Manganese	Mn	54.94
Mercury	Hg	200.59
Molybdenum	Mo	95.94
Nickel	Ni	58.70
Nitrogen	N	14.01
Oxygen	O	16.00
Phosphorus	P	30.97
Potassium	K	39.10
Silver	Ag	107.87
Sodium	Na	22.99
Sulfur	S	32.06

Example 5-1b   What is the gram molecular weight of NaOH?

The gram molecular weight of NaOH is the sum of the gram atomic weights of sodium, oxygen, and hydrogen. Therefore the gram molecular weight of NaOH is:

$$22.99 + 16.00 + 1.01 = 40.00$$

The gram molecular weight of NaOH is 40.00.

WHAT   Now let's move on to determining how many grams are in 1.0 mol of a compound.

HOW   ***Example 5-2***

How many grams are contained in 1 mol of potassium chloride?
The formula for a mol is as follows:

$$\frac{\text{No. grams of solute}}{\text{Gram molecular weight of solute}}$$

The question is asking for the quantity of grams in 1 mol of KCl. The gram molecular weight of the compound potassium chloride is calculated by adding the individual atomic weights of potassium and chloride. Potassium has an atomic weight of 39.10, and chloride has an atomic weight of 35.45. The gram molecular weight of potassium chloride then is 74.55. Next, the values that are known can be substituted into the mole equation:

$$1.0 \text{ mol KCl} = \frac{X \text{ g KCl}}{74.55 \text{ gmw KCl}}$$

Solving the equation, the result is 74.55 g KCl are contained in 1.0 mol of KCl.

Example 5-2a   How many grams are in 1.0 mol of HCl?

The gram molecular weight of HCl is 36.46. Using the formula for moles, the amount of grams of HCl can be determined:

$$1 \text{ mol HCl} = \frac{X \text{ g HCl}}{36.46 \text{ gmw HCl}}$$

Solving the equation, the result is 36.46 g of HCl are contained in 1.0 mol of HCl.

Example 5-2b   How many grams are in 1.0 mol of NaOH?

The gram molecular weight of NaOH is 40.00. Using the formula for moles, the result is 40.00 g of NaOH are contained in 1.0 mol of NaOH.

WHAT   ## Determining Molarity of a Solution

Now that you have learned to calculate a molar solution, use the molarity formula to determine the molarity of a solution.

HOW   **Example 5-3**

What is the molarity of a solution that contains 2.50 mol of hydrochloric acid in 1.00 L of solution?
    To solve this problem, use the formula for molarity. By substituting the numbers into the formula, the following equation is formed:

$$(X)(M) = \frac{2.50 \text{ mol HCl}}{1.00 \text{ L of solution}}$$

$$(X)(M) = 2.50$$

Therefore this solution has a concentration of 2.50 M, or stated another way, **the solution has a molarity of 2.50.**

Example 5-3a   What is the molarity of a solution that contains 3.0 mol of sodium hydroxide in 1.00 L of solution?

Using the formula for molarity, the equation will be:

$$(X)(M) = \frac{3.00 \text{ mol NaOH}}{1.00 \text{ L of solution}}$$

$$(X)(M) = 3.00$$

Therefore this solution has a molarity of 3.00.

Example 5-3b   What is the molarity of a solution that contains 4.5 mol of Na_2CO_3?

Using the formula for molarity and substituting in the value of 4.5 mol, the solution has a molarity of 4.5.

WHAT   Many compounds used in the laboratory consist of more than one or two elements. To calculate the correct mol concentration or molarity, you must first obtain the correct molecular weight of the compound.

HOW   ***Example 5-4***

What is the molecular weight of the compound Na_3PO_4?
    The first step is to list the gram atomic weight (gaw) of each individual element.

$$Na = 22.99 \text{ gaw}$$
$$P = 30.97 \text{ gaw}$$
$$O = 16.00 \text{ gaw}$$

Next, each element's gram atomic weight is multiplied by how many times that element is found in the compound.

Na: There are three sodium atoms in Na_3PO_4, so the 22.99 gaw of Na must be multiplied by 3 to reflect the true weight of Na in this molecule. Therefore the weight of Na in this molecule is 22.99×3, which equals 68.97 gaw.

P: There is only one phosphorus atom in Na_3PO_4, so the **30.97 gaw** of P is unchanged.

O: There are four oxygen atoms in Na_3PO_4. Therefore the 16.00 gaw of O must be multiplied by 4 to reflect the true weight of oxygen in this molecule. Thus, instead of 16.00, oxygen carries a weight of 64.00 gaw in this molecule.

Finally, the gram atomic weights for each element are added to obtain the gram molecular weight of the compound.
    The gram molecular weight of $Na_3PO_4 = 68.97 + 30.97 + 64.00 = 163.94$ gmw.

Example 5-4a   What is the gram molecular weight of H_3PO_4?

The gram molecular weight of H_3PO_4 is the sum of the gram atomic weights of hydrogen, phosphorus, and oxygen. There are three hydrogen atoms and four oxygen atoms in this molecule. Therefore the gram molecular weight of H_3PO_4 is:

$$(1.01 \times 3) + 30.97 + (16.0 \times 4) = 98.00$$

The gram molecular weight of H_3PO_4 is 98.00.

Example 5-4b   What is the gram molecular weight of $CaCl_2$?

The gram molecular weight of $CaCl_2$ is the sum of the gram atomic weights of calcium and chlorine. There is one calcium atom and two chlorine atoms in this molecule. Therefore the gram molecular weight of $CaCl_2$ is:

$$40.08 + (35.45 \times 2) = 110.98$$

The gram molecular weight of $CaCl_2$ is 110.98.

WHAT In this chapter you have been given examples of how to calculate the gram molecular weight of a compound, how to determine a molar quantity, and how to calculate molarity. As you learned, a solution with a molarity of 1.0 has 1.0 mol of solute in 1.0 L of solution. When making solutions you usually know the molarity that you want and the volume that you want. What needs to be calculated is how many grams of the solute you need.

HOW *Example 5-5*

Consider if you wanted to make 1.00 L of a 0.200 M solution of Na_3PO_4. How many grams of Na_3PO_4 would you need?

From Example 5-4, you already know that the gram molecular weight of the compound is 163.94. By substituting the quantities that are known into the molarity formula, you can solve for the amount of grams needed:

$$0.200 \text{ M} = \frac{X \text{ mol of } Na_3PO_4}{1.00 \text{ L of solution}} \quad 1 \text{ mol} = \frac{X \text{ g}}{gmw}$$

$$0.200 \text{ M} = \frac{\dfrac{X \text{ g } Na_3PO_4}{163.94 \text{ gmw } Na_3PO_4}}{1.00 \text{ L of solution}}$$

$$(0.200 \text{ M})(1.00 \text{ L}) = \frac{X \text{ g}}{163.94 \text{ gmw}}$$

$$0.200 = \frac{X \text{ g}}{163.94}$$

$$(0.200 \text{ M})(163.94) = X$$

$$32.79 = X$$

To prepare a 0.200 M solution of Na_3PO_4, 32.79 g of Na_3PO_4 are weighed, placed into a 1.00 L volumetric flask, dissolved in some water, and then qs to the 1.00 L calibration mark with additional water.

Example 5-5a How many grams of NaCl would you need to make a 0.300 M solution?

The gram molecular weight of NaCl is the sum of the atomic weights of sodium and chloride. The gram molecular weight is $22.99 + 35.45 = 58.44$. Substituting into the formula for molarity, the following equation is derived:

$$0.300 \text{ M} = \frac{\dfrac{X \text{ g NaCl}}{58.44 \text{ gmw NaCl}}}{1.00 \text{ L of solution}}$$

$$(0.300 \text{ M})(1.00 \text{ L}) = \frac{X \text{ g}}{58.44 \text{ gmw}}$$

$$0.300 = \frac{X}{58.44}$$

$$(0.300)(58.44) = X$$

$$17.53 = X$$

Therefore you would weigh out 17.53 g of NaCl, dissolve with some water in a 1.0 L volumetric flask, and then qs to the 1.0 L calibration mark with additional water to make a 0.3 M solution of NaCl.

Example 5-5b   How many grams do you need to make a 1.50 M solution of NaOH?

The gram molecular weight of NaOH is 40.00. Substituting into the formula for molarity, the result is 60.0 g of NaOH that must be added to a 1.0 L volumetric flask, dissolved with water if in powder form, and then qs to the 1.0 L calibration mark.

WHAT   Sometimes the amount of a solution needed is not 1.00 L but a different quantity, such as 100.0 mL or 2.5 L. Often calculations for solutions are modified to result in a quantity that is compatible with the type of laboratory glassware available. Because most solutes are measured by use of volumetric flasks, it makes little sense to calculate a quantity of solute that is not easily measured in the laboratory. For example, the stock of volumetric flasks in Laboratory A consists of a few 250 mL volumetric flasks, two 1 L flasks, and one 2 L flask. It would be very difficult to accurately measure 800.0 mL of solute with the supplies available. Therefore many calculations that deal with molarity use quantities of 50.0 mL, 100.0 mL, 250.0 mL, 500.0 mL, and 1.0 L in their equations because these are the most commonly used sizes of volumetric flasks.

HOW   ***Example 5-6***

If 250 mL of a 1.00 M solution of NaOH are needed, how many grams of NaOH are necessary to make this solution?
The first step is to calculate the molecular weight of NaOH.
From **Table 5-1**: Na = 22.99 gaw, O = 16.00 gaw, H = 1.01 gaw.
The gram molecular weight of NaOH = 22.99 + 16.00 + 1.01 = 40.00 gmw.

> **NOTE:** The problem calls for the solution to have a final volume of 250 mL. Molarity is based on a liter quantity (1000 mL), so the volume must be expressed in the formula in terms of liters.

Next, substitute into the molarity formula the items that are known.

$$1.00\,M = \frac{\left(\dfrac{X\ g\ NaOH}{40.00\ gmw\ NaOH}\right)}{0.250\ L\ of\ solution}$$

Next, using algebra, solve for X:

$$(1.00)(0.250) = \frac{X}{40.00}$$

$$0.250 = \frac{X}{40.00}$$

$$X = (40.00)(0.250)$$

$$X = 10.0\ g$$

The 1.00 M solution is prepared by dissolving 10.0 g of NaOH in a 250 mL volumetric flask with a small quantity of solvent (usually deionized water) and qs to the mark with solvent.

Example 5-6a How many grams of HCl are needed to make 500 mL of a 1.00 M solution?

From earlier examples you know that the gram molecular weight of HCl is 36.46. Substituting into the molarity formula the values for this problem, 18.23 g of HCl will be needed. Remember, the molarity formula is based on a 1.0 L volume, so 500 mL is 0.500 L. The answer is derived from multiplying 1.00 (the molar quantity) by 0.500, then multiplying that answer (0.500) by the molecular weight of 36.46.

Example 5-6b How many grams of NaCl are needed to make 2.0 L of a 1.00 M solution?

From earlier examples you know that the gram molecular weight of NaCl is 58.44. Substituting into the molarity formula the values for this problem, the answer is 116.88 g of NaCl.

WHAT **Putting It All Together**

In the preceding examples, the molarity of the solution was always 1.00. Let's see some examples when the total volume is not 1.0 L and the molarity of the solution is not 1.00.

HOW ***Example 5-7***

In Example 5-6 the amount of grams needed to make 250 mL of a 1.00 M solution of NaOH was determined. How many grams would be needed to make 250 mL of a 2.5 M solution?
    From Example 5-6 you know that the gram molecular weight of NaOH is 40.00. Substituting the new values into the molarity formula yields the following formula:

$$2.50 \text{ M} = \frac{\left(\dfrac{\text{X g NaOH}}{40.00 \text{ gmw NaOH}}\right)}{0.250 \text{ L of solution}}$$

Solving for X:

$$(2.50)(0.250) = \frac{\text{X}}{40.00}$$

$$0.625 = \frac{\text{X}}{40.00}$$

$$\text{X} = (40.00)(0.625)$$

$$\text{X} = 25.0 \text{ g}$$

Therefore 25.0 g of NaOH dissolved in 250 mL of water will make a 2.50 M solution.

Example 5-7a How many grams are needed to make 300 mL of a 3.20 M solution of HCl?

The gram molecular weight of HCl is 36.46. Substituting the values of this problem into the molarity formula yields a result of 35.0 g.

Example 5-7b How many grams of $CaCl_2$ are needed to make 1500.0 mL of a 0.5250 M solution?

The gram molecular weight of $CaCl_2$ is 110.98. Substituting the values of this problem into the molarity formula yields a result of 87.40 g of $CaCl_2$.

WHAT Sometimes in the laboratory a solution may be prepared, but the molarity of that solution may need to be confirmed. To confirm the molarity of a given solution, simply substitute into the basic molarity equation the items that are known and solve for the unknown molarity.

HOW *Example 5-8*

You weigh out 25.0 g of NaCl and dissolve them into 1.00 L of water. What is the molarity of the solution that you just made?

$$\text{Molarity} = \frac{\left(\dfrac{\text{grams of solute}}{\text{gram molecular weight of solute}}\right)}{1.00 \text{ L of solution}}$$

$$\text{Molarity} = \frac{\left(\dfrac{25.0 \text{ NaCl}}{58.44 \text{ gmw NaCl}}\right)}{1.00 \text{ L of solution}}$$

$$\text{Molarity} = 0.428$$

Therefore, by dissolving 25.0 g of NaCl in a 1.00 L volumetric flask with water and qs with water, a 0.428 M solution of NaCl is prepared.

Example 5-8a You weigh out 40.0 g of KCl and dissolve them into 500 mL of water. What is the molarity of the solution that you just made?

Using the molarity formula, the following equation is derived:

$$\text{Molarity} = \frac{\left(\dfrac{40.0 \text{ g KCl}}{74.55 \text{ gmw KCl}}\right)}{0.500 \text{ L of solution}}$$

$$\text{Molarity} = 1.07$$

Therefore, by dissolving **40.0 g** of KCl in 500 mL of water, you will prepare a 1.07 M solution.

Example 5-8b You weigh out 2.50 g of $CuSO_4$ and dissolve them into 0.100 L of water. What is the molarity of the solution that you just made?

The gram molecular weight of $CuSO_4$ is 159.61. The molarity of this solution is 0.16 moles/L.

WHAT Another term that is frequently used is millimolar. The millimolarity of a solution is calculated by the following formula:

$$1 \text{ mM solution} = \frac{1 \text{ mmol of solute}}{1 \text{ L of solution}}$$

$$1 \text{ mmol of solute} = \frac{\text{Number of milligrams of solute}}{\text{Gram molecular weight of solute}}$$

HOW *Example 5-9*

A solution contains 2.75 g of HCl in 1.00 L of solution. What is the millimolar concentration of this solution?

To solve this problem use the millimolar formula:

$$X \text{ mM solution} = \frac{\dfrac{2750 \text{ mg}}{36.46 \text{ gmw HCl}}}{1.00 \text{ L of solution}}$$

$$X \text{ mM solution} = 75.43$$

Therefore the millimolar concentration of this solution is 75.43.

Example 5-9a How many milligrams are needed to make 150 mL of a 10.0 mM solution of NaCl?

By substituting the values of this problem into the millimolar formula, the answer of 87.66 mg is derived.

Example 5-9b What is the millimolar concentration of a solution consisting of 25 mg of NaOH in 500 mL of water?

The millimolar concentration of this solution is 1.25 mM.

NOTE: Notice that the amount is in milligram and not gram. If you are given an amount in gram then you must convert it to milligrams if you are trying to determine the millimolar concentration.

WHAT **NORMALITY**

Another term used to quantify solutions is normality. Normality is different from molarity as normality accounts for the dynamics of the interaction of the dissolved solute with the solvent. The normality of a solution differs from the molarity because it is determined by the number of equivalent weights per liter, not the number of moles per liter. An equivalent weight is the amount of replaceable H^+ or OH^- ion or charge for the element or compound. This amount is usually reflected by the valence of the element or compound. The equivalent weight is calculated by dividing the gram molecular weight of an element or compound by the valence. Table 5-2 lists the valences of the most common elements used in the clinical laboratory. Some elements have more than one valence, depending on the oxidative state of that element. For elements with more than one valence, the most frequent valence is in bold.

HOW **Example 5-10**

What is the gram equivalent weight of HCl?
HCl has one replaceable hydrogen ion. Therefore the equivalent weight would be as follows:

$$\text{Gram equivalent weight} = \frac{\text{gmw}}{\text{valence}}$$

$$\text{Gram equivalent weight} = \frac{36.46}{1}$$

The gram equivalent weight of HCl = 36.46.

Example 5-10a What is the gram equivalent weight of NaOH?

NaOH has one replaceable hydroxyl ion. Therefore the gram equivalent weight of NaOH is the gram molecular weight of 40.0 divided by 1.0, or 40.0.

TABLE 5-2 Valences of the Most Common Elements Used in the Clinical Laboratory

Element Name	Element Abbreviation	Valence(s)
Aluminum	Al	+3
Calcium	Ca	+2
Carbon	C	+4, +2, −4
Chlorine	Cl	+7, +5, +3, +1, −1
Copper	Cu	+2, +1
Hydrogen	H	+1, −1
Iodine	I	+7, +5, +1, −1
Iron	Fe	+3, +2
Lead	Pb	+4, +2
Lithium	Li	−1
Magnesium	Mg	+2
Manganese	Mn	+2, +4. +7
Mercury	Hg	+2, +1
Molybdenum	Mo	+6, +4, +3
Nickel	Ni	+2
Nitrogen	N	+5, +4, +3, +2, +1, −3
Oxygen	O	−1, −2
Phosphorus	P	+5, +3, −3
Potassium	K	+1
Silver	Ag	+1
Sodium	Na	+1
Sulfur	S	+6, +4, +2, −2

Modified from Masterton WL, Slowinski EJ, Stanitski CL: *Chemical principles,* ed 5, Philadelphia, 1981, Saunders College.

Example 5-10b What is the gram equivalent weight of NaCl?

In this example, there is no hydrogen or hydroxyl group that is replaced. Instead, one atom of sodium combines with one atom of chloride to form sodium chloride. The gram equivalent weight of NaCl would be the same as its gram molecular weight, which is 58.44.

WHAT The previous examples have all had a valence of 1, and the gram equivalent weight was equal to the gram molecular weight. Now let's see examples when the valence does not have a value of 1.0.

HOW ***Example 5-11***

What is the gram equivalent weight of $CaCl_2$?

$$\text{Gram equivalent weight} = \frac{\text{gmw}}{\text{valence}}$$

The gram molecular weight of $CaCl_2$ is 110.98. There are two chloride ions that can react in solution; therefore the valence is 2.

$$\text{Gram equivalent weight} = \frac{110.98}{2}$$

$$\text{Gram equivalent weight} = 55.49$$

Therefore the gram equivalent weight of $CaCl_2$ is 55.49.

Example 5-11a   What is the gram equivalent weight of H_2SO_4?

To solve, first determine the valence. There are two hydrogen ions that can react in solution; therefore the valence is 2. The gram equivalent weight is equal to the gram molecular weight divided by 2, or 98.08 divided by 2, yielding 49.04.

Example 5-11b   What is the gram equivalent weight of H_3PO_4?

The gram equivalent weight is one-third of the gram molecular weight, as there are three replaceable hydrogen atoms in this compound. Therefore the gram equivalent weight of H_3PO_4 is 98.0 divided by 3, or 32.67.

WHAT   The normality of a solution is calculated using the following formula, which is not much different from that used to calculate molarity.

$$\text{Normality} = \frac{\left(\dfrac{\text{No. grams of solute}}{\text{gram equivalent weight of solute}}\right)}{1.00 \text{ L of solution}}$$

Remember that a gram equivalent weight of solute $= \dfrac{\text{gmw of solute}}{\text{valence}}$

Substituting into the first formula yields the following:

$$\text{Normality} = \frac{\dfrac{\text{No. grams of solute}}{\left(\dfrac{\text{gmw}}{\text{valence}}\right)}}{1.00 \text{ L of solution}} \text{(gram equivalent weight)}$$

To use this formula, first calculate the $\left(\dfrac{\text{gmw}}{\text{valence}}\right)$, then divide that number into the number of grams of solute. Last, divide the result of the equation by the number of liters of solution.

HOW   ***Example 5-12***

Calculate the normality of a solution containing 98.0 g of H_2SO_4 in 0.250 L of solution.

To solve this problem, first calculate the gram molecular weight of the compound. From **Table 5-1**, the gram molecular weight is equal to 98.08. Next, substitute all of the known numbers into the formula:

$$\text{Normality (X)} = \frac{98.0 \text{ g of solute}}{\dfrac{\left(\dfrac{98.08 \text{ gmw of } H_2SO_4}{\text{valence of 2[two replaceable hydrogen ions]}}\right)}{0.250 \text{ L of solution}}}$$

To solve this equation, first divide the gram molecular weight of solute by the valence:

$$\frac{98.08 \text{ gmw}}{2} = 49.04$$

Next, substitute the 49.04 g equivalent weight into the equation:

$$\text{Normality } (X) = \frac{\left(\dfrac{98.0 \text{ g of solute}}{49.04 \text{ geqw of solute}}\right)}{0.250 \text{ L of solution}}$$

Next, divide the grams of solute by the gram equivalent weight:

$$\frac{98.0}{49.04} = 2.00 \text{ equivalent weights}$$

Last, substitute the equivalent weights into the equation and solve for normality:

$$\text{Normality } (X) = \frac{2.00}{0.250}$$

$$\text{Normality } (X) = 8.00 \text{ Eq/L}$$

Therefore the normality of a solution containing 98.0 g of H_2SO_4 in 0.250 L of solution is 8.00 Eq/L.

Example 5-12a   What is the normality of a solution containing 65 g of HCl in 1.0 L of water?

The valence of HCl is 1.0. Using the normality formula yields the following:

$$\text{Normality } (X) = \frac{65.0 \text{ g of solute}}{\dfrac{\left(\dfrac{36.46 \text{ gmw of HCl}}{\text{valence of } 1[\text{one replaceable hydrogenion}]}\right)}{1.000 \text{ L of solution}}}$$

Solving for X:

$$\text{Normality} = 1.78 \text{ Eq/L}$$

Example 5-12b   What is the normality of a 1.00 L solution of 25.0 g of K_2CO_3?

The valence of this compound is 2; therefore the gram equivalent weight will be the gram molecular weight divided by 2, or 69.10. Substituting this value into the formula for normality yields:

$$\text{Normality } (X) = \frac{\left(\dfrac{25.0 \text{ g of solute}}{69.10 \text{ geqw of solute}}\right)}{1.00 \text{ L of solution}}$$

$$\text{Normality } (X) = 0.36 \text{ Eq/L}$$

Example 5-12c   How many grams of NaOH are required to prepare 2.00 L of a 0.750 N solution?

To solve this problem, first substitute all known values into the normality equation.

$$0.750 \text{ normal} = \frac{X \text{ g NaOH}}{\dfrac{\left(\dfrac{40.00 \text{ gmw of NaOH}}{\text{valence of } 1}\right)}{2.00 \text{ L of solution}}}$$

Because the valence is 1, the gram equivalent weight stays unchanged as 40.00.

Solving for X:

$$(2.00 \text{ L})(0.750 \text{ Eq/L}) = \frac{X}{40.00} \text{ gram equivalent weight}$$

$$1.50 \text{ Eq} = \frac{X}{40.00} \text{ gram equivalent weight}$$

$$(1.50)(40.00 \text{ g}) = X$$

$$60.0 \text{ g NaOH} = X$$

Therefore 60.0 g of NaOH are required to prepare 2.00 L of a 0.750 N solution of NaOH.

Example 5-12d   How many grams are needed to make 2.00 L of a 4.00 N solution of HCl?

The gram equivalent weight of HCl is the same as the gram molecular weight because the valence is 1.0. Substituting the given values into the normality formula yields the following equation:

$$4.00 \text{ Eq /L Normality} = \frac{\left(\dfrac{X \text{ g of solute}}{36.46 \text{ geqw of solute}} \right)}{2.00 \text{ L of solution}}$$

Solving for X:

$$(2.00 \text{ L})(4.00 \text{ Eq/L}) = \frac{X}{36.46} \text{ gram equivalent weight}$$

$$8.00 \text{ Eq} = \frac{X}{36.46} \text{ gram equivalent weight}$$

$$(8.00)(36.46 \text{ g}) = X$$

$$291.68 \text{ g HCl} = X$$

Therefore 292 g of HCl are needed to make 2.00 L of a 4 N solution.

Example 5-12e   How many grams are needed to make 1.00 L of a 1.50 N solution of H_2CO_3?

The valence of H_2CO_3 is 2, as there are two replaceable hydrogen ions. The gram molecular weight of H_2CO_3 is 62.03. Therefore the gram equivalent weight is 31.02. Substituting the values of the problem into the normality formula yields:

$$1.50 \text{ Eq/L Normality} = \frac{\left(\dfrac{X \text{ g of solute}}{31.02 \text{ geqw of solute}} \right)}{1.00 \text{ L of solution}}$$

$$(1.00 \text{ L})(1.50 \text{ Eq/L}) = \frac{X}{31.02} \text{ gram equivalent weight}$$

$$1.50 \text{ Eq} = \frac{X}{31.02} \text{ gram equivalent weight}$$

$$(1.50)(31.02 \text{ g}) = X$$

$$46.53 \text{ g } H_2CO_3 = X$$

Therefore 46.53 g of H_2CO_3 in 1.0 L of water will create a 1.50 N solution.

INTERCONVERSION BETWEEN MOLARITY AND NORMALITY

The formula for molarity and normality are very similar; the only difference is that the normality formula requires gram equivalent weights, and molarity requires gram molecular weights of the solute. A 1.0 normal solution has a concentration of 1.0 g Eq/L, whereas a 1.0 M solution has a concentration of 1.0 mol/L. Because of the similarity, the terms can be interconverted by using the following formula:

$$N = (n)(M)$$

Where: N = normality

n = valence

M = molarity

Example 5-13

Given a 2.50 M HCl solution, what is the normality of the solution?

$$\text{Remember: } N = (n)(M)$$

Use the following formula:

$$X\,N = (1[\text{valence}])(2.50)$$
$$X = 2.50\ N$$

Because HCl has a valence of 1, the molar solution is equal to the normal concentration.

Example 5-13a   Given a 0.750 M solution of NaCl, what is the normality of the solution?

NaCl has a valence of 1, and using the formula of $N = nM$, then,

$$X\,N = (1[\text{valence}])(0.750)$$
$$X = 0.750\ N$$

As the valence is equal to 1, the normality is equal to the molarity.

Example 5-13b   What is the normality of a 1.5 M solution of NaOH?

NaOH has a valence of 1, and using the formula of $N = (n)(M)$, then,

$$X\,N = (1[\text{valence}])(1.50)$$
$$X = 1.50\ N$$

Again, because the valence is 1.0, the normality is equal to the molarity.

Example 5-13c   Given a 1.75 M H_2SO_4 solution, what is the normality of the solution?

$$\text{Remember: } N = (n)(M)$$

Normality is based on the number of replaceable hydrogen ions or ions that will be used in a redox reaction. In a redox reaction, the hydrogen in H_2SO_4 is the reactant, whereas the oxygen is not. Therefore only the hydrogen ions need to be accounted for in a normality calculation.

Use the following formula:

$$X \, N = (2[\text{hydrogen valence}])(1.75)$$
$$X = 3.50 \, N$$

Notice that the normal concentration of this solution is double that of the molar concentration because of the cumulative hydrogen valence of 2.

Example 5-13d   What is the normality of a 3.25 M H_3PO_4 solution?

Remember: $N = (n)(M)$; therefore:

$$X \, N = (3[\text{hydrogen valence}])(3.25)$$
$$X = 9.75 \, N$$

Therefore a 3.25 M solution of H_3PO_4 is also a 9.75 N solution.

Example 5-13e   What is the normality of a 0.75 M solution of H_2CO_3?

A 0.75 M solution of H_2CO_3 is a 1.5 N solution.

Example 5-13f   What is the molarity of a 1.5 N solution of H_2SO_4?

$$\text{Remember, } N = (n)(M)$$
$$\text{Therefore, } 1.5 = 2 \, X$$
$$X = 0.75$$

Therefore a 1.5 N solution of H_2SO_4 has a molarity of 0.75.

Example 5-13g   What is the molarity of a 4.00 normal NaOH solution?

$$\text{Remember: } N = (n)(M)$$

In the molecule NaOH, the hydroxyl ion (OH) is replaced in a redox reaction. Use the following formula:

$$4.00 \, N = 1(\text{valence}) \times M$$
$$X = 4.00 \, M$$

Notice that the normality and molarity concentrations are the same because of the hydroxyl valence of 1.

Example 5-13h   What is the molarity of a 3.00 N KOH solution?

Remember: $N = (n)(M)$; therefore a 3.00 N KOH solution has a molarity of 3.00.

Example 5-13i   What is the normality of a 0.500 M NaOH solution?

The normality is 0.500.

Example 5-13j   What is the molarity of a 2.00 normal $CaCl_2$ solution?

In this molecule, calcium has a valence of +2, whereas chloride has a valence of −1. To balance this equation, two atoms of chloride are needed for every one atom of calcium.

$$\text{Remember: } N = (n)(M)$$

Use the following formula:

$$2.00\ N = 2(\text{calcium valence}) \times M$$
$$X = 1.00\ M$$

Notice that the molarity concentration is half that of the normality concentration owing to the calcium valence of 2.

Example 5-13k   What is the normality of a 0.40 M solution of H_2SO_4?

The normality would be twice that of the molarity, or 0.80 N.

Example 5-13l   What is the molarity of a 2.0 N solution of $MgSO_4$?

Magnesium has a valence of $+2$, therefore:

$$2.00\ N = 2(\text{valence}) \times M$$
$$X = 1.00\ M$$

A 2.0 N solution of $MgSO_4$ has a molarity of 1.00.

WHAT **MOLALITY**

In the laboratory, we sometimes measure the physical properties of solutions (e.g., when we measure the osmolality of serum or urine). Instead of measuring molar quantities of a solution, we measure molal quantities. A 1.0 molal solution is similar to a 1.0 molar solution. We know that a 1.0 molar solution is a solution with 1.0 mol of solute per 1.0 L of solution. A 1.0 molal solution is 1.0 mol of solute in 1.0 kg of solvent. Molal solutions are based on weight, not volume. A 1.0 molal solution in a 1.0 L volumetric flask may have a larger volume than a 1.0 molar solution, and the meniscus of the solution will be above the calibration line on the volumetric flask. FIGURE 5-1 and Example 5-14 illustrate the difference between a 1.0 molar solution in a 1.0 L volumetric flask compared with a 1.0 molal solution in a 1.0 L volumetric flask.

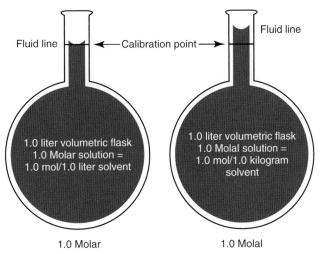

FIGURE 5-1 1.0 molar versus 1.0 molal solution.

HOW **Example 5-14**

A 1.0 molal solution of NaCl is prepared by dissolving 58.44 g of NaCl into 1000 g or 1.00 kg of water. A 1.0 M solution of NaCl is prepared by dissolving 58.44 g of NaCl into a total volume of 1000 mL or 1.0 L of water. The meniscus of the molal solution will be higher than the meniscus of the molar solution.

HOW **Example 5-15**

How many grams of NaOH are needed to make a 2.50 molal solution?

$$\text{Molality} = \frac{\left(\dfrac{\text{X grams of solute}}{\text{gram molecular weight of solute}}\right)}{1.00 \text{ kg of solvent}}$$

Referring to **Table 5-1**, the gram molecular weight of NaOH is 40.00. Next, substitute the known values into the formula and solve for the unknown (grams of NaOH).

$$2.50 \text{ molal} = \frac{\left(\dfrac{\text{X g of NaOH}}{40.00 \text{ gmw}}\right)}{1.00 \text{ kg of solvent}}$$

By using algebra, we can solve for X:

$$(2.50)(1.00) = \frac{X}{40.00}$$

$$2.50 = \frac{X}{40.00}$$

$$(2.50)(40.00) = X$$

$$100.0 = X$$

Therefore we need 100.0 g of NaOH to make a 2.50 molal solution.

Example 5-15a   How many grams of KCl are necessary to make a 1.24 molal solution?

Using the molality formula:

$$1.24 \text{ molal} = \frac{\left(\dfrac{\text{X g of KCl}}{74.55 \text{ gmw}}\right)}{1.00 \text{ kg of solvent}}$$

Solving for X:

$$(1.24)(1.00) = \frac{X}{74.55}$$

$$1.24 = \frac{X}{74.55}$$

$$(1.24)(74.55) = X$$

$$92.44 = X$$

Therefore 92.44 g of KCl are needed to make a 1.24 molal solution of KCl.

Example 5-15b How many grams of NaCl are needed to make a 0.75 molal solution?

Using the molality formula, 43.83 g of NaCl are necessary to make a 0.75 molal solution.

Example 5-15c What is the molality of a solution that contains 390 g of $CaCl_2$ per kilogram of solvent?

$$Molality = \frac{\left(\dfrac{\text{grams of solute}}{\text{gram molecular weight of solute}}\right)}{1.00 \text{ kg of solvent}}$$

Solving for X (molality), we derive the following equation:

$$X \text{ molality} = \frac{\left(\dfrac{390 \text{ g of } CaCl_2}{110.986 \text{ gmw}}\right)}{1.00 \text{ kg of solvent}}$$

Solving the equation, the result is as follows:

$$X = 3.51$$

Therefore we have a 3.51 molal solution of $CaCl_2$.

Example 5-15d What is the molality of a solution that contains 75 g of NaOH in 0.500 kg of solvent?

Using the molality formula, the following equation is derived:

$$X \text{ molality} = \frac{\left(\dfrac{75.0 \text{ g of NaOH}}{40.00 \text{ gmw}}\right)}{0.500 \text{ kg solvent}}$$

Solving for X, the result is 3.75 molality. Therefore 75.0 g of NaOH in 0.5 kg of solvent is a 3.75 molal solution.

Example 5-15e What is the molality of a solution that contains 116.88 g of NaCl in 1.0 kg of solvent?

Using the molality formula, this is a 2.0 molal solution.

WHAT INTERCONVERSION BETWEEN UNITS

In the clinical laboratory, the concentration of many analytes is expressed as milligrams per deciliter or, in the case of electrolytes, milliequivalents per liter. It is important to be able to convert concentrations of analytes from one type of expression to another.

HOW *Example 5-16*

How many milliequivalents per liter does a 15 mg/dL Ca^{+2} standard contain?
   This problem requires several steps to solve.
   First, convert deciliters to liters:

$$\left(\frac{15 \text{ mg}}{1.00 \text{ dL}}\right)\left(\frac{10 \text{ dL}}{1 \text{ L}}\right) = \frac{150 \text{ mg}}{1.00 \text{ L}}$$

Equivalents per liter is another term for normality. By using the normality equation, we can determine the equivalents per liter or the milliequivalents per liter of the 15.0 mg/dL standard:

$$\text{Normality (Eq/L)} = \frac{\dfrac{\text{grams of calcium per L}}{\left(\dfrac{\text{gram molecular weight of calcium}}{\text{Valence of 2}}\right)}}{1.00 \text{ L}}$$

Because we are using units of milligrams per liter, we can change the equation slightly to reflect this:

$$\text{Normality (mEq/L)} = \frac{\dfrac{\text{milligrams of calcium per L}}{\left(\dfrac{\text{gram molecular weight of calcium}}{\text{Valence of 2}}\right)}}{1.00 \text{ L}}$$

Now, substituting into the equation the numbers we know, we get the following:

$$\text{mEq/L} = \frac{\dfrac{150 \text{ mg Ca}}{\left(\dfrac{40.08 \text{ gmw}}{2 (\text{valence})}\right)}}{1.00 \text{ L}} = \frac{\left(\dfrac{150 \text{ mg}}{20.04 \text{ gEq}}\right)}{1.00 \text{ L}} = \frac{7.49 \text{mEq}}{1.00 \text{ L}}$$

Therefore the 15 mg/dL calcium standard is equal to 7.5 mEq/L (7.49 was rounded up to two significant figures).

Example 5-16a   How many milliequivalents per liter does a 2.5 mg/dL Mg^{+2} standard contain?

To solve, the 2.5 mg/dL is converted to 25.0 mg/L. Next, the gram atomic weight of magnesium (24.305) is divided by the valence of 2.0 to yield a gram equivalent weight of 12.15. Then the following formula is derived:

$$\text{mEq/L} = \frac{\left(\dfrac{25 \text{ mg}}{12.15 \text{ gEq}}\right)}{1.00 \text{ L}} = \frac{2.06 \text{ mEq}}{1.00 \text{ L}}$$

Therefore a 2.5 mg/dL Mg^{+2} standard contains 2.06 mEq/L.

Example 5-16b   How many milliequivalents per liter does a 4.0 mg/dL P^{+2} standard contain?

To solve, the 4.0 mg/dL is converted to 40 mg/L. Next, the gram atomic weight of P (30.974) is divided by the valence of 2.0 to yield a gram equivalent weight of 15.487. Then the following formula is derived:

$$\text{mEq/L} = \frac{\dfrac{40 \text{ mg}}{15.487 \text{ gEq}}}{1.00 \text{ L}} = \frac{2.58 \text{ mEq}}{1.00 \text{ L}}$$

Therefore a 4.0 mg/dL P^{+2} standard contains 2.58 mEq/L.

Example 5-16c   What is the concentration in milligrams per deciliter of a 140 mEq/L sodium standard?

This problem requires multiple unit conversion steps. You may find many different approaches to solving multiple unit conversion problems. In Example 5-16, the concentration was kept in terms of milliequivalents per liter. This example will be solved in units of equivalents per liter to demonstrate another approach to solving these types of problems.

First, convert milliequivalents per liter into equivalents per liter:

$$\frac{140\text{ mEq}}{1.00\text{ L}} = \frac{X\text{ Eq}}{1.00\text{ L}}$$

$$\left(\frac{140\text{ mEq}}{1.00\text{ L}}\right)\left(\frac{1\text{ Eq}}{1000\text{mEq}}\right) = \frac{0.140\text{ Eq}}{1.00\text{ L}}$$

Next, use the normality formula to determine grams per liter concentration of sodium:

$$0.140\text{ Eq} = \frac{\dfrac{X\text{ g Na}}{\left(\dfrac{22.99\text{ gmw}}{1(\text{valence})}\right)}}{1.00\text{ L}}$$

$$0.140\text{ Eq} = \frac{\left(\dfrac{X\text{ g}}{22.99\text{ gEq}}\right)}{1.00\text{ L}}$$

$$(0.140)(22.99) = 3.22\text{ g/L}$$

Next, convert 3.22 g/L to milligrams per deciliters:

$$\left(\frac{3.22}{1.00\text{ L}}\right)\left(\frac{1\text{ L}}{10\text{ dL}}\right) = \frac{0.322\text{ g}}{1.00\text{ dL}}$$

$$\left(\frac{0.322\text{ g}}{1.00\text{ dL}}\right)\left(\frac{1000\text{ mg}}{1\text{ g}}\right) = \frac{322\text{ mg}}{1.00\text{ dL}}$$

Therefore the 140 mEq/L sodium standard is equal to a concentration of 322 mg/dL.

Example 5-16d   What is the concentration in milligrams per deciliter of a 2.5 mEq/L Ca^{+2} standard?

First, convert the 2.5 mEq/L into equivalents per liter by dividing 2.5 by the conversion factor of 1000 or by moving the decimal point three places to the left. Therefore 2.5 mEq/L is equal to 0.0025 Eq/L. Next use the normality formula to determine the grams per liter concentration of calcium:

$$0.0025\text{ Eq} = \frac{\dfrac{X\text{ g Ca}}{\left(\dfrac{40.08\text{ gmw}}{2(\text{valence})}\right)}}{1.00\text{ L}}$$

$$0.0025\text{ Eq} = \frac{\left(\dfrac{X\text{ g}}{20.04\text{ gEq}}\right)}{1.00\text{ L}}$$

$$(0.0025)(20.04) = 0.0501\text{ g/L}$$

Next, convert 0.0501 g/L to milligrams per deciliters:

$$\left(\frac{0.0501 \text{ g}}{1.00 \text{ L}}\right)\left(\frac{1 \text{ L}}{10 \text{ dL}}\right) = \frac{0.00501 \text{ g}}{1.00 \text{ dL}}$$

$$\left(\frac{0.00501 \text{ g}}{1.00 \text{ dL}}\right)\left(\frac{1000 \text{ mg}}{1 \text{ g}}\right) = \frac{5.01 \text{ mg}}{1.00 \text{ dL}}$$

Therefore a 2.5 mEq/L Ca^{+2} standard is also equal to a concentration of 5.0 mg/dL.

Example 5-16e   What is the milligrams per deciliter concentration of a 5.0 mEq/L Mg^{+2} standard?

This is solved in the same manner as the previous calcium example. A 5.0 mEq/L Mg^{+2} standard is equal to a concentration of 6.1 mg/dL.

Example 5-16f   The gram molecular weight of the glucose molecule is 180.16. Given a 200 mg/dL glucose standard, what is the concentration in millimoles per liter?

Like the previous examples, this problem requires several steps to solve. First, convert 200 mg/dL to milligrams per liter:

$$\left(\frac{200 \text{ mg}}{\text{dL}}\right)\left(\frac{10 \text{ dL}}{1.00 \text{ L}}\right) = \frac{2000 \text{ mg}}{1.00 \text{ L}}$$

Next, to solve in terms of millimoles directly, use the millimoles per liter formula to solve for millimoles per liter:

$$\text{mmol/L} = \frac{\left(\dfrac{2000 \text{ mg per L of glucose}}{180.16 \text{ gmw glucose}}\right)}{1.00 \text{ L solution}}$$

$$\text{mmol/L} = 11.1$$

Therefore a 200 mg/dL glucose standard contains 11.1 mmol/L glucose.

Example 5-16g   The gram molecular weight of creatinine is 113.12. Given a 2.00 mg/dL creatinine standard, what is its concentration in millimoles per liter?

To solve, first convert the 2.00 mg/dL into milligrams per liter: 2.00 mg/dL is equal to 20.0 mg/L. Next use the molarity formula to determine the millimoles per liter concentration:

$$\text{mmol/L} = \frac{\left(\dfrac{20.0 \text{ mg per L of creatinine}}{113.12 \text{ gmw creatinine}}\right)}{1.00 \text{ L solution}}$$

$$\text{mmol/L} = 0.177$$

Therefore a 2.00 mg/dL creatinine standard contains 0.177 mmol/L creatinine.

Example 5-16h   The gram molecular weight of urea is 60.06. Given a 10.0 mg/dL urea standard, what is its concentration in millimoles per liter?

To solve, first convert the 10.0 mg/dL into milligrams per liter by moving the decimal place one place to the right; 10.0 mg/dL is equal to 100 mg/L. Next use the molarity formula to determine the millimoles per liter concentration:

$$mmol/L = \frac{\left(\dfrac{100 \text{ mg per L of urea}}{60.06 \text{ gmw urea}}\right)}{1.00 \text{ L solution}}$$

$$mmol/L = 1.66$$

Therefore a 10.0 mg/dL urea standard contains 1.66 mmol/L urea.

WHAT PERCENT SOLUTIONS

Solutions may be expressed in other concentrations besides molarity, molality, or normality. In the laboratory, solutions are sometimes expressed in terms of relative percent concentration of solute to solution. There are three types of percent concentrations that may be used in the laboratory. In all three types, the total volume of the solvent is based on a quantity of 100 mL or gram, not 1.00 L, as in molarity or normality concentrations.

WHAT Percent Weight/Weight

A percent weight/weight ($\%^{w/w}$) solution is calculated using the following formula:

$$\%^{w/w} = \frac{\text{Gram of solute}}{100.0 \text{ g of solution}} \text{ OR gram of solute per } 100.0 \text{ g of solution}$$

In this type of solution, the amounts of solute and solvents are weighed individually using a balance. It is important to note that as the total is based on 100.0 g of solution, the amount of solvent that must be weighed is determined by subtracting the quantity of solute needed from 100.0. A solution consists of solute + solvent. Once the amount of solvent is determined, the solvent and solute are combined and mixed together in a flask or beaker. In the clinical laboratory, deionized water is the most frequently used solvent. The $\%^{w/w}$ solutions are the most accurate because unlike $\%^{w/v}$, their concentrations do not fluctuate with temperature. However, the $\%^{w/w}$ solutions are not commonly prepared in the clinical laboratory.

HOW   *Example 5-17*

How many grams of NaOH and how many grams of solvent are needed to make a 30.0%$^{w/w}$ solution using deionized water as the solvent?

To solve this problem, remember the basic formula for $\%^{w/w}$, and substitute the numbers that are known.

$$30.0\%^{w/w} = X \text{ g of solute in 100 g of solution}$$

$$X = 30.0 \text{ g of NaOH}$$

To make this solution: 100 g total weight − amount of solute = amount of solvent or 100 − 30.0 g NaOH = 70.0 g solvent. Therefore, to make this solution, 30.0 grams of NaOH are needed and dissolved into 70.0 grams of deionized water.

Example 5-17a   How many grams of HCl are necessary to make a 10.0% HCl$^{w/w}$ solution using deionized water as the solvent?

Using the formula for %$^{w/w}$, 10.0 g of HCl would be dissolved in 90.0 g of H_2O in a beaker or flask.

Example 5-17b   How much solvent would be needed to make a 20.0%$^{w/w}$ solution of $CuSO_4$?

To make this solution, 80.0 g of solvent would be needed. This question asked for the amount of solvent, not the amount of solute ($CuSO_4$).

WHAT   Percent Weight/Volume

A percent weight/volume (%$^{w/v}$) solution is calculated by the following formula:

$$\%^{w/v} = \frac{g \text{ of solute}}{100.0 \text{ mL of solution}} \text{ OR g of solute per 100.0 mL of solution}$$

The %$^{w/v}$ solution is the most frequently used percent solution in the clinical laboratory. For this solution, the amount of solute is weighed on a balance and then placed into a 100 mL volumetric flask in which there is a small amount of solvent to dissolve the solute. Once the solute is dissolved, the remaining solvent (which in most cases in the clinical laboratory is deionized water) is then added to the volumetric flask to the calibrated mark. The Latin term *quantis satis*, or "quantity sufficient" (qs) is often used in the laboratory to describe the addition of the solvent to the calibrated mark. For example, you may be instructed to add a determined amount of solute to a volumetric flask and then qs it to the calibration mark with the appropriate solvent.

HOW   *Example 5-18*

What is the %$^{w/v}$ of a solution that has 25.0 g of NaCl dissolved into a total volume of 100.0 mL deionized water?
    To solve this problem, use the formula for %$^{w/v}$:

$$X\%^{w/v} = \frac{25.0 \text{ g NaCl}}{100.0 \text{ mL of solution}}$$

$$X = 25.0\%^{w/v}$$

Therefore a solution with 25.0 g of NaCl dissolved into a total volume of 100.0 mL of water has a %$^{w/v}$ concentration of 25.0%.

Example 5-18a   How many grams of NaOH would be needed to make a 40.0%$^{w/v}$ solution using deionized water as the solvent?

To make a 40.0%$^{w/v}$ solution, 40.0 g of NaOH would be dissolved into 100.0 mL of water.

Example 5-18b   How many grams of $CaCl_2$ would be needed to make a 10.0%$^{w/v}$ solution using deionized water as the solvent?

To make a 10.0%$^{w/v}$ solution, 10.0 g of $CaCl_2$ would be dissolved into 100.0 mL of water.

WHAT **Percent Volume/Volume**

A percent volume/volume ($\%^{v/v}$) solution uses volume, or liquid, measurements for both the solute and the solvent.

A $\%^{v/v}$ solution is calculated by the following formula:

$$\%^{v/v} = \frac{\text{mL of solute}}{100.0 \text{ mL of solution}} \text{ OR milliliter of solute per 100.0 mL of solution}$$

Percent $^{v/v}$ is similar to $\%^{w/w}$ in that the total volume of the solution is 100 mL. Therefore the amount of solvent is determined by the following formula:

$$100.0 \text{ mL total volume} - \text{amount of solute} = \text{amount of solvent}$$

HOW **Example 5-19**

How many milliliters of ethanol (EtOH) are needed to make a $75.0\%^{v/v}$ solution using deionized water as the solvent?

This problem is solved in the same manner as solving for $\%^{w/w}$ and $\%^{w/v}$. Using the formula for $\%^{v/v}$ and substituting in the appropriate given numbers, the following equation is derived:

$$75.0\%^{v/v} \text{ EtOH} = \text{X mL EtOH in 100.0 mL of solution}$$
$$\text{X} = 75.0 \text{ mL EtOH}$$

How many milliliters of water are necessary for this solution?
The amount of water needed is determined by the following formula:

$$\text{Amount of solvent} = 100.0 - \text{amount of solute}$$
$$\text{X} = 100.0 - 75.0$$
$$\text{X} = 25.0$$

Therefore 75.0 mL of EtOH would be added to 25.0 mL of deionized water to produce a solution of $75.0\%^{v/v}$ EtOH.

Example 5-19a   How many milliliters of HCl are needed to make a $10.0\%^{v/v}$ solution using deionized water as the solvent?

To make a $10.0\%^{v/v}$ solution, 10.0 mL of HCl are added to 90.0 mL of deionized water.

Example 5-19b   How many milliliters of H_2SO_4 are needed to make a $2.5\%^{v/v}$ solution using deionized water as the solvent?

To make a $2.5\%^{v/v}$ solution, 2.5 mL of H_2SO_4 are added to 97.5 mL of deionized water.

WHAT **Conversion of Percentage Calculations to Molarity**

In the laboratory, sometimes a chemical solution may be labeled in terms of relative percentage, but you may need to know the molarity of that solution. By using both molarity and percentage formulas, you can interchange between the two types of concentrations.

HOW   *Example 5-20*

Suppose you found a bottle labeled 0.85%$^{w/v}$ NaCl in your laboratory. What is the molarity of this solution?

To solve this problem, first use the percent formula to determine the concentration of NaCl in the solution. A %$^{w/v}$ solution is calculated by the number of g of solute dissolved in 100.0 mL of solvent. As we have a 0.85%$^{w/v}$ solution, we know that there are 0.85 g of NaCl dissolved in 100.0 mL of water. Because molarity is based on the concentration in 1.00 L of solute, we need to determine the quantity of NaCl present in 1.00 L. We can use a simple ratio formula to determine this:

$$\frac{0.85 \text{ g NaCl}}{100.0 \text{ mL}} = \frac{X \text{ g NaCl}}{1000.0 \text{ mL}}$$

Using algebra and crossmultiplying, we derive the following:

$$(0.85 \text{ g})(1000.0 \text{ mL}) = (X \text{ g})(100.0 \text{ mL})$$
$$850 = 100.0 \text{ X}$$
$$X = 8.50 \text{ g}$$

Next, use the molarity formula to determine the molarity of this solution. We know that there are 8.50 g of NaCl present per liter of solvent in this solution. The molecular weight of NaCl is 58.44. Next, substitute all of the known values to determine the molarity of this solution:

$$M = \frac{\left(\dfrac{\text{gram of solute}}{\text{gmw of solute}}\right)}{1.00 \text{ L of solution}}$$

$$\text{Molarity of } 0.850\%^{w/v} \text{ NaCl solution} = \frac{\left(\dfrac{8.50 \text{ g NaCl}}{58.44 \text{ gmw}}\right)}{1.00 \text{ L of solution}}$$

$$\text{Molarity} = \frac{8.50}{58.44} = 0.14 \text{ molar}$$

Therefore an 0.85%$^{w/v}$ NaCl solution has a molarity of 0.14 mol/L.

Example 5-20a   What is the molarity of a 40.0%$^{w/v}$ NaOH solution made with deionized water as the solvent?

To solve, first determine how many grams of NaOH are in the 40.0%$^{w/v}$ solution. You know that a 40.0%$^{w/v}$ solution of NaOH contains 40.0 g of NaOH in 100.0 mL of water. In Example 5-20 the decimal point was moved one place to the right to convert 0.85 g/100.0 mL to 8.5 g/1000.0 mL. Therefore, by moving the decimal point one place to the right in this example, 40.0 g NaOH in 100.0 mL of water is the same as 400.0 g of NaOH in 1000.0 mL of water. Next, determine the gram molecular weight of NaOH by determining the sum of the gram atomic weights of Na, O, and H. The gram molecular weight of NaOH is 40.00. Next, substitute the values obtained so far in this problem into the molarity formula:

$$\text{Molarity of 40.0\%}^{\text{w/v}} \text{ NaOH solution} = \frac{\left(\dfrac{400 \text{ g NaOH}}{40.0 \text{ gmw}}\right)}{1.00 \text{ L of solution}}$$

$$\text{Molarity} = \frac{400}{40.0} = 10.0 \text{ molar}$$

Therefore a 40.0%$^{\text{w/v}}$ NaOH solution has a molarity of 10.0 mol/L.

Example 5-20b   What is the molarity of a 10.0%$^{\text{w/v}}$ $CaCl_2$ solution?

To solve, 10.0%$^{\text{w/v}}$ is equal to 10.0 g/100 mL or 100 g/1000 mL. The gram molecular weight of $CaCl_2$ is 110.98. Therefore,

$$\text{Molarity of 10.0\%}^{\text{w/v}} \text{ } CaCl_2 \text{ solution} = \frac{\left(\dfrac{100.0 \text{ g } CaCl_2}{110.98 \text{ gmw}}\right)}{1.00 \text{ L of solution}}$$

$$\text{Molarity} = \frac{100.0}{110.98} = 0.90 \text{ M}$$

Therefore a 10%$^{\text{w/v}}$ $CaCl_2$ solution has a molarity of 0.90 mol/L.

Example 5-20c   What would be the normality of a solution of 15.0%$^{\text{w/v}}$ H_2SO_4?

To solve this problem, remember that

$$\%^{\text{w/v}} = \frac{\text{No. gram of solute}}{100.0 \text{ mL of solution}}$$

$$\text{Therefore, } 15.0\%^{\text{w/v}} = \frac{15.0 \text{ g of solute}}{100.0 \text{ mL of solution}}$$

To determine the amount of g in 1.00 L:

$$\frac{15.0 \text{ g } H_2SO_4}{100.0 \text{ mL}} = \frac{\text{X g } H_2SO_4}{1000.0 \text{ mL}}$$

Crossmultiplying the equations results in the following:

$$(15.0)(1000.0) = (\text{X})(100.0)$$
$$15,000 = (100.0)(\text{X})$$
$$\text{X} = 150.0 \text{ g}$$

Next, use the normality formula to determine the normality of the solution.

$$\text{N} = \frac{150 \text{ g } H_2SO_4}{\left(\dfrac{98.08 \text{ gmw}}{2 \text{ valence}}\right)}{1.00 \text{ L of solution}}$$

$$\text{N} = \frac{\dfrac{150 \text{ g } H_2SO_4}{49.04 \text{ Eq}}}{1.00 \text{ L of solution}}$$

$$\text{N} = 3.06 \text{ Eq/L}$$

Therefore a 10.0%$^{\text{w/v}}$ H_2SO_4 solution has a normality of 3.06 Eq/L.

Example 5-20d   What is the normality of a 12.5%$^{w/v}$ NaOH solution?

To solve, use the normality formula after determining the number of grams per liter and the gram equivalent weight of NaOH.

$$N = \frac{125 \text{ g NaOH}}{\dfrac{\left(\dfrac{40.0 \text{ gmw}}{1 \text{ valence}}\right)}{1.00 \text{ L of solution}}}$$

$$N = \frac{\left(\dfrac{125 \text{ g NaOH}}{40.00 \text{ Eq}}\right)}{1.00 \text{ L of solution}}$$

$$N = 3.12 \text{ Eq/L}$$

Therefore a 12.5%$^{w/v}$ solution of NaOH has a normality of 3.12 Eq/L.

Example 5-20e   What is the normality of a 10.0%$^{w/v}$ H$_2$CO$_3$ solution?

To solve, use the normality formula after determining the number of grams per liter and the gram equivalent weight of H$_2$CO$_3$.

$$N = \frac{100.0 \text{ g H}_2\text{CO}_3}{\dfrac{\left(\dfrac{62.03 \text{ gmw}}{2 \text{ valence}}\right)}{1.00 \text{ L of solution}}}$$

$$N = \frac{\left(\dfrac{100.0 \text{ g H}_2\text{CO}_3}{31.02 \text{ Eq}}\right)}{1.00 \text{ L of solution}}$$

$$N = 3.22 \text{ Eq/L}$$

Therefore a 10.0%$^{w/v}$ H$_2$CO$_3$ solution has a normality of 3.22 Eq/L.

WHAT CONCENTRATION CALCULATIONS

Sometimes, in the clinical laboratory, a concentrated solution must be diluted to make a less concentrated solution. The following formula can be used whenever a calculation involves changing concentrations between two solutions:

$$C1V1 = C2V2$$

In which:

C1 = the stock concentration
V1 = the volume of stock required
C2 = the concentration of the new solution
V2 = the volume of the new solution

Because this is a derivation of a ratio and proportion formula, if three of the four items are known, then the fourth item can be calculated.

HOW   **Example 5-21**

A solution with 350.0 mL of a 2.0%$^{w/v}$ sodium chloride is needed. In the stock room is a 5.0%$^{w/v}$ solution of sodium chloride. How many milliliters of the 5.0%$^{w/v}$ sodium chloride solution are necessary to make the 2.0% solution?

Using the formula for concentrations, the following equation can be derived:

$$C1V1 = C2V2 \ \text{Where}: C1 = 5.0\%^{w/v}$$
$$V1 = X$$
$$C2 = 2.0\%^{w/v}$$
$$V2 = 350.0 \ \text{mL}$$

As long as the same units are used in both sides of the equation, units do not have to be included in the equation.

$$(5.0)(X) = (2.0)(350.0)$$
$$(5.0)(X) = 700.0$$
$$X = 140.0 \ \text{mL}$$

140.0 mL of the 5.0%$^{w/v}$ solution are diluted with water (or qs) to a total volume of 350 mL.

Example 5-21a   500.0 mL of a 20.0%$^{v/v}$ EtOH solution is needed. In the stock room is a bottle of 80.0%$^{v/v}$ EtOH. How many milliliters of the 80.0% EtOH are needed?

Using the formula for concentration calculations, $C1V1 = C2V2$, and substituting into it the values of this problem, the following equation is derived:

$$(80.0)(X) = (20.0)(500.0)$$
Solving for X:
$$X = 125.0$$

Therefore 125 mL of the 80.0%$^{v/v}$ EtOH are diluted with water to a total volume of 500.0 mL and a concentration of 25.0%$^{v/v}$ EtOH.

Example 5-21b   If you have a 10.0% acetic acid solution, how much of it will you need to make 200.0 mL of a 5.0% acetic acid solution?

You would need to take 100.0 mL of the 10.0% solution and qs to 200.0 mL with water.

Example 5-21c   If you had 15.0%$^{w/v}$ KCl solution, how much of it will you need to make 100.0 mL of a 10.0%$^{w/v}$ KCl solution?

You would need to take 66.7 mL of the 15.0%$^{w/v}$ KCl solution and qs to 100.0 mL.

Example 5-21d   Twenty milliliters of a 2.00 M solution are diluted to 100.0 mL in a 100 mL volumetric flask. What is the concentration of the new solution?

Using the concentration formula:

$$C1V1 = C2V2 \text{ Where : } C1 = 2.00 \text{ M}$$
$$V1 = 20.0 \text{ mL}$$
$$C2 = X$$
$$V2 = 100.0 \text{ mL}$$
$$(2.00)(20.0) = (X)(100.0)$$
$$40.0 = (X)(100.0)$$
$$0.40 \text{ M} = X$$

The new solution has a molarity of 0.40 M.

Example 5-21e   100.0 mL of a 1.5 M solution are diluted to 250.0 mL in a 250.0 mL volumetric flask. What is the concentration of the new solution?

To solve, use the concentration formula:

$$(1.50)(100.0) = (X)(250.0)$$
$$150.0 = (X)(250.0)$$
$$0.60 \text{ M} = X$$

The new solution has a concentration of 0.60 M.

Example 5-21f   75.0 mL of a 3.0 M solution are diluted to 150.0 mL. What is the concentration of the new solution?

To solve, use the concentration formula:

$$(3.00)(75.0) = (X)(150.0)$$
$$225 = (X)(150.0)$$
$$1.50\text{M} = X$$

The new solution has a concentration of 1.50 M.

Example 5-21g   250.0 mL of a 4 M solution are diluted to 1.00 L. What is the concentration of the new solution?

Using the concentration formula:

$$(4.00)(250.0) = (X)(1000)$$
$$1000.0 = (X)(1000)$$
$$1.00 \text{ M} = X$$

The new solution has a concentration of 1.00 M.

Example 5-21h   If there are 100.0 mL of a 6.00 M NaOH solution but a 5.00 M solution is needed, how much water should be added to the 6.00 M solution to dilute it to 5.00 M?

Using the concentration formula:

$$C1V1 = C2V2 \text{ Where} : C1 = 6.00 \text{ M}$$
$$V1 = 100.0 \text{ mL}$$
$$C2 = 5.00 \text{ M}$$
$$V2 = X$$
$$(6.00)(100.0) = (5.00)(X)$$
$$600.0 = (5.00)(X)$$
$$120.0 = X$$

The problem asked for how much water should be added to the 6.00 M solution. We see that 120.0 mL will form a 5.00 M solution; therefore **20.0 mL** of water should be added to the 100 mL of the 6.00 M solution to dilute it to 5.00 M.

Example 5-21i   There are 250.0 mL of a 0.5 M HCl solution available. You need a 0.250 M HCl solution. How much water can you add to the 0.5 M solution to dilute it to 0.250 M?

To solve, use the concentration formula:

$$(0.50)(250.0) = (0.250)(X)$$
$$125.0 = (0.250)(X)$$
$$500 \text{ mL} = X$$

Therefore, you would add 250 mL of water to the original 250 mL solution.

Example 5-21j   If you had 1.00 L of a 4.0 M KCl solution but needed a 3.5 M KCl solution, how much water could you add to the 4.0 M KCl solution?

Use the concentration formula:

$$(4.0)(1000.0) = (3.5)(X)$$
$$4000.0 = (3.5)(X)$$
$$1143 \text{ mL} = X$$

Therefore 143 mL are added to the 1.00 L of the 4.0 M solution to dilute it to a 3.5 M solution.

Example 5-21k   If you had 100.0 mL of a 1.5 M HCl solution but needed a 1.25 M HCl solution, how much water could you add to the 1.5 M HCl solution?

Use the concentration formula:

$$(1.50)(100.0) = (1.25)(X)$$
$$150.0 = (1.25)(X)$$
$$120 \text{ mL} = X$$

Therefore 20 mL of water are added to the 1.5 M HCl solution to dilute it to 1.25 M.

Example 5-2ll   A 250.0 mL stock HCl solution is placed in a volumetric flask and diluted to a total volume of 1.00 L. The concentration of the diluted specimen is 2.00 M. What is the concentration of the stock HCl?

Use the following concentration formula:

$$C1V1 = C2V2 \quad \text{Where}: C1 = X$$
$$V1 = 250.0 \text{ mL}$$
$$C2 = 2.00 \text{ M}$$
$$V2 = 1000 \text{ mL}$$
$$(X)(250.0) = (2.00)(1000)$$
$$(250.0)(X) = 2000$$
$$X = 8.00$$

Therefore the stock solution has a concentration of 8.00 M.

Example 5-21m   200.0 mL of a stock NaOH solution was diluted to a total volume of 1.0 L. The concentration of the diluted solution is 1.0 M. What was the concentration of the stock NaOH?

Using the concentration formula:

$$(X)(200.0) = (1.00)(1000)$$
$$(200.0)(X) = 1000$$
$$X = 5.00$$

Therefore the stock NaOH had a molarity of 5.00 M.

Example 5-21n   500.0 mL of a stock KCl solution was diluted to a total volume of 2.0 L. The concentration of the diluted solution is 1.75 M. What was the concentration of the stock KCl?

Using the concentration formula:

$$(X)(500.0) = (1.75)(2000.0)$$
$$(500.0)(X) = 3500.0$$
$$X = 7.00$$

The molarity of the stock KCl was 7.00 M.

WHAT **EXAMPLE PROBLEMS**

This section is designed to be useful to both the student and the laboratory professional. Students can use the additional problems to master the material. The laboratory professional can use the examples as templates for solving laboratory calculations. By finding an example similar to the problem that you need to solve, substitute the numbers appropriate to your calculation into the equation.

1. **Q.** What is the molecular weight of HCl?
   A. The molecular weight of a molecule is the sum of the molecular weight of the individual atoms that comprise the molecule. From the Periodic Table on p. **146**, the atomic weight of hydrogen is 1.01, whereas the atomic weight of chlorine is 35.45. Thus the molecular weight of $HCl = 1.01 + 35.45 = 36.46$ gmw.

2. **Q.** What is the molecular weight of H_2SO_4?

    A. The atomic weights of the atoms in this molecule are hydrogen $= 1.01$, sulfur $= 32.06$, oxygen $= 16.00$.

    The molecular weight of the molecule is the sum of the atoms of the molecule. Thus, because there are two hydrogen atoms, the atomic weight of hydrogen in this molecule is 2.02; because there is only one sulfur atom, its atomic weight contribution stays at 32.06. There are four oxygen atoms in this molecule; therefore the contribution of oxygen is $16.0 \times 4 = 64.0$ g atomic weight, and the total gram molecular weight for this molecule is:

$$2.02 + 32.06 + 64.00 = 98.08 \text{ gmw}$$

3. **Q.** What is the molecular weight of potassium permanganate $(KMnO_4)$?

    A. The molecular weight of potassium permanganate is 158.03.

4. **Q.** What is the molecular weight of AgCl?

    A. The molecular weight of AgCl is 143.32.

5. **Q.** What is the molecular weight of H_2CO_3?

    A. The molecular weight of H_2CO_3 is 62.02.

6. **Q.** How many grams of NaCl are necessary to make a 2.75 M solution in a total volume of 1.00 L?

    A. To determine the answer to this problem, it is helpful to understand the components of the molarity formula. The formula $M =$ moles per liter contains the term *mole*. What is a mole? The number of moles of a solute is equal to the number of grams of solute divided by the gram molecular weight of the solute. In other words, 1 mol of a substance is the weight in grams of the substance that is the same as its gram molecular weight. This is so the two weights cancel out to yield the value of 1. In this example, the gram molecular weight of NaCl is equal to 58.44. By substituting all known values into the molarity formula, the following equation is derived:

$$2.75 \text{ M solution} = \frac{\left(\dfrac{X \text{ g of NaCl}}{58.44 \text{ gmw NaCl}}\right)}{1.00 \text{ L of solution}}$$

Using algebra to solve this equation yields the following:

$$(2.75)(1.00) = \frac{X}{58.44}$$

$$(2.75)(58.44) = X$$

$$160.71 \text{ g} = X$$

Therefore a 2.50 M solution of NaCl in 1.00 L of solution contains 160.71 g of NaCl.

7. **Q.** How many grams of KCl are necessary to make 1000 mL of a 4.00 M solution?

    A. This problem is solved similarly to question 6. The gram molecular weight of KCl is 74.55. Remember that 1000 mL is equal to 1.00 L. Using the molarity formula and substituting into it the known values for this problem yields:

$$4.00 \text{ M solution} = \frac{\left(\dfrac{X \text{ g of KCl}}{74.55 \text{ gmw KCl}}\right)}{1.00 \text{ L of solution}}$$

Solving for X:

$$(4.00)(1.00) = \frac{X}{74.55}$$

$$(4.00)(74.55) = X$$

$$298.20 \text{ g} = X$$

Therefore 298.20 g are necessary to make a 4.0 M solution of KCl in 1000 mL.

8. **Q.** How many grams of NaOH are needed to make a 1.00 L quantity of a 1.8 M solution?
   A. 72.0 g are necessary to make a 1.8 M solution of NaOH in 1.00 L.

9. **Q.** How many grams of Na_2CO_3 are needed to make a 1.00 L quantity of a 0.75 M solution?
   A. 79.499 g are necessary to make 1.00 L of a 0.75 M Na_2CO_3 solution.

10. **Q.** What is the molarity of a solution that contains 3.0 mol of sodium chloride in 1.00 L of solution?
    A. The formula for molarity is M = 1.00 mol of solute in 1.00 L of solution. Substituting the numbers from the equation into the formula yields M = 3.00 mol of solute (NaCl) in 1.00 L of solution.
    Therefore the molarity equals 3.00 mol/L.

11. **Q.** What is the molarity of a solution that contains 0.75 mol HCl in 1.00 L of water?
    A. The molarity of this solution equals 0.75 mol/L.

12. **Q.** What is the molarity of a solution that contains 4.00 mol of HCl in 250.0 mL of solution?
    A. M = moles per liter, but as the solution volume is only 250 mL, not 1.00 L, this difference must be accounted for; 0.250 L is equivalent to 250.0 mL. Therefore the equation to solve this problem is M = 4.00 mol/0.250 L, which is equal to M = 16.0 mol/L.

13. **Q.** How many grams of $CaCl_2$ are necessary to prepare 500 mL of a 1.50 M solution?
    A. Use the molarity formula to solve this problem. Remember that only 500 mL of the solution, not 1.00 L, is to be used. The molecular weight of $CaCl_2$ is:

$$40.08 + 35.45 + 35.45 = 110.98 \text{ gmw}$$

Substituting the numbers that we know into the molarity formula yields:

$$1.50 \text{ M} = \frac{\left(\dfrac{X \text{ g CaCl}_2}{110.98 \text{ gmw CaCl}_2}\right)}{0.500 \text{ L of solution}}$$

Solving this formula for X yields the following:

$$(1.50)(0.500) = \frac{X}{110.98}$$

$$0.750 = \frac{X}{110.98}$$

$$(0.750)(110.98) = X$$

$$83.24 \text{ g} = X$$

Therefore 83.2 g of $CaCl_2$ must be weighed and qs to 500 mL of water to form a 1.50 M solution.

14. **Q.** What is the molarity of a solution that contains 120.0 g of NaOH in 1.00 L?

A. The gram molecular weight of NaOH is 40.00. Substituting into the molarity formula, the data that are known yield the following equation:

$$XM = \frac{\left(\dfrac{120.0 \text{ g NaOH}}{40.00 \text{ gmw NaOH}}\right)}{1.00 \text{ L of solution}}$$

Solving the equation yields the following:

$$X = \frac{3.00 \text{ mol}}{1.00 \text{ L}}$$

$$X = 3.00 \text{ M}$$

Therefore a solution containing 120.0 g of NaOH in 1.00 L of water has a molarity of 3.00 mol/L.

15. **Q.** What is the molarity of a 400 mL solution that contains 20.0 g of NaOH?

A. The gram molecular weight of NaOH is 40.00. Substituting the data into the molarity formula yields the following:

$$XM = \frac{\dfrac{20.0 \text{ g NaOH}}{40.00 \text{ gmw NaOH}}}{0.400 \text{ of solution}}$$

Solving the equation yields the following:

$$(0.400)(X) = \frac{20.0}{40.0}$$

$$(0.400)(X) = 0.500$$

$$X = \frac{0.500}{0.400}$$

$$X = 1.25 \text{ M}$$

Therefore a solution that contains 20.0 g of NaOH in 400 mL has a molarity of 1.25 mol/L.

16. **Q.** Into how many milliliters of water should 7.00 g of $MgSO_4$ be dissolved to make a 0.400 M solution?

A. In the previous examples, all of the parameters of the molarity formula have been solved for except for volume. Use the molarity formula to solve for volume. The gram molecular weight of $MgSO_4$ is 120.36. Substituting into the molarity formula the numbers from this problem yields the following equation:

$$0.400 \text{ M} = \frac{\left(\dfrac{7.00 \text{ g MgSO}_4}{120.36 \text{ gmw}}\right)}{X \text{ L of solution}}$$

Solving the equation yields the following:

$$(0.400 \text{ mol/L})(XL) = 0.0582 \text{ mol}$$

$$XL = \frac{0.0582 \text{ mol}}{0.400 \text{ mol/L}}$$

$$XL = 0.145 \text{ L or } 145.0 \text{ mL}$$

Thus, to prepare a 0.400 M solution of $MgSO_4$, 7.00 g of $MgSO_4$ are dissolved in water and qs to 145.0 mL.

17. **Q.** Into how much water should 9.32 g of KCl be dissolved to prepare a 0.500 M solution?
    A. The gram molecular weight of KCl is 74.55. Using the molarity formula, and substituting into it the data from the problem, the following equation is derived:

$$0.500 \text{ M} = \frac{\left(\dfrac{9.32 \text{ gKCl}}{74.55 \text{ gmw}} \right)}{X \text{ L of solution}}$$

Solving the equation yields the following:

$$(0.500 \text{ mol/L})(X) = 0.125 \text{ mol}$$

$$X = \frac{0.125 \text{ mol}}{0.500 \text{ mol/L}}$$

$$X = 0.250 \text{ L or } 250.0 \text{ mL}$$

Therefore 9.32 g of KCl are dissolved in solvent and qs to 250.0 mL to prepare a 0.500 M solution.

18. **Q.** What is the gram equivalent weight of NaOH?
    A. The gram equivalent weight is calculated by dividing the gram molecular weight of NaOH by the number of replaceable OH ions in the molecule. In NaOH, there is only one replaceable hydroxyl ion. Therefore the gram molecular weight would be divided by 1, resulting in an identical gram equivalent weight. The gram molecular weight of NaOH is 40.00; therefore the gram equivalent weight of NaOH is also 40.00.

19. **Q.** What is the gram equivalent weight of KCl?
    A. The gram equivalent weight is equal to 74.55, the same as the gram molecular weight since the valence of K is 1.0.

20. **Q.** What is the gram equivalent weight of H_2SO_4?
    A. In this molecule, there are two replaceable hydrogen ions. Therefore the gram molecular weight of this molecule would be divided by 2 to yield the gram equivalent weight of the molecule. The gram molecular weight of H_2SO_4 is 98.08. The gram equivalent weight of H_2SO_4 is equal to 49.04.

21. **Q.** What is the gram equivalent weight of H_3PO_4?
    A. The gram equivalent weight of H_3PO_4 is 32.7, or the gram molecular weight of 98 divided by 3.

22. **Q.** What is the normality of a solution that contains 20.0 g NaOH in 1.00 L of solution?

    A. The normality formula is similar to the molarity formula. The formula for normality is as follows:

$$1.00 \text{ N} = \frac{1.00 \text{ Eq}}{1.00 \text{ L}}$$

$$1.00 \text{ Eq} = \frac{\text{gram of solute}}{\text{gram equivalent weight of solute}}$$

$$\text{One gram equivalent weight} = \frac{\text{gram molecular weight}}{\text{valence}}$$

Combined together, the formula for normality is:

$$\text{Normal} = \frac{\dfrac{\text{No. gram of solute}}{\left(\dfrac{\text{gmw of solute}}{\text{valence of reactant solute}}\right)}}{1.00 \text{ L of solution}}$$

The gram molecular weight of NaOH is 40.00. There is only one hydroxyl ion that can react, so the valence is 1. Substituting into the normality formula, the data from the problem yields the following formula:

$$\text{XN} = \frac{\dfrac{20.0 \text{ g NaOH}}{\left(\dfrac{40.00 \text{ gmw}}{\text{valence of 1}}\right)}}{1.00 \text{ L of solution}}$$

Solving the formula yields the following:

$$\text{XN} = \frac{\left(\dfrac{20.0 \text{ g NaOH}}{40.00 \text{ gram equivalent weight}}\right)}{1.00 \text{ L of solution}}$$

$$\text{XN} = \frac{0.500 \text{ Eq}}{1.00 \text{ L of solution}}$$

$$\text{X} = 0.50 \text{ normal solution}$$

The solution has a normality of 0.50 Eq/L.

23. **Q.** What is the normality of a solution that contains 173.0 g H_2SO_4 in 1.00 L of solution?

    A. The gmw of H_2SO_4 is 98.08. Because there are two hydrogens that can react in an oxidation reduction reaction, the valence is 2. Substituting into the normality equation all of the data from the problem yields the following:

$$\text{XN} = \frac{\dfrac{173.0 \text{ g } H_2SO_4}{\left(\dfrac{98.08 \text{ g molecular weight}}{\text{valence of 2}}\right)}}{1.00 \text{ L of solution}}$$

Solving the equation:

$$XN = \frac{\left(\dfrac{173.0 \text{ g H}_2\text{SO}_4}{49.04 \text{ gmw}}\right)}{1.00 \text{ L of solution}}$$

$$XN = \frac{3.53 \text{ Eq}}{1.00 \text{ L of solution}}$$

$$X = 3.53 \text{ N solution}$$

The normality of this solution is 3.53 Eq/L.

24. **Q.** How do you prepare 300.0 mL of a 0.250 normal NaOH solution?
    A. What this question is asking for is how many grams of NaOH are needed to make this solution. The gram molecular weight of NaOH is 40.00. Since there is only one hydrogen, the valence will be 1. Using the normality formula, the following formula is derived:

$$0.250 \text{ N} = \frac{X \text{ g NaOH}}{\left(\dfrac{40.00 \text{ gmw NaOH}}{\text{valence of 1}}\right)}{0.300 \text{ L of solution}}$$

Solving the equation:

$$0.250 \text{ N} = \frac{\left(\dfrac{X \text{ g NaOH}}{40.00 \text{ g Eq weight NaOH}}\right)}{0.300 \text{ L of solution}}$$

$$(0.250 \text{ Eq/L})(0.300 \text{ L}) = \frac{X}{40.00 \text{ g Eq}}$$

$$(0.075 \text{ Eq}) = \frac{X}{40.00 \text{ g Eq}}$$

$$(0.075 \text{ Eq})(40.00 \text{ gEq}) = X$$

$$X = 3.00 \text{ g}$$

3.00 g of NaOH are weighed, dissolved in some water, and qs to 300 mL to prepare a 0.250 N solution.

25. **Q.** Given a 1.50 M HCl solution, what is the normality of the solution?
    A. The formula, N = (n)(M), is useful to quickly convert between normality and molarity concentrations for a solution. The formula is defined as follows:
    N = Normality
    n = valence
    M = Molarity
    Using the formula, and substituting into it the known data:

$$N = (1)(1.50)$$

$$N = 1.50$$

Notice that the normality is the same as the molarity. This is true of any solution in which the equivalent weight is the same as the gram molecular weight.

26. **Q.** Given a 3.00 M H_2SO_4 solution, what is the normality?

   A. The problem can be solved by using the formula $N = (n)(M)$. In this situation, there are two hydrogens that can react; therefore the valence (or n) is 2. Therefore:

$$X \text{ normality} = (2)(3.00 \text{ M})$$
$$X \text{ normality} = 6.00$$

Notice that the normality is twice that as the molarity. This is because the equivalent weight is half that of the gram molecular weight.

27. **Q.** Given a 2.00 normal $CaCl_2$ solution, what is the molarity?

   A. The formula $N = (n)(M)$ can be used to solve this problem. The "n" is equal to 2, as the valence of calcium is +2. Therefore:

$$2.00 \text{ N} = (2.00)(XM)$$
$$X = 1.00 \text{ M}$$

28. **Q.** What is the molality of a solution that contains 300.0 g of a compound per 1.00 kg of water? The compound has a molecular weight of 241.

   A. The formula for molality is similar to that of molarity. A 1.00 molal solution is quantitated as a solution that contains 1.00 mol of solute in 1.00 kg of solvent. The formula is as follows:

$$1.00 \text{ molal} = \frac{1.00 \text{ mol of solute}}{1.00 \text{ kg of solvent}}$$

Substituting into the formula the data that are known yields the equation:

$$X \text{ molal} = \frac{\left(\dfrac{300.0 \text{ g of solute}}{241 \text{ gmw of solute}}\right)}{1.00 \text{ kg of solvent}}$$

Solving for X:

$$(X \text{ mol/kg})(1.00 \text{ kg}) = \frac{300.0 \text{ g}}{241 \text{ gmw}}$$
$$X = 1.24 \text{ molal}$$

The molality of the solution is 1.24 mol/kg.

29. **Q.** What is the molality of a NaCl solution that contains 145.0 g of NaCl per 0.500 kg of water?

   A. The gram molecular weight of NaCl is 58.44. Using the molality formula, and substituting into it the data from the problem, the following equation is derived:

$$X \text{ molal} = \frac{\left(\dfrac{145 \text{ g NaCl}}{58.44 \text{ gmw}}\right)}{0.500 \text{ kg}}$$

Solving the equation yields:

$$X \text{ molal} = \frac{2.48 \text{ mol}}{0.500 \text{ kg}}$$

$$X = 4.96 \text{ molal}$$

Therefore the molality of the solution is 4.96 mol/kg.

30. **Q.** How many milligrams per deciliter are contained in 145 mEq/L of Na^+?

A. To convert milliequivalents per liter to milligrams per deciliter, first convert milliequivalents per liter to equivalents per liter:

$$\frac{145 \text{ mEq}}{1.00 \text{ L}} = \frac{X \text{ Eq}}{1.00 \text{ L}}$$

$$\left(\frac{145 \text{ mEq}}{1.00 \text{ L}}\right)\left(\frac{1 \text{ Eq}}{1000 \text{ mEq}}\right) = \frac{0.145 \text{ Eq}}{1.00 \text{ L}}$$

Next, use the normality formula to determine grams per liter concentration of sodium:

$$0.145 \text{ Eq} / L = \frac{X \text{ g Na}}{\left(\dfrac{22.99 \text{ atomic weight Na}}{1(\text{valence})}\right)}{1.00 \text{ L of solution}}$$

Solving the equation:

$$0.145 \text{ Eq}/L = \frac{\left(\dfrac{X \text{ g Na}}{22.99 \text{ gEq}}\right)}{1.00 \text{ L of solution}}$$

$$(0.145)(1.00) = \frac{X}{22.99}$$

$$(0.145)(22.99) = X$$

$$3.33 \text{ g}/L = X$$

Last, convert 3.33 g/L to milligrams per deciliter:

$$\left(\frac{3.33 \text{ g}}{1.00 \text{ L}}\right)\left(\frac{1 \text{ L}}{10 \text{ dL}}\right) = \frac{0.333 \text{ g}}{1.00 \text{ dL}}$$

$$\left(\frac{0.333 \text{ g}}{1.00 \text{ dL}}\right)\left(\frac{1000 \text{ mg}}{1 \text{ g}}\right) = \frac{333 \text{ mg}}{1.00 \text{dL}}$$

Therefore the 145 mEq/L sodium solution is equal to a concentration of 333 mg/dL.

31. **Q.** How many milligrams per deciliter are contained in a 1.50 mEq/L Mg^{+2} standard?

A. Another way to convert milligrams per deciliter to milliequivalents per liter is to keep all terms in the "milli" quantity. This saves a few steps, but do not use this method if it confuses you. (It is better to take a little longer to get a problem right than to use a shortcut and get it wrong.) The valence for magnesium is 2, and the atomic weight of magnesium is 24.30. Using the normality formula, the following formula is derived:

$$1.50 \text{ mEq} / L = \dfrac{X \text{ mg}}{\left(\dfrac{24.30 \text{ atomic weight Mg}}{2(\text{valence})}\right)} \Big/ 1.00 \text{ L of solution}$$

Solving the equation:

$$1.50 = \dfrac{\left(\dfrac{X \text{ mg}}{12.15 \text{ equivalent weight}}\right)}{1.00 \text{ L of solution}}$$

$$(1.50)(1.00 \text{ L}) = \dfrac{X \text{ mg}}{12.15 \text{ equivalent weight}}$$

$$(1.50)(12.15) = X \text{ mg/L}$$

$$18.22 \text{ mg/L} = X$$

Next, convert milligrams per liter to milligrams per deciliter:

$$\left(\dfrac{18.2 \text{ mg}}{1.00 \text{ L}}\right)\left(\dfrac{1 \text{ L}}{10 \text{ dL}}\right) = \left(\dfrac{1.82 \text{ mg}}{1.00 \text{ dL}}\right)$$

Therefore a 1.50 mEq/L standard of Mg^{+2} contains 1.82 mg/dL of Mg^{+2}.

32. **Q.** How many milliequivalents per liter does an 8.00 mg/dL Ca^{+2} standard contain?
    A. To solve this problem, use the normality formula. First, convert the 8.00 mg/dL quantity to grams per liter:

$$\left(\dfrac{8.00 \text{ mg}}{1.00 \text{ dL}}\right)\left(\dfrac{1 \text{ g}}{1000 \text{ mg}}\right)\left(\dfrac{10 \text{ dL}}{1 \text{ liter}}\right) = \dfrac{0.0800 \text{ g}}{1.00 \text{ L}}$$

Next, use the normality formula to determine equivalents per liter:

$$X \text{ Eq} / L = \dfrac{0.0800 \text{ g calcium}}{\left(\dfrac{40.08 \text{ atomic weight}}{2(\text{valence})}\right)} \Big/ 1.00 \text{ L of solution}$$

Solving the equation:

$$X \text{ Eq/L} = \dfrac{\left(\dfrac{0.0800 \text{ g}}{20.04 \text{ Eq}}\right)}{1.00 \text{ L of solution}}$$

$$X \text{ Eq/L} = \dfrac{0.004 \text{ Eq}}{1.00 \text{ L of solution}}$$

$$X = 0.004 \text{ Eq/L}$$

Finally, convert equivalents per liter to milliequivalents per liter:

$$\left(\dfrac{0.004 \text{ Eq}}{1.00 \text{ L}}\right)\left(\dfrac{1000 \text{ mEq}}{1 \text{ Eq}}\right) = \dfrac{4.00 \text{ mEq}}{1.00 \text{ L}}$$

Therefore an 8.00 mg/dL calcium standard contains 4.00 mEq/L calcium.

33. Q. How are 100 g of a 30.0%$^{w/w}$ solution of MgSO$_4$ prepared?
   A. The definition of a %$^{w/w}$ solution is the number of grams of solute per 100 g of solution (solute + solvent). A 30.0%$^{w/w}$ solution of MgSO$_4$ would be prepared by weighing 30.0 g of MgSO$_4$ and adding it to 70.0 g of solvent (usually deionized water) to make a total solution weight of 100 g.

34. Q. How many grams of NaOH are needed for a 10%$^{w/w}$ solution?
   A. 10 g of NaOH would be added to 90 g of solvent.

35. Q. How many grams of CaCl$_2$ are needed to prepare 100 mL of a 15.0%$^{w/v}$ solution using deionized water as the solvent?
   A. The definition of a %$^{w/v}$ solution is the number of grams of solute dissolved in 100 mL of solution. Therefore 15.0 g of CaCl$_2$ would be added and dissolved in a small amount of water in a 100 mL volumetric flask, and then additional water would be added to qs to the 100 mL mark on the volumetric flask.

36. Q. How many grams of HCl are needed to prepare 100 mL of a 20%$^{w/v}$ solution?
   A. 20 g of HCl are needed to make this solution.

37. Q. How many grams of KCl are actually present in 5.00 mL of a 20.0%$^{w/v}$ solution of KCl?
   A. As, by definition, a 20.0%$^{w/v}$ solution contains 20.0 g in 100.0 mL, by using ratio and proportion the amount present in 5.00 mL can be determined:

$$\frac{20.0 \text{ g}}{100.0 \text{ mL}} = \frac{X \text{ g}}{5.00 \text{ mL}}$$

By crossmultiplying, the following equation is derived:

$$(20.0)(5.00) = (100.0)(X)$$
$$100 = 100.0 \text{ X}$$
$$1.00 \text{ g} = X$$

Therefore there is 1.00 g of KCl present in 5.00 mL of a 20.0%$^{w/v}$ solution.

38. Q. How is a 10.0%$^{v/v}$ solution of glacial acetic acid prepared using deionized water as the solvent?
   A. By definition, a %$^{v/v}$ solution is the number of mL of solute per 100.0 mL of solution. Therefore a 10.0%$^{v/v}$ solution of glacial acetic acid would contain 10.0 mL glacial acetic acid added to 90.0 mL of water to make a total solution volume of 100.0 mL.

39. Q. How many milliliters of ethanol (EtOH) are needed to prepare a 75.0%$^{v/v}$ solution using deionized water as the diluent?
   A. A 75%$^{v/v}$ solution of EtOH contains 75.0 mL EtOH in 25.0 mL of water. Therefore 75.0 mL of EtOH are necessary for this preparation.

40. Q. What is the molarity of a 20.0%$^{w/v}$ glucose solution?
   A. By definition, there are 20.0 g of glucose in 100.0 mL of solution. By ratio and proportion, the amount of grams of glucose per liter can be determined:

$$\frac{20.0 \text{ g}}{100.0 \text{ mL}} = \frac{X \text{ g}}{1000.0 \text{ mL}}$$

Crossmultiplying the equation yields:

$$(20.0)(1000.0) = (100.0)(X)$$
$$20,000 = (100.0)(X)$$
$$200.0 \text{ g} = X$$

Therefore, there are 200.0 g of glucose in 1.00 L of water. Next, use the molarity formula to solve the problem:

$$X \text{ M} = \frac{\left(\dfrac{200.0 \text{ g glucose}}{180.16 \text{ g}}\right)}{1.00 \text{ L of solution}}$$

$$(X)(1.00 \text{ L}) = 1.11 \text{ mol glucose}$$

$$X = 1.11 \text{ M}$$

Therefore a $20.0\%^{w/v}$ glucose solution has a molarity of 1.11.

41. **Q.** What is the normality of a $15.0\%^{w/v}$ $CaCl_2$ solution? Note: gmw CaCl2 = 110.98.

   A. A $15.0\%^{w/v}$ solution contains 15.0 g per 100.0 mL of solution and therefore contains 150 g of $CaCl_2$ per 1000.0 mL of solution. $CaCl_2$ has a valence of 2, and using the normality formula, the equation becomes:

$$X \text{ Normal} = \frac{150.0 \text{ g CaCl}_2}{\left(\dfrac{110.98 \text{ gmw}}{\text{valence of 2}}\right)}{1.00 \text{ L of solution}}$$

$$X \text{ Normal} = \frac{\left(\dfrac{150.0 \text{ g CaCl}_2}{55.49 \text{ gEq}}\right)}{1.00 \text{ L of solution}}$$

$$X \text{ Normal} = 2.70 \text{ Eq/L}$$

Therefore a $15.0\%^{w/v}$ $CaCl_2$ solution has a normality of 2.70 Eq/L.

42. **Q.** A 250.0 mL, $45.0\%^{v/v}$ ethanol (EtOH) solution is needed. In the stock room is a bottle of $75.0\%^{v/v}$ EtOH. How much of the $75.0\%^{v/v}$ EtOH should you use to prepare the 250.0 mL solution?

   A. This problem is solved using a simple ratio and proportion calculation. The formula is as follows:

$$C1V1 = C2V2$$

In which:
C1 = the stock concentration
V1 = the volume of stock required
C2 = the concentration of the new solution
V2 = the volume of the new solution
By substituting into the equation the items that are given, the following equation is derived:

$$(75.0\%)(X) = (45.0\%)(250.0 \text{ mL})$$
$$(75.0)(X) = 11,250.0$$
$$X = 150.0 \text{ mL}$$

Therefore 150.0 mL of the stock solution is added to a 250.0 mL volumetric flask. The remainder of the solution is deionized water (solvent), of which 100.0 mL is added to make the total volume 250.0 mL.

43. **Q.** A 125.0 mL, 3.50 M solution is diluted to 500.0 mL in a 500.0 mL volumetric flask. What is the concentration of the new solution?

   A. The formula C1V1 = C2V2 is used to solve this problem.

$$(3.50 \text{ M stock})(125.0 \text{ mL}) = (X)(500.0 \text{ mL})$$

$$437.5 = (500.0)(X)$$

$$\frac{437.5}{500.0} = 0.88 \text{ M}$$

Therefore the new solution has a molarity of 0.88.

WHAT **PRACTICE PROBLEMS**

Solve the following practice problems to further master the material. Answers and explanations to some problems can be found in the Answer Key.

Determine the molecular weight of the following molecules according to **Table 5-1**.

1. KOH

2. $MgSO_4$

3. H_2PO_4

4. $AlCl_3$

5. H_3SO_4

6. $CuSO_4$

7. NiO

Determine the molarity of the following solutions.

8. 3.50 mol NaCl in 1.00 L of solution

9. 1.50 mol HCl in 800.0 mL of solution

10. 85.0 g of NaOH in 1.00 L of solution

11. 6.50 g of $NaHCO_3$ in 500.0 mL of solution

How would you prepare the following solutions?

12. 200.0 mL of 0.750 M KCl

13. 75.0 mL of 0.400 M NaCl

14. 500.0 mL of 0.400 M $MgSO_4$

15. 0.600 L of 2.50 M KCl

16. 500.0 mL of 0.40 M HCl

17. 0.200 L of 0.600 M NaOH

Calculate the gram equivalent weights for the following molecules.

18. HCl

19. NaOH

20. $AlCl_3$

21. H_3SO_4

22. $CaCl_2$

Determine the normality of the following solutions.

23. 4.00 g NaOH in 750.0 mL of solution

24. 24.5 g of H_3PO_4 in 1.500 L of solution

25. 200 g of K_3PO_4 in 250.0 mL of solution

26. 12.0 g H_2SO_4 in 750.0 mL of solution

27. 5 g HCl in 100.0 mL of solution

Convert the following molar solutions to normal solutions.

28. 5.50 M HCl

29. 2.50 M H_2SO_4

30. 1.75 M H_3PO_4

31. 0.85 M $CaCl_2$

32. 2.5 M NaOH

33. 1.5 M KOH

Convert the following normal solutions to molar solutions.

34. 3.50 N NaOH

35. 0.02 N $MgSO_4$

36. 3.00 N H_2SO_4

37. 0.15 N HCl

38. 2.50 N K_3PO_4

39. What is the molality of a solution containing 75 g NaCl in 1.00 kg of water?

40. What is the molality of a solution containing 35 g KCl in 1.00 kg of water?

41. How many grams of KCl are needed to make a 3.00 molal solution in 0.750 kg of water?

Convert the following units.

42. 10.0 mg/dL calcium standard to milliequivalents per liter

43. 4.00 mg/dL magnesium standard to milliequivalents per liter

44. 145 mEq/L sodium standard to milligrams per deciliter

45. 115 mEq/L chloride standard to milligrams per deciliter

46. 135 mEq/L sodium standard to millimoles per liter

47. 4.00 mEq/L HCl solution to millimoles per liter

48. 500.0 mg/dL glucose standard to millimoles per liter

49. 7.5 mmol/L glucose standard to milligrams per deciliter

50. 12.0 mg/dL creatinine standard to millimoles per liter

Solve the following problems.

51. Calculate the quantity of grams found in a 12.0%$^{w/w}$ solution of NaCl.

52. Calculate the quantity of milliliters found in 100 mL of a 10.0%$^{v/v}$ solution of HCl.

53. Calculate the quantity of grams found in 100 mL of a 15.0%$^{w/v}$ solution of NaOH.

54. Calculate the quantity of grams found in 10.0 mL of a 20.0%$^{w/v}$ KCl solution.

55. Calculate the quantity of grams found in 50.0 mL of a 35%$^{w/v}$ HCl solution.

56. What is the molarity of a 15.0%$^{w/v}$ KCl solution?

57. What is the molarity of a 2.5%$^{w/v}$ HCl solution?

58. Calculate the molarity of a 30.0%$^{w/v}$ CaCl$_2$ solution.

59. Determine the quantity of stock 75.0%$^{v/v}$ EtOH required to prepare 500.0 mL of a 25.0%$^{v/v}$ EtOH solution.

60. Determine the concentration of a solution if 300.0 mL of a 15.0%$^{w/v}$ tris buffer solution was diluted to a final volume of 1000 mL.

61. Determine the quantity of stock 25%$^{v/v}$ acetic acid required to prepare 150 mL of a 10%$^{v/v}$ acetic acid solution.

QUICK NOTES

- A **solution** contains two parts: **the solute and the solvent**. The solvent is the liquid into which the solute is diluted. Usually in the clinical laboratory the solvent is deionized water, and the solute can be a liquid or a solid such as a dry chemical.
- The term **qs** is a Latin term that means "the quantity is sufficient."
- The gram molecular weight of a molecule is the sum of its gram atomic weights.
- One mol of a solution is equal to the number of grams of solute divided by the gram molecular weight of the solute.
- A 1.0 molar solution is determined by dividing 1.0 mol of a solute into 1.0 liter of solution.
- The normality of a solution is determined by the following formula: $N = nM$, where N = normality, n = gram equivalent weight of the solute, and M = molarity.
- In the human body, there are only three elements that laboratory science students and laboratory professionals may have to use in a normality calculation. They are H, Mg, and Ca.

- Hydrogen can have an equivalent weight of either 1, 2, or 3 depending on the amount of hydrogen atoms in the molecule. Magnesium and calcium have equivalent weights of 2.0.
- Molality solutions are based on weight, so the formula is slightly different than the molarity calculations. Molality = mol of solute in 1.0 kilogram of solvent.
- When converting analytes from mg/dL to mEq/L, only the dL has to be converted to liters, but since both numerators are in milli units, the units do not have to be converted to grams from mg or equivalents from milliequivalents.
- Percent solutions are based on a unit of 100 and not 1000 as are molarity solution calculations.
- The most common percent solution is $\%^{w/v}$ or number of grams of solute dissolved into 100.0 mL of solvent.
- C1V1 = C2V2 calculation is used when you have a more concentrated solution and you need to dilute it to a lower concentration. All concentration units have to be the same; you cannot have a normality solution and then use this formula to determine the amount of a molar solution you might need. Either convert both to normality or both to molarity.

Periodic Table of the Elements

IA	IIA	IIIB	IVB	VB	VIB	VIIB		VIIIB		IB	IIB	IIIA	IVA	VA	VIA	VIIA	VIIIA
1 **H** 1.0079																	2 **He** 4.0026
3 **Li** 6.941	4 **Be** 9.0122											5 **B** 10.81	6 **C** 12.011	7 **N** 14.007	8 **O** 15.999	9 **F** 18.998	10 **Ne** 20.179
11 **Na** 22.990	12 **Mg** 24.305											13 **Al** 26.982	14 **Si** 28.086	15 **P** 30.974	16 **S** 32.06	17 **Cl** 35.453	18 **Ar** 39.948
19 **K** 39.098	20 **Ca** 40.08	21 **Sc** 44.956	22 **Ti** 47.88	23 **V** 50.942	24 **Cr** 51.996	25 **Mn** 54.938	26 **Fe** 55.847	27 **Co** 58.933	28 **Ni** 58.69	29 **Cu** 63.546	30 **Zn** 65.38	31 **Ga** 69.72	32 **Ge** 72.59	33 **As** 74.922	34 **Se** 78.96	35 **Br** 79.904	36 **Kr** 83.80
37 **Rb** 85.468	38 **Sr** 87.62	39 **Y** 88.906	40 **Zr** 91.22	41 **Nb** 92.906	42 **Mo** 95.94	43 **Tc** (98.906)[a]	44 **Ru** 101.07	45 **Rh** 102.91	46 **Pd** 106.42	47 **Ag** 107.87	48 **Cd** 112.41	49 **In** 114.82	50 **Sn** 118.69	51 **Sb** 121.75	52 **Te** 127.60	53 **I** 126.90	54 **Xe** 131.29
55 **Cs** 132.91	56 **Ba** 137.33	57 **La*** 138.91	72 **Hf** 178.49	73 **Ta** 180.95	74 **W** 183.85	75 **Re** 186.21	76 **Os** 190.2	77 **Ir** 192.22	78 **Pt** 195.08	79 **Au** 196.97	80 **Hg** 200.59	81 **Tl** 204.38	82 **Pb** 207.2	83 **Bi** 208.98	84 **Po** (209.98)[a]	85 **At** (209.99)[a]	86 **Rn** (222.02)[a]
87 **Fr** (223.02)[a]	88 **Ra** (226.03)[a]	89 **Ac†** (227.03)[a]	104 **?**[b] (261)[a]	105 **Ha**[b] (262)[a]													

* Lanthanoid Series

58 **Ce** 140.12	59 **Pr** 140.91	60 **Nd** 144.24	61 **Pm** (144.91)[a]	62 **Sm** 150.36	63 **Eu** 151.96	64 **Gd** 157.25	65 **Tb** 158.93	66 **Dy** 162.50	67 **Ho** 164.93	68 **Er** 167.26	69 **Tm** 168.93	70 **Yb** 173.04	71 **Lu** 174.97

† Actinoid Series

90 **Th** 232.04	91 **Pa** (231.04)[a]	92 **U** 238.03	93 **Np** (237.05)[a]	94 **Pu** (244.06)[a]	95 **Am** (243.06)[a]	96 **Cm** (247.07)[a]	97 **Bk** (247.07)[a]	98 **Cf** (251.08)[a]	99 **Es** (252.08)[a]	100 **Fm** (257.10)[a]	101 **Md** (256.09)[a]	102 **No** (259.10)[a]	103 **Lr** (260.11)[a]

[a] Value in parentheses denotes mass number of most stabel known isotope.

[b] Name and symbol are not officially accepted. Kurchatovium, Ku, has been proposed by Russian investigators and rutherfordium, Rf, by American investigators for element 104.

Atomic weights have been updated according to Holden, N. E. and Martin, R. L.: Atomic weights of the elements, 1981. Pure and Appl. Chem., 55(7): 1011–1118, 1983.

From Burtis C, Ashwood E: *Tietz Fundamentals of Clinical Chemistry*, 4th ed. Philadelphia, W.B. Saunders, 1996.

Clinical Chemistry Laboratory

OBJECTIVES

At the end of this chapter, the reader should be able to do the following:

1. Convert between absorbance and transmittance values.
2. Calculate the concentration of unknown samples using Beer's law.
3. Calculate the concentrations of unknown samples by multiple standards and millimolar absorptivity methods.
4. Calculate the concentration of enzyme unknown samples using the principles of kinetic analysis.
5. Calculate the pH of solutions using the Henderson-Hasselbalch equation.

6. Calculate bicarbonate, pH, and pCO_2 of unknown samples using the derivation of the Henderson-Hasselbalch equation.
7. Interpret a patient's acid–base status.
8. Calculate the anion gap of unknown samples.
9. Calculate serum and urine osmolality concentrations.
10. Calculate the osmol gap in patient samples.
11. Calculate the concentration of LDL and VLDL cholesterol.

WHAT **SPECTROPHOTOMETRY**

It is beyond the scope of this book to go into great detail about spectrophotometry and spectrophotometric techniques. Some manual methodologies that are taught to MLT and MLS students have been moved to Appendix A, as these are no longer performed in the laboratory. In general, spectrophotometry is used to quantify the concentration of various analytes based on the amount of light that the analyte absorbs. It is based on the theory of Beer's law, which states that the amount of absorbance of a solution is directly proportional to the solution's concentration. In practical terms, the darker the solution, the higher the absorbance and the more concentrated the solution.

Beer's law: $\quad A = abc \quad$ where: $\quad$ A = absorbance
a = absorptivity coefficient
b = pathlength
c = concentration

The absorptivity coefficient (a) is the amount of light absorbed by an analyte at a specific wavelength and is constant for a particular analyte at a particular wavelength if certain conditions such as temperature, solvent, and pH remain constant. The pathlength (b) is the distance that light travels through the solution and (if the analysis is performed correctly) is also a constant. Thus by removing the two constants in the equation, the following equation is derived:

Beer's law: $A \alpha c$

which states that absorbance is directly proportional to concentration. By using Beer's law, many instruments can rapidly calculate the concentration of many different analytes.

Beer's law is possible because of the concept of transmittance. As depicted in Figure 6-1, a cuvette containing the solution to be analyzed is placed within a basic spectrophotometer so that light can be shown through it. The solution will absorb some of the light (absorbance), and the remainder will be transmitted through the cuvette to the photodetector. Notice that the arrow to the right of the cuvette, which represents the transmitted light, is smaller than the arrow to the left of the cuvette, which represents the incident light. The ratio of the amount of transmitted light divided by the amount of incident light is known as *transmittance*. This is demonstrated mathematically as follows:

$$\text{Transmittance} = \left(\frac{L_T}{L_I}\right)$$

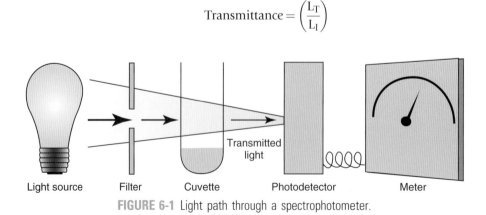

Light source $\qquad$ Filter $\qquad$ Cuvette $\qquad$ Photodetector $\qquad$ Meter

FIGURE 6-1 Light path through a spectrophotometer.

where:

$$L_T = \text{Transmitted light}$$
$$L_I = \text{Incident light}$$

Transmittance ratios range from 0.000 to 1.000. By multiplying by 100, percent transmittance values can be obtained, ranging from 0.00 to 100.00 on a linear scale. If all of the light is transmitted through a solution—that is, no light is absorbed by the solution—the transmittance ratio is 1.00 and the percent transmittance is 100%. Conversely, if no light is transmitted through the solution (i.e., there is 100% absorbance of the light by the solution), the transmittance ratio is 0.000, or 0% transmittance. Mathematically, transmittance and absorbance are related by the following formula:

$$A = -\log T$$

This can be manipulated to the following formula:

$$A = \log\left(\frac{1}{T}\right)$$

The formula can be converted from T to % T:

$$A = \log\left(\frac{1}{T}\right)\frac{100\%}{100\%}$$

$$A = \frac{\log 100\%}{\%T}$$

Solving this equation:

$$A = \log 100\% - \log \%T$$

OR

$$A = 2.00 - \log \%T$$

In contrast to transmittance ratios, absorbance values range from 0.000 to infinity on a logarithmic scale. Figure 6-2 illustrates an absorbance and percent transmittance meter. Notice

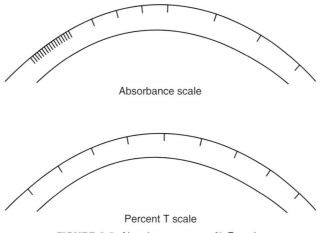

Absorbance scale

Percent T scale

FIGURE 6-2 Absorbance versus % T scale.

how much easier it is to interpret the linear percent transmittance scale versus the logarithmic absorbance scale.

By convention, absorbance values are reported to the third decimal place (0.000), whereas percent T values are reported to the nearest tenth (0.0% T).

HOW   *Example 6-1*

A manual creatinine assay was performed using the Jaffé method in a MLT student lab. A 45% T reading was obtained for the cuvette containing the level 1 creatinine control and reagent. What is the absorbance value?

To solve this problem, use the following formula:

$$A = 2.00 - \log\%T$$

Substituting in the % T value, the following equation is derived:

$$A = 2.00 - \log 45$$

Using a calculator or the logarithm table in Appendix 2-A, determine the log of 45.

$$\log 45 = 1.653$$
$$A = 2.00 - 1.653$$
$$A = 0.347$$

Therefore the % T value of 45% is equal to an absorbance value of 0.347.

Example 6-1a   Given a 60% T reading on a spectrophotometer, what is the absorbance value?

To solve, use $A = 2.00 - \log\% T$:

$$A = 2.00 - \log 60$$
$$A = 2.00 - 1.778$$
$$A = 0.222$$

Therefore the % T value of 60% is equal to an absorbance value of 0.222.

Example 6-1b   Given a 30% T reading, what is the absorbance value?

Using the same $A = 2.00 - \log\% T$, and solving for A, the absorbance value is 0.523.

Example 6-1c   Given a transmittance ratio of 0.400, what is the absorbance value?

To solve this problem, first convert the transmittance ratio to a percent transmittance value.

$$0.400 \text{ transmittance} \times 100 = 40.0\% \text{ transmittance}$$

Next, substitute 40.0% T into the conversion formula:

$$A = 2.00 - \log 40.0$$

Using a calculator or the logarithm table in Appendix 2-A, determine the log of 40:

$$\log 40.0 = 1.602$$
$$A = 2.00 - 1.602$$
$$A = 0.398$$

Therefore the transmittance ratio of 0.400 is equal to an absorbance value of 0.398.

Example 6-1d Given a transmittance ratio of 0.125, what is the absorbance value?

To solve, first convert the ratio of 0.125 into percentage by multiplying by 100. The % T result is 12.5%. Next, use the absorbance formula to convert the % T value to absorbance:

$$A = 2.00 - \log 12.5$$
$$A = 0.903$$

Therefore a transmittance ratio of 0.125 is equal to an absorbance value of 0.903.

Example 6-1e Given a transmittance ratio of 0.775, what is the absorbance value?

Using the formula $A = 2.00 - \log \%T$, the absorbance value is 0.111.

Example 6-1f Given an absorbance value of 0.875, what is the %T value?

Using the formula and substituting into it the given values, the following equation is derived:

$$0.875 = 2.00 - \log \%T$$

Solving this equation leads to the following:

$$0.875 - 2.00 = -\log \%T$$
$$-1.125 = -\log \%T$$

The negative signs in this equation can be removed because they are found on both sides of the equation.

$$1.125 = \log \%T$$

Next, find the antilog of 1.125 from the logarithm table or by using a calculator. The antilog of a number is determined on many calculators by pressing INV and then LOG. Some calculators require another key be pressed before the LOG key. Follow the manufacturer's directions for determining antilogarithms for your calculator.

The antilog of 1.125 is 13.34.

% T = 13.34 or log using significant rules, 13.3

To verify this result, use 13.34 as % T and determine the absorbance.

$$A = 2.00 - \log 13.34$$
$$A = 2.00 - 1.125$$
$$A = 0.875$$

Example 6-1g   Given an absorbance value of 1.125, what is the % T value?

This problem can be solved just like Example 6-1f.

$$1.125 = 2.00 - \log \%T$$
$$1.125 - 2.00 = -\log \%T$$
$$-0.875 = -\log \%T$$
$$0.875 = \log \%T$$

The antilog of 0.875 is 7.50.

$$\%T = 7.50$$

Can you work this problem backwards to prove that 7.50 is the correct answer?

Example 6-1h   Given an absorbance value of 0.837, what is the % T value?

The % T value is 14.6.

WHAT   Just measuring the absorbance or % T values of solutions will not result in any meaningful results. When analytes are measured, "standards" are used within the analysis. Standards are known quantities of the chemical that is to be analyzed. By including standards within an analysis, the patient specimens can be compared with the standards for quantification. We know before we analyze the standards what the concentrations of the standards are and within the analysis we measure the absorbance of the standards. Once the standards and patient specimens' absorbance values are measured, there are three techniques to determine the concentration of the analyte in the patient's specimen. Two of these techniques, the single-standard method and the factor method, are discussed in Chapter 15.

WHAT **Standard Curve Method for Determining the Concentration of Unknowns**

Most assays do not use a single standard to quantify unknowns. Instead, four to six standards of different concentrations are used that are spread evenly across the linear range of the method. In this manner, more of the linear range of the assay is covered by the standards compared with the single-standard method. On many automated instruments, a series of standards, or calibrators, are used to "set" the standard curve that is stored in the instrument's computer. The electronic signal generated by the transmittance value of a sample is compared with the computer's standard curve for the analyte being measured in the sample. The computer then generates a quantitative result for that sample's analyte that can then be sent to the instrument's computer and/or printer.

Students of clinical laboratory science often learn the concept of a standard curve by graphing on linear graph paper the concentrations of standards on the x axis and the absorbance of the standards on the y axis. A "standard curve" is shown in Figure 6-3. The following brief discussion of manually produced standard curves is designed to assist the students of medical laboratory science to better understand what is happening inside the "black box" of an automated instrument.

In a manual assay that follows Beer's law, and using linear graph paper, the standard curve of the absorbances obtained from the standards should be a straight line. The concentrations of the standards should range between the highest and lowest linear range and two to three concentrations evenly spaced between the two outermost limits. The standard curve line should be a "best fit" line, not "point to point" or "connect the dots." The line should begin at 0,0 and never extend beyond the highest standard. Patient samples that have absorbances higher than the highest concentration of standard must be diluted so the absorbance obtained falls

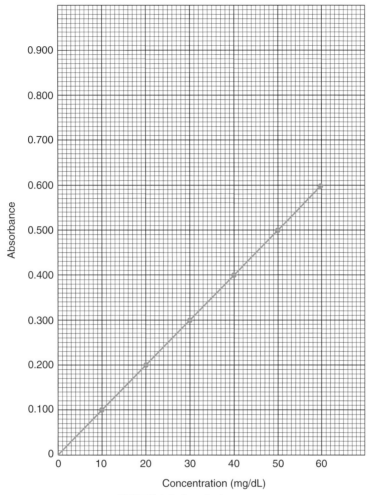

FIGURE 6-3 Standard curve.

within the linear range and reanalyzed. Standard curves are not limited to the chemistry laboratory; they are also used in the hematology laboratory.

A standard curve of the percent transmittance values of the standards can also be plotted. However, if plotted on linear graph paper, the % T standard curve is curvilinear, as shown in Figure 6-4. To form a straight line, % T values must be plotted on semilogarithm graph paper, as shown in Figure 6-5.

HOW   *Example 6-2*

A manual glucose assay was performed using 50 mg/dL, 100 mg/dL, 200 mg/dL, and 300 mg/dL standards. The following is a list of the absorbance values of each standard.

STANDARD CONCENTRATION	ABSORBANCE
50 mg/dL	0.150
100 mg/dL	0.300
200 mg/dL	0.600
300 mg/dL	0.900

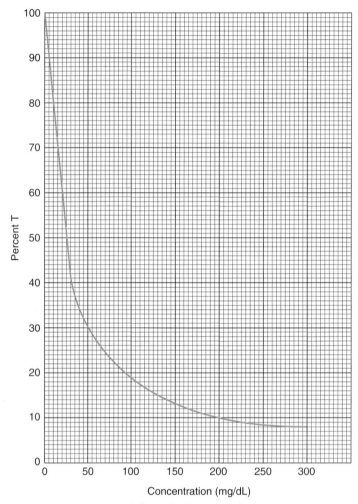

FIGURE 6-4 % T standard curve on linear paper.

Using the absorbance values and the concentration of each standard, the following standard curve (Figure 6-6A) can be produced. Notice that the line does not extend beyond the 300 mg/dL standard concentration and intersects 0,0.

If a patient sample was also analyzed at the same time that the standards were analyzed and had an absorbance value of 0.400, what would the glucose concentration of the sample be?

To solve this problem, use the graph of the standard curve (see Figure 6-6A). Find on the *y* axis scale 0.400 absorbance (see Figure 6-6B).

Next, using a ruler or straightedge, a line is drawn across the graph until it intersects the standard curve line. Now a line is drawn straight down to the *x* axis (see Figure 6-6C).

The point where the vertical line intersects the *x* axis is the concentration of the patient sample with an absorbance of 0.400. This glucose value from Figure 6-6C is 135 mg/dL.

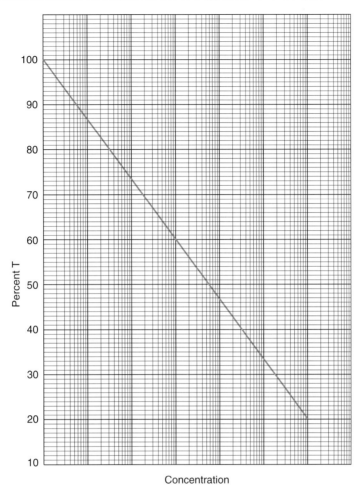

FIGURE 6-5 % T standard curve on semilogarithm paper.

Example 6-2a   Using the same glucose graph as in Example 6-2, what would the concentration be if the patient's absorbance value had been 0.690?

By following the absorbance readings up to 0.690, then going across the graph until the line intersects with the standard curve line, then by reading down to the glucose concentration, the glucose concentration would have been 230 mg/dL.

Example 6-2b   Again by using the same graph, what if the absorbance had been 0.200?

The result would have been 70 mg/dL.

Example 6-2c   A total protein assay was performed using four protein standards, two quality control specimens, and five patient specimens. The absorbance values for each of the standards, quality control specimens, and patient specimens are listed here:

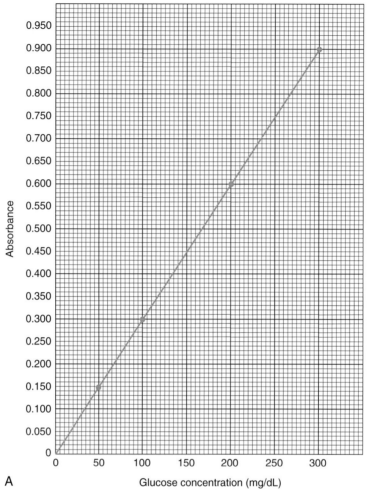

A

Glucose concentration (mg/dL)

FIGURE 6-6 (A) to (C) Standard curve of glucose assay.

SAMPLE	ABSORBANCE
3.00 g/dL standard	0.195
4.50 g/dL standard	0.290
7.50 g/dL standard	0.480
15.00 g/dL standard	0.960
QC level 1	0.270
QC level 2	0.440
Patient 1	0.580
Patient 2	0.170
Patient 3	0.260
Patient 4	0.490
Patient 5	0.900

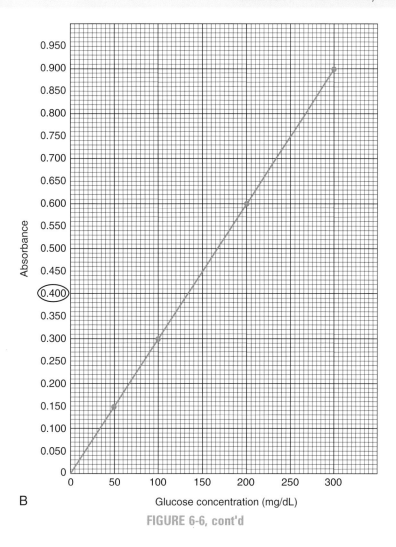

B

Glucose concentration (mg/dL)

FIGURE 6-6, cont'd

Figure 6-7 is a graph of the standards. From the standard curve line obtained, what are the concentrations of the quality control materials and each of the patient specimens?

The absorbance of QC level 1 is 0.270. Find the absorbance on the y axis, and draw a horizontal line until it intersects the standard curve line. Next, draw a vertical line from the intersection of the horizontal line with the standard curve to the x axis. The concentration of QC level 1 is found at the point on the x axis at which the vertical line intersects the x axis. In this example, the total protein concentration of QC level 1 is 4.20 g/dL. QC level 2 is found in the same manner. QC level 2 has an absorbance of 0.440 that corresponds from the graph to a concentration of 6.80 g/dL. The total protein concentration of each patient is listed here:

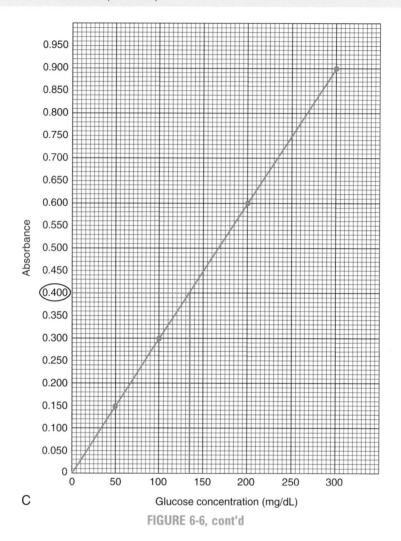

C

FIGURE 6-6, cont'd

PATIENT NO.	CONCENTRATION
1	9.00 g/dL
2	2.70 g/dL
3	4.00 g/dL
4	7.70 g/dL
5	14.00 g/dL

Example 6-2d   Using the total protein graph in Figure 6-7, what would the protein value be for an unknown with an absorbance of 0.160?

The protein value would be 2.50 g/dL.

Example 6-2e   Using the protein graph again, what would the protein value be if the unknown had a value of 0.840?

The result is 13.00 mg/dL.

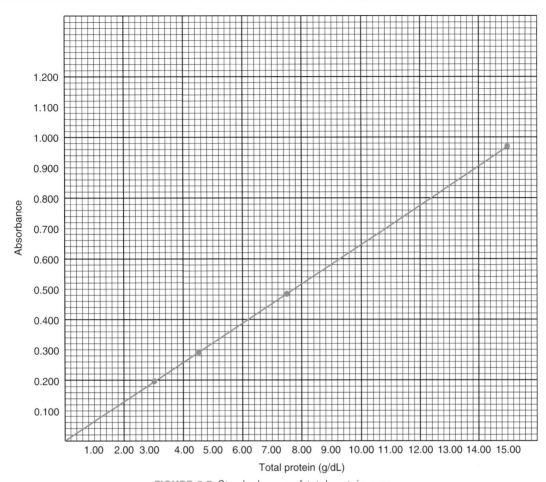

FIGURE 6-7 Standard curve of total protein assay.

WHAT   **Molar Absorptivity Method for Determining the Concentration of Unknowns**

Another method for determining the concentration of analytes is by using the molar absorptivity of the analyte. Some automated methods may calculate the concentration of analytes using this method, but the concept is presented here for the benefit of students of clinical laboratory science. The molar absorptivity for a compound is constant at a given wavelength and when conditions, such as temperature, remain constant. Remember that Beer's law states that A = abc. If the absorbance, pathlength, and molar absorptivity of an analyte are known, the concentration of the analyte can be determined.

HOW   *Example 6-3*

The molar absorptivity of nicotinamide adenine dinucleotide and hydrogen (NADH) is $6.22 \times 10^3 \ M^{-1} \ cm^{-1}$ at 340 nm. If an assay of an analyte using NADH as an indicator was performed using a 1 cm light path and a measured absorbance of NADH of 1.650, what would be the concentration of the NADH?

Using Beer's law that A = abc, substitute the known data into it:

$$1.650 = \left(6.22 \times 10^3 \text{ M}^{-1} \text{ cm}^{-1}\right)(1 \text{ cm})(\text{X M})$$

$$\frac{1.650}{\left(6.22 \times 10^3 \text{ M}^{-1}\right)} = \text{XM}$$

$$\text{X} = 2.65 \times 10^{-4} \text{ M}$$

Therefore the concentration of the compound is 2.65×10^{-4} M.

Example 6-3a   Using the information about NADH in Example 6-3, what would be the concentration of an analyte measured using NADH at 340 nm using a 1 cm light path and a measured absorbance of NADH of 0.584?

By substituting the value of 0.584 into the equation instead of 1.650, the concentration of the analyte is 9.39×10^{-5} M.

Example 6-3b   A different analyte was measured with the same parameters as in Example 6-3a, but the measured absorbance of NADH was 1.244. What is the analyte's concentration?

The concentration of the analyte is 2.00×10^{-4} M.

WHAT **END-POINT VERSUS KINETIC REACTIONS**

Chemical reactions in the clinical chemistry laboratory may be end-point or kinetic. End-point assays measure the absorbance of the reaction at the completion of the reaction. Many manual wet chemistry assays performed by students of clinical laboratory science are end-point assays with an incubation period from 15 to 20 minutes to allow for completion of the reaction.

End-point assays can use a single standard, a standard curve, or the molar absorptivity method to calculate the concentration of patient samples. End-point assays may use enzymes within the reaction as part of the reagent, but analyses of enzymes are not performed as end-point reactions. In many laboratories, analytes are measured by large multichannel random access analyzers. In the quest for increased speed, kinetic reactions were developed. A kinetic reaction differs from an end-point assay in that the reaction does not go to completion; rather, absorbances are taken at certain intervals for short periods. Some analyzers continuously monitor the absorbance readings instead of monitoring at fixed intervals to improve accuracy. In any reaction, kinetic or end-point, there may be three phases: the lag phase, in which the reactant and reagents are first reacting together; the reacting phase, during which the product is formed; and the reagent depletion phase (Figure 6-8).

In the lag phase, the absorbance of the product is not constant; in the reacting phase, the absorbance steadily changes. If there is more reactant than the reagent can react with, the third phase (reagent depletion) occurs. In this phase, the absorbance values remain the same. In an end-point assay, the reagents are in such excess that the reagent depletion phase should not occur. Rather, the reaction is allowed to proceed past the reacting phase until all of the reactant is exhausted. At this point, the absorbance is stable. In a kinetic reaction, the absorbance readings are taken during the second phase. In a kinetic reaction, the change in absorbance, or delta absorbance, is measured.

WHAT **ENZYME KINETICS**

This section will feature a broad overview of enzyme kinetics and the associated calculation. This section is designed to help the student of medical laboratory science rather than the laboratory professional, as manual enzyme assays are no longer (thankfully!) performed in the clinical laboratory but may be performed by students during their didactic training.

Kinetic reactions may be "first order" or "zero order" as shown in Figure 6-9.

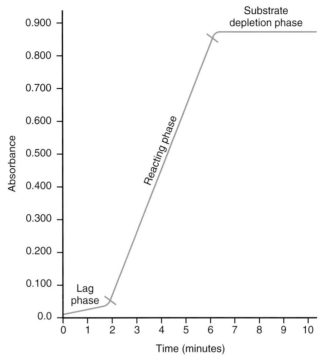

FIGURE 6-8 Three phases of a reaction.

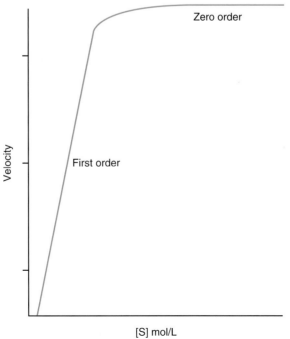

FIGURE 6-9 Kinetic reactions.

First-Order Reactions

First-order reactions are reactions in which the enzyme is in excess and the substrate concentration (the concentration of the analyte to be measured) is the limiting factor. In a first-order reaction, the substrate concentration is low relative to the enzyme concentration. At low substrate concentrations, the rate of the reaction is dependent on the substrate concentration. First-order reactions tend to be used when nonenzyme analytes are measured and enzymes are used in the reaction sequence as a reagent.

Zero-Order Kinetics

When the activity of an enzyme needs to be measured, conditions of the assay are maintained to allow zero-order kinetics to occur. In zero-order kinetics, the rate of the reaction is directly proportional to the enzyme concentration and independent of the substrate concentration. The following reaction occurs when measuring enzyme activity:

$$E + S \leftrightarrow ES \rightarrow E + P$$

where:
E = enzyme
S = substrate
ES = enzyme-substrate complex
P = product

In a zero-order kinetic assay, the substrates are kept in excess; the rate-limiting factor is the concentration of the enzyme being analyzed. All other secondary enzymes used in the reaction are also kept in excess. Temperature, pH, and other variables are kept constant during the reaction. The rate of the reaction can be calculated by the Michaelis-Menten equation:

$$v = \frac{(V_{max}[S])}{K_m + [S]}$$

where:
v = velocity or rate of reaction (which is equal to the enzyme activity)
V_{max} = the maximum velocity when the enzyme is saturated with substrate
[S] = substrate concentration
K_m = Michaelis-Menten constant

The curve of velocity versus substrate concentration for zero-order kinetics (Figure 6-10) can be used to illustrate this equation.

The Michaelis-Menten constant, K_m, is the molar substrate concentration at which the velocity of the reaction is $1/2V_{max}$. The K_m is specific for a particular enzyme-substrate complex under defined conditions. The substrate concentration typically is kept at least 10 to 20 times higher than the K_m of the reaction to ensure zero order kinetics.

Historically, the units used to quantitate enzyme activity were arbitrary because they were based on the specific enzyme that was measured. In an effort to standardize the unit of enzyme activity, the Enzyme Commission of the International Union of Biochemistry established the international unit (IU) as the unit of enzyme activity in 1964. Thus 1 IU is defined as the amount of enzyme that will catalyze the reaction of 1 µmol of substrate per minute (µmol/min) of

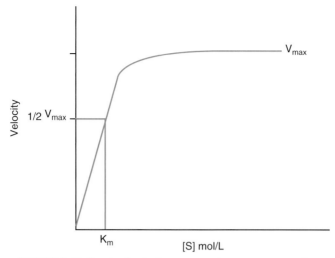

FIGURE 6-10 Graph of velocity versus substrate concentration.

reaction under defined conditions, such as temperature, pH, and substrate. The World Health Organization, as part of their Système Internationale, adopted the katal, abbreviated K, as the unit of enzyme activity. Thus 1 katal is defined as the activity of the enzyme that changes the substrate by 1 mol per second under defined conditions of temperature, pH, and substrate. The katal is not widely used in the United States. The katal and the international unit are mathematically related by the following:

$$1.0 \text{ IU} = 16.7 \text{ nK}$$

Unlike other chemistry analytes, standards for many enzymes are not available. Instead, the activity of an enzyme is measured using zero-order kinetics. By using the following formula, it is possible to determine the activity of a particular enzyme without a standard:

$$\left(\frac{\Delta \text{Absorbance of unknown}}{\in \varepsilon \times d}\right) (10^6) \left(\frac{1}{T}\right) \left(\frac{V_T}{V_S}\right) = \text{IU/L}$$

where:
ΔAbsorbance of unknown = delta absorbance per minute of unknown
ε = molar absorptivity constant for product in units of $M^{-1}cm^{-1}$
D = pathlength (usually 1 cm)
10^6 = conversion factor to convert mole per liter to μmol/liter
T = time in minutes
V_T = total volume (reagents + sample)
V_S = sample volume

NOTE: If the extinction coefficient is in units of mM^{-1} cm^{-1}, then the conversion factor will be 10^3, not 10^6.

Many clinical chemistry enzyme assays use the oxidation of NADH or the reduction of NAD^+ as part of a coupled indicator reaction. NADH will absorb at 340 nm, whereas NAD^+

does not. Therefore, in an indicator reaction in which NADH is oxidized to NAD^+, the absorbance values of the reaction will decrease over time. Conversely, if the indicator reaction reduces NAD^+ to NADH, the absorbance values will increase over time. The molar extinction coefficient for NADH is 6.22×10^3 $M^{-1}cm^{-1}$ at 340 nm. The millimolar extinction coefficient for NADH is 6.22 $mM^{-1}cm^{-1}$.

HOW   **Example 6-4**

A kinetic creatine kinase assay was performed manually. The method used the coenzyme NADP as the reaction indicator. The reagent volume used was 2.8 mL, and the sample volume was 60.0 mcL. Absorbance readings were taken every 30 seconds for 2 minutes. The light path of the spectrophotometer was 1 cm, and the delta absorbance for the level 1 QC was 0.019. The molar extinction coefficient for NADH is 6.22×10^3 $M^{-1}cm^{-1}$. What is the concentration in IU/L of the level 1 QC?

To solve this problem, use the formula for determining enzyme activity:

$$\left(\frac{\Delta \text{Absorbance of unknown}}{\epsilon\varepsilon \times d}\right)(10^6)\left(\frac{1}{T}\right)\left(\frac{V_T}{V_S}\right) = \text{IU/L}$$

Substituting into the formula the data from the problem, the following equation is derived:

$$\left(\frac{0.019}{(6.22 \times 10^3 \text{ mol}^{-1} \text{ cm}^{-1})(1 \text{ cm})}\right)(10^6)\left(\frac{1}{0.5 \text{ min}}\right)\left(\frac{2.86 \text{ mL}}{0.060 \text{ mL}}\right)$$
$$= (3.055 \times 10^{-6} \text{ mol}^{-1})(10^6 \text{ μmol/mol})(\times 2)(47.66) = 291 \text{ IU/L}$$

Example 6-4a   An enzyme experiment was performed using NADH as the reaction indicator with a molar extinction coefficient for NADH of 6.22×10^3 $M^{-1}cm^{-1}$. The sample volume was 0.5 mL, and the reagent used was 1.5 mL. The reaction was timed at 30 second intervals for 3 minutes. The delta absorbance was 0.064. What is the IU concentration of the enzyme?

Substituting into the formula the values of this problem yields the following:

$$\left(\frac{0.064}{(6.22 \times 10^3 \text{ mol}^{-1} \text{ cm}^{-1})(1 \text{ cm})}\right)(10^6)\left(\frac{1}{0.5 \text{ min}}\right)\left(\frac{2.00 \text{ mL}}{0.50 \text{ mL}}\right)$$
$$= (1.029 \times 10^{-5} \text{ mol}^{-1})(10^6 \text{ μmol/mol})(\times 2)(4.0) = 82.3 \text{ IU/L}$$

Example 6-4b   Assume that the units for the extinction coefficient were in millimolar units. The problem would be set up as follows:

$$\left(\frac{0.064}{(6.22 \text{ mol}^{-1} \text{ cm}^{-1})(1 \text{ cm})}\right)(10^3)\left(\frac{1}{0.5 \text{ min}}\right)\left(\frac{2.00 \text{ mL}}{0.50 \text{ mL}}\right)$$
$$= (1.029 \times 10^{-2} \text{mol}^{-1})(10^3 \text{ μmol/mol})(\times 2)(4.0) = 82.3 \text{ IU/L}$$

WHAT Remember that when the extinction units are in millimolar units, the conversion of 10^3 is used, not 10^6.

Just as a factor can be used to shorten calculations for assays following Beer's law (see Appendix A), so can a factor be determined for an enzyme calculation. From the previous formula, the only item that is variable is the delta absorbance change of the sample. All other items are established and not variable. By multiplying all items except the delta absorbance value, a factor can be established. Therefore the formula for a factor is:

$$\left(\frac{1}{\varepsilon \times d}\right)(10^6)\left(\frac{1}{T}\right)\left(\frac{V_T}{V_S}\right) = \text{enzyme factor}$$

HOW **_Example 6-5_**

Using the data from Example 6-4, calculate a factor that could be used to determine the activity of creatine kinase in other samples analyzed in the same assay.

Substituting into the formula the data from Example 6-4, the following equation is derived:

$$\left(\frac{1}{(6.22 \times 10^3 \text{ mol}^{-1} \text{ cm}^{-1})(1 \text{ cm})}\right)(10^6)\left(\frac{1}{0.5 \text{ min}}\right)\left(\frac{2.86 \text{ mL}}{0.060 \text{ mL}}\right) = \text{Factor}$$

$$\text{Combining the equation}: \frac{2.86 \times 10^6}{(6.22 \times 10^3)(0.5)(0.06)} = \text{Factor}$$

$$\text{Factor} = 15327$$

The result from Example 6-4 can be determined using the factor method by multiplying the delta absorbance of 0.019 by the factor 15327, which equals 291 IU/L, the same result calculated by using the entire enzyme kinetic equation.

WHAT # BUFFER CALCULATIONS

Buffers are solutions of weak acids or bases and their salts that resist changes in pH. For example, during serum protein electrophoresis procedures, the pH of the solution that conducts the current is maintained by a buffer. Buffers are used in other areas of the clinical laboratory as well, including the molecular diagnostics laboratory. The pH of any solution is determined by its acidity. A simple definition of an acid is that of a substance that will donate a hydrogen ion (or a proton). A base is a substance that will accept the hydrogen ion or donate a hydroxyl ion. This definition is known as the _Bronsted theory_. A Bronsted acid that has donated a hydrogen ion will then become a Bronsted base.

The acid is termed a _conjugate acid_ and the newly formed base is termed the _conjugate base_. Some examples of conjugate acid-conjugate base pairs are the H_2CO_3/HCO_3^- (carbonic acid/bicarbonate) buffer system and the phosphate buffer system H_2PO_4/HPO_4^{-2}. An acid or base is termed _strong_ or _weak_ depending on its tendency to dissociate. Strong acids or bases will completely dissociate when in solution. HCl is a strong acid. When placed in water, it will completely dissociate to H^+ and Cl^- ions. The dissociation constant K_a determines the relative strength of an acid or base. The K_a for a weak acid or base can be calculated by the following equation:

$$K_a = \frac{([H^+][A^-])}{[HA]}$$

where:
$[H^+]$ = hydrogen ion concentration (mol/L)
$[A^-]$ = salt of the acid (mol/L) (also called the conjugate base)
$[HA]$ = undissociated acid (mol/L)

By manipulating the formula, the following formulas are derived:

$$[H^+] = K_a \left(\frac{[HA]}{[A^-]}\right)$$

This can be rearranged further:

$$\log[H^+] = \log K_a + \log\left(\frac{[HA]}{[A^-]}\right)$$

By definition, $pH = -\log[H^+]$ in units of moles/liter; therefore, if both sides of the equation are multiplied by -1, we have:

$$-\log[H^+] = -\log K_a - \log\left(\frac{[HA]}{[A^-]}\right)$$

Substituting pH for $-\log[H^+]$:

$$pH = -\log K_a - \log\left(\frac{[HA]}{[A^-]}\right)$$

By definition, $-\log K_a = pK_a$, therefore substituting pK_a into the equation yields:

$$pH = pK_a - \log\left(\frac{[HA]}{[A^-]}\right)$$

Using the rules of logarithms, the negative sign can be changed to a positive sign if the equation is inverted. Thus:

$$pH = pK_a + \log\left(\frac{[A^-]}{[HA]}\right)$$

This equation is termed the *Henderson-Hasselbalch equation* and it is used to determine arterial or venous pH.

If the ratio of salt to acid is 1, then $pH = pK_a$, and the buffer is at maximal buffering capacity. In an acid solution, raising the pH above the pK_a will increase the dissociation of the acid and increase the amount of $[H^+]$ and lower the pH. In a basic solution, if the pH is below the pK_a, more hydroxyl (OH^-) ions will be released, lowering the pH. The pK_a for acids and bases can be found in the appendixes of many chemistry textbooks.

WHAT   The simplest calculation of pH is that it is the negative logarithm of the hydrogen ion concentration. Sometimes the pH is determined of molar solutions.

HOW   *Example 6-6*

What is the pH of a solution of 0.200 M HCl?

The definition of pH is that it is the negative logarithm of the hydrogen ion concentration. Therefore:

$$pH = -\log [0.200]$$
$$pH = -(-0.699)$$
$$pH = 0.699$$

Example 6-6a   What is the pH of a solution of 0.150 M HCl?

Using the formula for pH, the pH of this solution is 0.824.

Example 6-6b   What is the pH of a solution of 0.018 M HCl?

Using the formula for pH, the pH of this solution is 1.745.

WHAT   Based on the dissociation constant of water, the pH scale ranges from 0 to 14. A pH of 7.0 is neutral. Solutions with a pH below 7.0 are acidic and those with a pH above 7.0 are basic. By definition:

$$pH + pOH = 14$$
$$[H^+][OH^-] = 10^{-14} \text{ M}$$

HOW   *Example 6-7*

What is the pH of a 0.150 M solution of NaOH?

The base NaOH contains 0.150 M hydroxide ions (OH^-) in solution. By definition, $[H^+][OH^-] = 10^{-14}$ M. Therefore:

$$[H^+] = \frac{10^{-14}}{[OH^-]}$$

$$[H^+] = \frac{10^{-14}}{0.150}$$

$$[H^+] = 6.67 \times 10^{-14}$$

$$pH = -\log(6.67 \times 10^{-14})$$

$$pH = 13.176$$

Example 6-7a   What is the pH of a 0.200 M KOH solution?

Using the same pH formula as in Example 6-7, the pH is 13.301.

Example 6-7b   What is the pH of a 0.080 M KOH solution?

Using the same pH formula as in Example 6-7, the pH is 12.903.

Example 6-7c   A technologist prepared a phosphate buffer by adding 5.874 g of KH_2PO_4 and 1.191 g of its salt K_2HPO_4 qs to 1.00 L of water. What is the pH of the phosphate buffer? The pK_a for the buffer is 7.2.

The Henderson-Hasselbalch equation can be used to determine the pH of the buffer solution. In this problem, the KH_2PO_4 is the conjugate acid, and K_2HPO_4 is the conjugate base. Thus:

$$pH = pK_a + \log\left(\frac{[A^-]\,(\text{conjugate base})}{[HA]\,(\text{conjugate acid})}\right)$$

$$pH = 7.2 + \log\left(\frac{[K_2HPO_4]}{[KH_2PO_4]}\right)$$

Next, determine the molarity of each compound based on the quantity of grams of each. The gram molecular weight of K_2HPO_4 is 174.14, and the gram molecular weight of KH_2PO_4 is 136.05. Using the molarity formula, the molarity of each compound can be determined:

$$\text{Molarity of } K_2HPO_4 = \frac{\left(\frac{1.191\text{ g}}{174.14\text{ gmw}}\right)}{1.00\text{ L}}$$

$$\text{Molarity of } K_2HPO_4 = 6.839 \times 10^{-3}$$

$$\text{Molarity of } KH_2PO_4 = \frac{\left(\frac{5.874\text{ g}}{136.05}\right)}{1.00\text{ L}}$$

$$\text{Molarity of } KH_2PO_4 = 4.318 \times 10^{-2}$$

Next, use the Henderson-Hasselbalch equation to solve for pH:

$$pH = 7.2 + \log\left(\frac{[K_2HPO_4]}{[KH_2PO_4]}\right)$$

$$pH = 7.2 + \log\left(\frac{6.839 \times 10^{-3}}{4.318 \times 10^{-2}}\right)$$

Using the rules of logarithms:

$$pH = 7.2 + \left(\log 6.839 \times 10^{-3} - \log 4.318 \times 10^{-2}\right)$$
$$pH = 7.2 + (-2.1650 - (-1.3647))$$
$$pH = 7.2 + (-2.1650 + 1.3647)$$
$$pH = 7.2 + (-0.8003)$$
$$pH = 6.3997$$

WHAT ACID–BASE CALCULATIONS

The pH of the body is strictly controlled by the carbonic acid–bicarbonate buffer system:

$$dCO_2 + H_2O \leftrightarrow \underset{\text{carbonic acid}}{H_2CO_3} \leftrightarrow \underset{\text{bicarbonate}}{HCO_3^-} + H^+$$

The waste product of cell metabolism, CO_2, is carried within the plasma from our tissues to our lungs in several forms. The three most important are as a gas dissolved in the plasma, dCO_2, or as bicarbonate, and the third is in the form of carbaminohemoglobin ($HbCO_2$) within the red blood cells.

This system depends on the actions of the lungs and kidneys to adjust for deviations in pH. The Henderson-Hasselbalch equation can be used to describe the relationship:

$$pH = pK_a + \log\left(\frac{[HCO_3^-]}{[H_2CO_3]}\right)$$

The pK_a for the carbonic acid/bicarbonate buffer system is 6.10 at 37°C. The ratio of bicarbonate to carbonic acid is 20:1. The pH of the blood is directly affected by the concentration of bicarbonate, but inversely affected by the concentration of carbonic acid. The pH of the blood can be measured; however, carbonic acid and bicarbonate cannot be directly measured. In equilibrium, there is a tendency for carbonic acid to dehydrate and form water and dissolved CO_2. By definition of Henry's law, the amount of a soluble dissolved gas is proportional to the partial pressure of the gas. With blood gas instruments, the partial pressure of CO_2 can be measured (pCO_2). The relationship between dCO_2 and pCO_2 can be mathematically stated as follows:

$$dCO_2 = \alpha\, pCO_2$$

The term α is the solubility coefficient of pCO_2 and has a value of 0.0306 mmol/L/mm Hg (millimoles per liter per millimeter of mercury). Because carbonic acid forms dCO_2 under equilibrium conditions, the term dCO_2 can be substituted into the Henderson-Hasselbalch equation:

$$pH = pK_a + \log\frac{[HCO_3^-]}{[dCO_2]}$$

As dCO_2 is equal to $\alpha\, pCO_2$, the equation can further be changed to the following:

$$pH = pK_a + \log\left(\frac{[HCO_3^-]}{[\alpha\, pCO_2]}\right)$$

Because pH and pCO_2 can be measured, the concentration of bicarbonate can be calculated.

HOW   *Example 6-8*

Given a pCO_2 of 40.0 mm Hg and a pH of 7.45, calculate the bicarbonate concentration. The $pK_a = 6.10$.

To solve this problem, use the derived Henderson-Hasselbalch formula:

$$pH = pK_a + \log\left(\frac{[HCO_3^-]}{\alpha\, pCO_2}\right)$$

Substituting into the equation the data from the problem, the following equation is derived:

$$7.45 = 6.10 + \log\left(\frac{[HCO_3^-]}{(0.0306 \text{ mmol/L/mm Hg})(40.0 \text{ mm Hg})}\right)$$

$$\log\left(\frac{[HCO_3^-]}{(0.0306 \text{ mmol/L/mm Hg})(40.0 \text{ mm Hg})}\right) = 7.45 - 6.10$$

$$\left(\frac{[HCO_3^-]}{(0.0306 \text{ mmol/L/mm Hg})(40.0 \text{ mm Hg})}\right) = \text{antilog}(7.45 - 6.10)$$

$$[HCO_3^-] = [(0.0306 \text{ mmol/L/mm Hg})(40.0 \text{ mm Hg})][\text{antilog}(7.45 - 6.10)]$$

$$[HCO_3^-] = (1.224 \text{ mmol/L})(\text{antilog } 1.35)$$

$$[HCO_3^-] = (1.224 \text{ mmol/L})(22.39)$$

$$[HCO_3^-] = 27.4 \text{ mmol/L}$$

Example 6-8a   Given a whole blood sample with a pCO_2 of 32 mm Hg and a bicarbonate of 24 mmol/L, calculate the pH. The $pK_a = 6.10$.

$$pH = 6.10 + \log\frac{24 \text{ mmol/L}}{(0.0306 \text{ mmol/L/mm Hg})(32 \text{ mm Hg})}$$

$$pH = 6.10 + 1.39$$

$$pH = 7.49$$

To determine the total CO_2 concentration in the blood, the following formula is used:

$$tCO_2 = dCO_2 + [HCO_3^-] + [H_2CO_3]$$

The actual concentration of H_2CO_3 is quite small, and the term is usually ignored. In addition, dCO_2 can be written in terms of αpCO_2. Therefore the equation becomes:

$$tCO_2 = \alpha pCO_2 + [HCO_3^-]$$

Example 6-8b   Given a pH of 7.42, a bicarbonate of 22 mmol/L, and a pCO_2 of 35 mm Hg, calculate the total CO_2.

Use the Henderson Hasselbalch and substitute into it the values given to solve this problem:

$$tCO_2 = (0.0306 \text{ mmol/L/mm Hg})(35 \text{ mm Hg}) + [22]$$

$$tCO_2 = 23.1 \text{ mmol/L}$$

The calculations for pH, bicarbonate, and total carbon dioxide are rarely performed manually today in most clinical chemistry laboratories. Instead, these calculations are performed by the blood gas analyzers. It is important, though, that clinical laboratory professionals still know how these results are actually obtained and could manually calculate them if they needed to.

WHAT ACID–BASE DISORDERS

The pH of the blood is normally between 7.35 and 7.45. When the pH is below 7.35, the condition is termed *acidosis*. When the pH of the blood is above 7.45, the condition is termed *alkalosis*. By reviewing the Henderson-Hasselbalch equation, changes in the acid–base status and their effect on pH can be visualized.

$$\text{Remember: pH} = pK_a + \log\left(\frac{[HCO_3^-]}{[H_2CO_3]}\right)$$

Another way of visualizing the relationship between bicarbonate and carbonic acid is as follows:

$$pH = pK_a + \log\frac{\text{kidney}}{\text{lung}}$$

Another way of looking at it is the ratio of base/acid because bicarbonate is a base and CO_2 is an acid. The lungs are responsible for removing CO_2 and therefore control the level of CO_2 in the blood, whereas the kidneys can control the level of bicarbonate. The lungs can react immediately while it can take the kidneys up to 3 days to adjust, or compensate. The reference interval for pCO_2 is usually 35 to 45 mm Hg for adults, and the reference interval for bicarbonate is 22 to 29 mmol/L[1]. This is normally a 20:1 ratio of bicarbonate to carbonic acid. There are four conditions that can occur that will affect the pH of the blood.

WHAT Respiratory Acidosis

As the name implies, the pH of the blood is acidotic (i.e., below 7.35). The first term, *respiratory*, refers to the major cause of the acidosis. If the lungs cannot adequately remove CO_2, the CO_2 will build up in the blood and pCO_2 levels will increase. This will result in a lowering of the pH because there is a reciprocal relationship between CO_2 concentration and pH. Therefore, if the CO_2 level goes down (e.g., hyperventilation), the pH goes up; if the CO_2 level rises (e.g., hypoventilation as seen in asthma and COPD), the pH goes down. In an effort to retain the 20:1 ratio, the kidneys will try to compensate by retaining bicarbonate in an effort to neutralize the acidic condition. The respiration rate of the lungs will increase in an effort to remove CO_2.

The effects of the action of the lungs are much faster than that of the kidneys. It may take days for the kidneys to fully compensate a respiratory acidosis.

WHAT Respiratory Alkalosis

In this condition, the CO_2 levels are decreased, resulting in a rise in pH. Compensation is either by decreasing the respiration rate or by the kidneys retaining H^+.

WHAT Metabolic Acidosis

In this condition, the primary cause is metabolic. Many conditions can lead to the increase of acids (including carbonic acid) in the blood. The most common condition is seen in diabetic ketoacidosis in which ketoacids build up in the blood. The body compensates by increasing the respiration rate to remove CO_2 and therefore raise the pH. The kidneys respond by increasing acid excretion and bicarbonate retention.

WHAT **Metabolic Alkalosis**

This condition is caused primarily by an excess of bicarbonate. The excess may be due to insufficient excretion of bicarbonate by the kidney or increased ingestion of bicarbonate such as antacids. Severe vomiting will lead to the loss of hydrogen ions and a buildup of bicarbonate. The lungs will compensate by slowing respiration to retain CO_2, and the kidneys may compensate by excreting more bicarbonate.

Determining Acid–Base Status and Compensation Status

To determine the acid–base status, first look at the pH. If it is above 7.45, the patient is *alkalotic*; if it is below 7.35, the patient is *acidotic*. Next, look at the bicarbonate values. Does it fit the pH? You know that bicarbonate values move in the same direction as the pH (i.e., when the bicarbonate goes up, the pH goes up). So, if the pH was alkalotic, is the bicarbonate elevated above normal? If the pH is acidotic, is the bicarbonate below normal? Next, look at the pCO_2 values. Are they what you would expect to find given the pH that you have? For example, if the pH is alkalotic, is the pCO_2 decreased? Or if the pH is acidotic, is the pCO_2 increased?

When there is a problem metabolically and the pH is affected, the lungs react immediately to bring the pH back into the normal range. The kidneys take longer to get the pH back into the normal range. This is called *compensation*. A good rule of thumb is to remember that *the body never overcompensates!* The body has compensated when the pH is back in the normal range. The bicarbonate and pCO_2 levels could be very abnormal, but as long as the pH is in the normal range again, the body has compensated. To determine what caused the initial problem and what had to compensate, a good rule of thumb to remember is that the analyte that has moved in the anticipated direction of the pH is the culprit, whereas the analyte that has moved opposite of what you would expect to see of the pH is the compensator.

Let's look at some simplified acid–base situations to better understand the concept.

HOW **Example 6-9**

A patient arrives in the emergency room (ER) having an asthma attack and is experiencing trouble exhaling. Blood gas results reveal a pCO_2 of 28 mm Hg, a bicarbonate of 24 mmol/L, and a pH of 7.55. What is this patient's acid–base status? Has the patient compensated for their acid–base status?

Since the pH is 7.55, the patient is alkalotic and has not yet brought the pH into the normal range. The pCO_2 is abnormally low, but the bicarbonate is normal. Based on the patient's asthma condition that makes it difficult to exhale, this patient has uncompensated respiratory alkalosis.

Example 6-9a   A patient with diabetes presents to the doctor's office with a glucose meter reading of HI, which means that it is over the linear range of the meter (600 mg/dL). The patient is admitted to the hospital. The admission results reveal a plasma glucose of 780 mg/dL, a pH of 7.26, a bicarbonate of 11 mmol/L, and a pCO_2 of 25 mm Hg. What is this patient's acid–base status, and is it fully compensated, uncompensated, or partially compensated?

Since the pH is 7.26, the pH is not fully compensated. The bicarbonate is very low, which fits with the pH in the acidic range. However, the pCO_2 is also low. You would expect that if the pCO_2 is low that the pH would be high; in this case the pCO_2 is trying to compensate for the metabolic problem of ketoacidosis. Therefore this is a case of partially compensated metabolic acidosis.

Example 6-9b   A patient's blood gas results are pH 7.50, pCO_2 57 mm Hg, and HCO_3^- 40 mmol/L. What is this patient's blood gas status, and is it fully compensated, uncompensated, or partially compensated?

The patient is alkalotic, and because the pH is not in the reference range, the blood gas status is not fully compensated. Both the pCO_2 and the HCO_3^- are elevated. Because the pH will decrease as the pCO_2 rises, the pCO_2 is partially compensating for the metabolic alkalosis demonstrated by the increased bicarbonate.

Example 6-9c   A patient's blood gas results are pH 7.25, pCO_2 57 mm Hg, and HCO_3^- 40 mmol/L. What is this patient's blood gas status, and is it fully compensated, uncompensated, or partially compensated?

This patient is acidotic because the pH is below 7.35. You might notice that the pCO_2 and HCO_3^- are the same values as in Example 6-9b. However, this patient has partially compensated respiratory acidosis based on the increased bicarbonate that is trying to neutralize the increased pCO_2. Remember, the value of pCO_2 or HCO_3^- that moves opposite of what you would expect to see of the pH is the compensator analyte.

WHAT **ANION GAP**

Just as the body strives to maintain a 20:1 balance between bicarbonate and carbonic acid, the body tries to maintain electrolyte neutrality. The concentration of anions should equal the concentration of cations in the body. The measurement of this balance is by the anion gap. The anion gap does not measure all anions or cations in the body, merely those of the highest concentration to significantly alter the balance. The cation found in highest concentration in the blood is sodium. Chloride is the most abundant anion in the blood. In addition, bicarbonate also is an anion and is included in the anion gap. Some laboratories include potassium in the anion gap. However, the concentration of potassium is relatively low compared with the other electrolytes. The anion gap is calculated as follows:

$$[Na^+] - ([Cl^-] + [HCO_3^-])$$

OR

$$([Na^+] + [K^+]) - ([Cl^-] + [HCO_3^-])$$

The reference range for the anion gap calculated without potassium is 8 to 16 mmol/L, whereas the reference range for the anion gap calculated with potassium is 10 to 20 mmol/L[1]. The anion gap is useful to detect changes in the concentration of the unmeasured anions and cations. For example, when the anion gap is elevated, the elevation is due to the presence of other anions, such as proteins, or, most commonly, acids such as ketoacids. A decreased anion gap may be seen when there is an increase in unmeasured cations, such as magnesium or calcium. In addition, the anion gap may be used as a quality assurance measurement to ensure the reliability of the electrodes that determine electrolyte concentration.

Example 6-10

A 58-year-old insulin-dependent woman with diabetes is admitted to the ER in a comatose state. Her electrolyte profile is as follows:

	REFERENCE RANGES
Sodium = 140 mmol/L	Sodium = 136–145 mmol/L
Potassium = 3.5 mmol/L	Potassium = 3.5–5.1 mmol/L
Chloride = 105 mmol/L	Chloride = 98–107 mmol/L
Bicarbonate = 17 mmol/L	Bicarbonate = 19–24 mmol/L

Calculate the anion gap using both formulas.

$$Anion\ gap = 140 - (105 + 17)$$
$$Anion\ gap = 140 - 122$$
$$Anion\ gap = 18\ mmol/L\ (reference\ range: 8 - 16\ mmol/L)$$
$$Anion\ gap = (140 + 3.5) - (105 + 17)$$
$$Anion\ gap = 143.5 - 122$$
$$Anion\ gap = 22\ mmol/L\ (reference\ range: 10 - 20\ mmol/L)$$

Example 6-10a Calculate the anion gap given the following values: Na = 143 mmol/L, K = 4.3 mmol/L, Cl = 108 mmol/L, bicarbonate = 27 mmol/L.

The anion gap using potassium in the calculation is 12 mmol/L. The anion gap without potassium is 8 mmol/L.

Example 6-10b Calculate the anion gap given the following values: Na = 141 mmol/L, K = 3.8 mmol/L, Cl = 110 mmol/L, bicarbonate = 30 mmol/L.

The anion gap with potassium in the equation is 5 mmol/L; without potassium it is 1 mmol/L.

WHAT **CALCULATED OSMOLALITY AND OSMOLALITY GAP**

Calculated Osmolality

The osmolality of a solution is based on the number of dissolved particles in a solution, not on the size, weight, or ionic activity of the particles. A 1 molal solution of glucose is also a 1 osmolal solution because glucose does not dissociate, whereas a 1 molal solution of sodium chloride is equal to a 2 osmolal solution because the sodium chloride dissociates into both sodium particles and chloride particles. Osmolality measures the total concentration of all ions and molecules present in serum or urine. Sodium, glucose, and urea are major contributors to the total osmolality of serum. Because the major contributors to serum osmolality are tightly regulated, the osmolality of serum can be calculated.

$$\text{Calculated osmolality (mOsmol / kg } H_2O) = 1.86[Na^+] + \frac{[\text{glucose}]}{18} + \frac{[BUN]}{2.8}$$

The number 1.86 is used because each sodium ion is balanced by an anion, but there is not a perfect dissociation; 18 is used because the molecular weight of glucose is approximately 180, and the factor of 18 converts milligrams per deciliter to millimoles per liter. The molecular weight of blood urea nitrogen (BUN) is approximately 28; thus 2.8 is used. This formula cannot be used for calculating urine osmolality because the concentration of particles varies too greatly depending on the state of hydration.

HOW
Example 6-11

A 78-year-old man was admitted to the ER suffering from heat stroke. The laboratory results were as follows:

Sodium = 160 mEq/L
Potassium = 5.5 mEq/L
Glucose = 110 mg/dL
BUN = 16 mg/dL

What is the patient's serum osmolality?
To calculate the serum osmolality, use the following formula and substitute into it the data from the problem:

$$\text{Calculated osmolality (mOsmol/kg } H_2O) = 1.86 [Na^+] + \frac{[\text{glucose}]}{18} + \frac{[BUN]}{2.8}$$

$$\text{Calculated osmolality (mOsmol/kg } H_2O) = (1.86)(160) + \frac{110}{18} + \frac{16}{2.8}$$

$$\text{Calculated osmolality} = 298 + 6.1 + 5.7$$

$$\text{Calculated serum osmolality} = 310 \text{ mOsmol/kg } H_2O$$

$$\text{(reference range for patients} > 60 = 280 - 301 \text{ mOsm/kg)}$$

The calculated serum osmolality is elevated above the reference range and reflects the patient's dehydration status.

Example 6-11a   Calculate the serum osmolality given the following values: Na = 145 mmol/L, glucose = 155 mg/dL, BUN = 30 mg/dL.

Using the osmolality formula, the serum osmolality is 289 mOsmol/kg H_2O.

Example 6-11b   Calculate the serum osmolality given the following values: Na = 155 mmol/L, glucose = 550 mg/dL, BUN = 80 mg/dL.

Using the osmolality formula, the serum osmolality is 347 mOsmol/kg H_2O.

WHAT   **Osmolal Gap**

This is the difference between the calculated osmolality and the measured osmolality. The average osmolal gap is 0 to 10 mOsm/kg H_2O. When the gap is elevated, it is usually due to other particles besides sodium, glucose, or BUN. The presence of ketones or alcohols such as ethanol in the serum can elevate the osmolal gap. The osmolal gap may also be useful as a quality assurance measurement to detect technical errors.

HOW   ***Example 6-12***

A 54-year-old woman was found unconscious and was admitted to the hospital. Her laboratory results were as follows:

Sodium = 145 mEq/L
Potassium = 4.5 mEq/L
Glucose = 95 mg/dL
BUN = 12 mg/dL
Serum osmolality = 320 mOsm/kg
Serum EtOH = 185 mg/dL

What is the patient's osmolal gap?
To calculate the osmolal gap, first calculate the osmolality:

$$\text{Calculated osmolality (mOsmol/kg } H_2O) = 1.86[Na^+] + \frac{[\text{glucose}]}{18} + \frac{[\text{BUN}]}{2.8}$$

$$\text{Calculated osmolality (mOsmol/kg } H_2O) = (1.86)(145) + \frac{95}{18} + \frac{12}{2.8}$$

$$\text{Calculated osmolality} = 270 + 5.3 + 4.3$$

$$\text{Calculated osmolality} = 280 \text{ mOsm/kg}$$

$$\text{Osmolal gap} = \text{Difference between calculated and measured osmolality}$$

$$\text{Osmolal gap} = 320 \text{ mOsm/kg} - 280 \text{ mOsm/kg}$$

$$= 40 \text{ mOsm/kg}$$

The osmolal gap, 40 mOsm/kg, is indicative of the presence of other dissolved particles in the serum. The elevated ethanol concentration most likely is the cause of the increased osmolal gap.

HOW   **LIPID CALCULATIONS**

Coronary artery disease (CAD) is one of the leading causes of death today. Consequently, patients and their physicians have interest in laboratory tests that can detect risk factors for developing CAD. The measurements of total cholesterol, high-density lipoprotein (HDL) cholesterol, low-density lipoprotein (LDL) cholesterol, and triglycerides are commonly performed to determine such risk. At present there are only a few methods that measure LDL directly. Instead, the LDL cholesterol is calculated. The Friedewald formula for determining LDL cholesterol is as follows:

$$\text{LDL cholesterol} = \text{Total cholesterol} - \left[HDL + \left(\frac{\text{Triglycerides}}{5} \right) \right]$$

The fraction, triglycerides/5, is an estimation of very-low-density lipoprotein (VLDL) cholesterol. This formula is not accurate if the triglyceride concentration is greater than 400 mg/dL and assumes no other source of triglycerides such as chylomicrons. Because chylomicrons are the major transporter of dietary fat and are so rich in (exogenous) triglycerides, patients must be fasting to eliminate the presence of chylomicrons.

HOW

Example 6-13

A 43-year-old man with a family history of coronary artery disease (CAD) has the following lipid profile analysis performed. Calculate the patient's LDL cholesterol result.

Total cholesterol = 280 mg/dL
Triglycerides = 150 mg/dL
HDL cholesterol = 50 mg/dL

To calculate the quantity of LDL cholesterol, use the formula given previously:

$$\text{LDL cholesterol} = \text{Total cholesterol} - \left[\text{HDL} + \left(\frac{\text{Triglycerides}}{5}\right)\right]$$

$$= 280 \text{ mg/dL} - (50 \text{ mg/dL} + [150 \text{ mg/dL} \div 5])$$

$$= 280 \text{ mg/dL} - (50 \text{ mg/dL} + 30 \text{ mg/dL})$$

$$= 280 \text{ mg/dL} - 80 \text{ mg/dL}$$

$$= 200 \text{ mg/dL}$$

The National Cholesterol Education Program has established the acceptable ranges for triglycerides and cholesterol to reduce the incidence of CAD. Total cholesterol values below 200 mg/dL are desirable; those between 200 and 240 mg/dL are considered to be borderline high risk; cholesterol values above 240 mg/dL place the patient in the high-risk group for developing CAD. In addition, a LDL cholesterol of less than 130 mg/dL is desirable; those between 130 and 150 mg/dL are considered to be borderline high risk, and patients with LDL cholesterol values above 150 mg/dL are considered to be in the high-risk group for developing CAD. This patient has both elevated total cholesterol and LDL cholesterol, which places him in the high-risk group for developing CAD.

Example 6-13a

Given a total cholesterol value of 250 mg/dL, a triglyceride value of 350 mg/dL, and an HDL cholesterol of 40 mg/dL, calculate the patient's LDL cholesterol.

$$\text{LDL cholesterol} = \text{Total cholesterol} - \left[\text{HDL} + \left(\frac{\text{Triglycerides}}{5}\right)\right]$$

$$= 250 \text{ mg/dL} - (40 \text{ mg/dL} + 350 \text{ mg/dL} \div 5)$$

$$= 250 \text{ mg/dL} - (40 \text{ mg/dL} + 70 \text{ mg/dL})$$

$$= 250 \text{ mg/dL} - 110 \text{ mg/dL}$$

$$= 140 \text{ mg/dL}$$

The LDL cholesterol is 140 mg/dL.

Example 6-13b   Given a total cholesterol of 400 mg/dL, a triglyceride value of 380 mg/dL, and an HDL cholesterol of 50, calculate the patient's LDL cholesterol.

Using the LDL cholesterol formula, the patient's LDL cholesterol is 274 mg/dL.

WHAT   ## ADDITIONAL CLINICAL CHEMISTRY CALCULATIONS

There are a few additional calculations that are performed in the clinical chemistry laboratory, but they are usually computer generated. However, it is good laboratory practice to be able to check the accuracy of these calculations.

WHAT   ### Serum Protein Electrophoresis Calculations

When a serum protein electrophoresis is performed, an electrophoretogram is produced where the protein fractions that were separated by the electrophoresis are quantitated. Figure 6-11 shows a normal electrophoretogram with the separated protein fractions. There are five major protein classes that are separated in a serum protein electrophoresis: albumin, alpha-1, alpha-2, beta, and gamma. A total protein is always performed, so after the percentage of each fraction has been determined, the concentration of each individual fraction can be determined by densitometry.

HOW   ***Example 6-14***

A serum protein electrophoresis was performed by a medical laboratory scientist student. The area of each protein fraction was determined; based on the total protein value and the individual percentages of each separated protein, the quantity in grams per deciliter of each separated protein can be determined.

	%	G/DL
Albumin	61.8	____
Alpha-1	3.8	____
Alpha-2	9.4	____
Beta	15.2	____
Gamma	9.8	____
	Total Protein	7.1 g/dL

To determine the g/dL of each fraction, first divide each fraction by 100 because the result is in a percentage, and then multiply each fraction by 7.1.

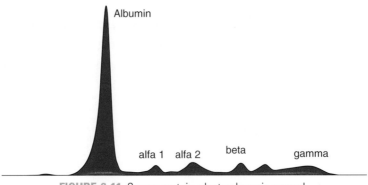

FIGURE 6-11 Serum protein electrophoresis normal.

$$\text{Example: Albumin} = 61.8/100 = 0.618 \times 7.1 = 4.39 \text{ g/dL}$$

Continue with each fraction to determine its concentration. The answers can be found at the end of the chapter.

> **NOTE:** The total of all five fractions should be 7.1 g/dL.

WHAT Calculation of A/G Ratio

The A/G ratio is a ratio of albumin to globulins and is useful when a patient might have liver or kidney disease. The normal ratio is 0.8 to 2.0. Albumin makes up 50% to 60% of the total protein and can be decreased because of diet or disease. The globulins are our immune proteins and can be elevated in infections or other diseases. Globulins are calculated by subtracting the albumin value from the total protein value. To calculate the A/G ratio, simply divide the albumin value by the obtained globulin value.

HOW Example 6-15

A patient's total protein was 7.4 g/dL. The albumin value was 4.5 g/dL. Calculate the A/G ratio.

$$\text{A/G Ratio} = (4.5)/(7.4 - 4.5)$$
$$\text{A/G Ratio} = 4.5/2.9$$
$$\text{A/G Ratio} = 1.6$$

WHAT Calculation of % CK-MB/CK Index

Although % CK-MB and total CK are no longer the gold standard for evaluating a patient's status concerning whether they are experiencing a myocardial infarction, both tests are still ordered. CK-MB is an isoenzyme of creatine kinase and is found in the heart and skeletal muscle, as well in other organs. Normal % CK-MB values are very low but may rise when the cardiac muscle is damaged, as occurs in a myocardial infarction. An index value greater than 3 may indicate cardiac muscle damage. To calculate the index, divide the CK-MB value by the total CK value and multiply by 100.

HOW Example 6-16

A patient is admitted into the emergency department with chest pains. Total CK is 250 IU/L and CK-MB is 5 IU/L. What is the CK-MB index?

$$\text{CK} - \text{MB Index} = (5/250) \times 100$$
$$\text{CK} - \text{MB Index} = 2\%$$

WHAT Calculation of Indirect Bilirubin

Indirect bilirubin is bilirubin that is unconjugated and not water soluble. To calculate, subtract the direct bilirubin measurement from the total bilirubin (which contains both direct and indirect) measurement.

HOW **Example 6-17**

A hepatitis C patient's total bilirubin was 20.5 mg/dL and the direct bilirubin was 4.7 mg/dL. Calculate the indirect bilirubin value.

Indirect bilirubin = Total bilirubin 20.5 mg/dL − Direct bilirubin 4.7 mg/dL = 15.8 mg/dL.

HOW **EXAMPLE PROBLEMS**

This section is designed to be useful to both the student and the laboratory professional. Students can use the additional problems to master the material. The laboratory professional can use the examples as templates for solving laboratory calculations. By finding an example similar to the problem that you need to solve, substitute the numbers appropriate to your calculation into the equation.

1. **Q.** A 35% T reading was obtained for a solution of albumin. What is the absorbance value?
   A. To solve the problem, use the following formula:
   Absorbance = 2.00 − log % transmittance
   Substituting into the equation the data from the problem yields the following:

$$\text{Absorbance} = 2.00 - \log 35$$
$$\text{Absorbance} = 2.00 - 1.544$$
$$\text{Absorbance} = 0.456$$

2. **Q.** A 67% T reading was obtained for a solution of a compound. What is the absorbance value?
   A. Using the formula, A = 2.00 − log % T, and substituting it into the data from the problem yields the following:

$$A = 2.00 - \log 67$$
$$A = 2.00 - 1.826$$
$$A = 0.174$$

3. **Q.** Given a 45% T reading, what is the absorbance?
   A. The absorbance is 0.347.

4. **Q.** What is a 0.41 transmittance ratio in terms of absorbance?
   A. First convert transmittance to % transmittance:
   transmittance × 100 = % transmittance
   0.41 transmittance × 100 = 41% transmittance
   Next, use the same formula in problems 1 and 2 to determine the absorbance value:

$$A = 2.00 - \log 41$$
$$A = 2.00 - 1.613$$
$$A = 0.387$$

5. **Q.** Given a 0.82 transmittance ratio, what is its absorbance?
   A. The absorbance is 0.086.

6. **Q.** What will the absorbance value of 0.385 be in terms of % T?

   A. Using the absorbance formula, and substituting it into the data from the problem yields the following:

   $0.385 = 2.00 - \log \% \text{ T}$

   Solving the equation:

   $$0.385 - 2.00 = -\log \% \text{ T}$$
   $$-1.615 = -\log \% \text{ T}$$

   The negative signs from both sides of the equation can be removed, and the antilog of 1.615 can be determined.

   Antilog of $1.615 = 41.2\%$ T

   Therefore the absorbance value of 0.385 is equal to a 41.2% T value.

7. **Q.** What is the % T value for a sample with an absorbance value of 1.490?

   A. Using the absorbance formula, substitute into it the data from the problem:

   $$1.490 = 2.00 - \log \% \text{ T}$$
   $$-0.51 = -\log \% \text{ T}$$
   $$0.51 = \log \% \text{ T}$$
   $$\text{antilog } 0.51 = 3.24$$
   $$1.490 \text{ Absorbance} = 3.24\% \text{ T}$$

8. **Q.** Given an absorbance value of 0.648, what is the % T value?

   A. The % T value is 22.5% T.

9. **Q.** Given that the molar absorptivity of NADH is 6.22×10^3 M^{-1} cm^{-1} at 340 nm, if an assay of an analyte using NADH as an indicator was performed using a 1 cm light path and a measured absorbance of NADH of 0.560, what would be the concentration of the NADH?

   A. Beer's law states that $A = abc$, where "A" is equal to the absorbance of the compound measured, "a" is equal to the absorptivity coefficient of the compound, "b" is the pathlength in centimeters, and "c" equals the concentration of the compound. Given three of the four parameters, the fourth can be calculated. In this example, the formula is as follows:

   $$0.560 = \left(6.22 \times 10^3 \text{ } M^{-1} \text{ } cm^{-1}\right)(1 \text{ cm})(X)$$

   $$0.560 = \left(6.22 \times 10^3 \text{ } M^{-1}\right)(X)$$

   $$\frac{0.560}{6.22 \times 10^3 \text{ } M^{-1}} = X$$

   $$9.00 \times 10^{-5} \text{ M} = X$$

   Therefore the concentration of the compound is 9.00×10^{-5} M.

10. **Q.** The molar absorptivity of a compound is 11,000 M^{-1} cm^{-1}. What is the absorbance of this compound, which has a concentration of 2.00×10^{-6} M and is in a cuvette with a 1 cm pathlength?

    A. Using the Beer's law formula and substituting into it the values from the problem yields the following:

    $$\text{Absorbance} = \left(11,000 \text{ } M^{-1} \text{ } cm^{-1}\right)(1 \text{ cm})\left(2.00 \times 10^{-6} \text{ M}\right)$$
    $$\text{Absorbance} = 0.0220$$

11. **Q.** A kinetic enzyme assay was performed using NADH as the reaction indicator. The molar absorptivity of NADH is 6.22×10^3 M^{-1} cm^{-1}. Absorbance readings were taken every 30 seconds with a ΔAbs./min of 0.052. The sample volume was 50.0 mcL and the reagent volume was 1.5 mL. The lightpath was 1.0 cm. What is the activity of the enzyme?

   A. The activity of enzymes may be calculated by the following formula:

$$\left(\frac{\Delta Abs.\ of\ unk}{\varepsilon \times d}\right)(10^6)\left(\frac{1}{T}\right)\left(\frac{V_T}{V_S}\right) = IU/L$$

where:

ΔAbs. of unk = ΔAbs. per minute of unknown

ε = molar absorptivity constant for product in units of M^{-1} cm^{-1}

d = pathlength (usually 1 cm)

10^6 = conversion factor to convert mol/L to μmol/L

T = time in minutes

V_T = total volume (reagents + sample)

V_S = sample volume

NOTE: If the extinction coefficient is in units of mM^{-1} cm^{-1}, then the conversion factor will be 10^3, not 10^6.

Substituting into the formula the data from the problem yields the following:

$$\left(\frac{\Delta 0.052\ Abs./min}{(6.22 \times 10^3\ M^{-1}\ cm^{-1})(1\ cm)}\right)(10^6)\left(\frac{1}{1\ min}\right)\left(\frac{1.55\ mL}{0.050\ mL}\right)$$

$$= (8.36 \times 10^{-6}\ mol^{-1})(10^6\ \mu mol / mol)(31) = 259\ IU / L$$

12. **Q.** A manual enzyme assay was performed to determine the activity of alanine aminotransferase in five samples. NADH, with a millimolar absorptivity of 6.22 mM^{-1} cm^{-1}, was used as the assay indicator. The sample volume was 300.0 mcL, and the reagent volume was 3.0 mL. The pathlength of the spectrophotometer is 1 cm. What is the factor that, given the delta absorbance values of each sample, can be used to quickly calculate the activity of AST in each sample?

   A. When performing calculations to determine the activity of a number of samples, a factor can be calculated from the fixed items in the enzyme calculation formula. Once the factor has been established, the activity of each sample is obtained by multiplying the delta absorbance of each sample by the factor. The calculation of a factor eliminates tedious calculations and may reduce mathematical errors. The formula to calculate a factor for enzyme analysis is as follows:

$$\left(\frac{1}{\varepsilon \times d}\right)(10^3)\left(\frac{1}{T}\right)\left(\frac{V_T}{V_S}\right) = factor$$

Substituting into the equation the data from the problem yields the following:

$$\left(\frac{1}{(6.22 \text{ mM}^{-1} \text{ cm}^{-1})(1 \text{ cm})}\right)(10^3)\left(\frac{1}{1 \text{ min}}\right)\left(\frac{3.30 \text{ mL}}{0.300 \text{ mL}}\right)$$

Solving the equation:

$$\left(\frac{1}{(6.22 \text{ mM}^{-1} \text{ cm}^{-1})(1 \text{ cm})}\right)(10^3)\left(\frac{1}{1 \text{ min}}\right)(11) = \left(\frac{11000}{6.22 \text{ mM}^{-1} \text{ cm}^{-1}(1 \text{ cm})}\right) = 1768$$

The factor is 1768. Notice that 10^3 was used in the calculation instead of 10^6. This is because the millimolar absorptivity, not the molar absorptivity, of NADH was used.

13. **Q.** Using the factor calculated in example problem 12, and given the delta absorbance values for five samples analyzed for AST activity, what is the activity of AST in each sample?

SAMPLE	ΔABS./MIN
1	0.015
2	0.037
3	0.011
4	0.093
5	0.020

   A. The factor for this assay was calculated to be 1768. By multiplying the delta absorbance of each sample by the factor, the AST activity of each sample can be determined:

$$\text{Sample } 1 = 0.015 \times 1768 = 26 \text{ IU/L}$$
$$\text{Sample } 2 = 0.037 \times 1768 = 65 \text{ IU/L}$$
$$\text{Sample } 3 = 0.011 \times 1768 = 19 \text{ IU/L}$$
$$\text{Sample } 4 = 0.093 \times 1768 = 164 \text{ IU/L}$$
$$\text{Sample } 5 = 0.020 \times 1768 = 35 \text{ IU/L}$$

14. **Q.** What is the pH of a 0.150 M solution of HCl?
    A. By definition, pH is the negative log of the hydrogen ion concentration (i.e., $pH = -\log[H^+]$). Hydrochloric acid is a strong acid that, in solution, will completely dissociate into hydrogen and chloride ions. Therefore the pH of the 0.150 M solution of HCl will be as follows:

$$pH = -\log[0.150]$$
$$pH = 0.824$$

15. **Q.** What is the pH of a 0.250 M solution of NaOH?
    A. By definition: $pH + pOH = 14$ and $[H^+] + [OH^-] = 10^{-14}$ M. Therefore the equation for this problem is as follows:

$$[H^+] = \frac{10^{-14} \text{ M}}{OH^-}$$

Substituting into the equation the data from the problem yields:

$$[H^+] = \frac{10^{-14} \text{ M}}{0.250 \text{ M}}$$

$$[H^+] = 4 \times 10^{-14}$$

$$pH = -\log[H^+]$$

$$pH = -\log 4 \times 10^{-14}$$

$$pH = 13.4$$

16. **Q.** What is the pH of a 1 L solution of sodium acetate buffer prepared by combining 0.25 M of acetic acid with 0.45 M of sodium acetate? The pK_a of acetic acid is 4.77.

    A. The Henderson-Hasselbalch equation can be used to solve this problem.

    $$pH = pK_a + \log\left(\frac{[A^-](\text{conjugate base})}{[HA^-](\text{conjugate acid})}\right)$$

    $$pH = 4.77 + \log\left(\frac{0.45 \text{ M}}{0.25 \text{ M}}\right)$$

    $$pH = 4.77 + 0.255$$

    $$pH = 5.02$$

17. **Q.** What is the pH of a patient with a bicarbonate of 20 mmol/L and a pCO_2 of 38 mm Hg?

    A. The Henderson-Hasselbalch formula is used to determine the pH of whole blood samples. The formula is as follows:

    $$pH = pK_a + \log\left(\frac{[HCO_3^-]}{[H_2CO_3]}\right)$$

    The pK_a for the carbonic acid/bicarbonate buffer system is 6.1 at 37°C. In the body, the majority of the carbonic acid is in the form of dissolved CO_2 gas (dCO_2). Blood gas instruments can measure the partial pressure of CO_2 in whole blood. Mathematically, the partial pressure of carbon dioxide and the quantity of dissolved carbon dioxide gas in the blood can be related by the following formula:

    $$dCO_2 = \alpha pCO_2$$

    Where α is the solubility coefficient of pCO_2 and has a value of 0.0306 mmol/L/mm Hg. By combining the knowledge that most of the carbonic acid is in the form of dissolved carbon dioxide gas, and the relationship between dissolved carbon dioxide gas and the partial pressure of carbon dioxide, the following formula can be produced:

    $$pH = pK_a + \log\left(\frac{[HCO_3^-]}{[\alpha \, pCO_2]}\right)$$

Substituting into the equation the data from the problem yields the following equation:

$$pH = 6.1 + \log\left(\frac{20}{(0.0306 \text{ mmol/L/mm Hg})(38 \text{ mm Hg})}\right)$$

$$pH = 6.1 + \log 17.2$$

$$pH = 6.1 + 1.24$$

$$pH = 7.34$$

18. **Q.** Given a patient's pCO_2 of 35 mm Hg and a pH of 7.25, what is the bicarbonate concentration?

    A. Using the Henderson-Hasselbalch equation for pH, the following equation is derived:

$$7.25 = 6.1 + \log\left(\frac{[HCO_3^-]}{(0.0306 \text{ mmol/L/mm Hg})(35 \text{ mm Hg})}\right)$$

$$1.15 = \log\left(\frac{[HCO_3^-]}{(0.0306 \text{ mmol/L/mm Hg})(35 \text{ mm Hg})}\right)$$

$$\frac{[HCO_3^-]}{(0.0306)(35)} = \text{antilog } 1.15$$

$$\frac{[HCO_3^-]}{1.07 \text{ mmol/L}} = 14.12$$

$$[HCO_3^-] = (14.12)(1.07 \text{ mmol/L})$$

$$[HCO_3^-] = 15 \text{ mmol/L}$$

19. **Q.** What is the pCO_2 content of a sample of whole blood that had a pH of 7.35 and a bicarbonate concentration of 35 mmol/L?

    A. Using the Henderson-Hasselbalch equation, the following equation is derived:

$$7.35 = 6.1 + \log\left(\frac{35 \text{ mmol/L}}{(0.0306 \text{ mmol/L/mm Hg})(X)}\right)$$

$$1.25 = \log\left(\frac{35 \text{ mmol/L}}{(0.0306 \text{ mmol/L/mm Hg})(X)}\right)$$

$$\text{antilog } 1.25 = \frac{35 \text{ mmol/L}}{(0.0306 \text{ mmol/L/mm Hg})(X)}$$

$$17.78 = \frac{35 \text{ mmol/L}}{(0.0306 \text{ mmol/L/mm Hg})(X)}$$

$$(17.78)(0.0306 \text{ mmol/L/mm Hg})(X) = 35 \text{ mmol/L}$$

$$(0.544)(X) = 35 \text{ mmol/L}$$

$$X = \frac{35 \text{ mmol/L}}{0.544 \text{ mmol/L/mm Hg}}$$

$$X = 64 \text{ mm Hg}$$

20. **Q.** Given a patient's pH of 7.31, what is the patient's acid–base status?
    A. The patient is acidotic. The pH is below the normal level of 7.35 to 7.45.

21. **Q.** Given a patient's pH of 7.51, what is the patient's acid–base status?
    A. The patient is alkalotic. The pH is above the normal level of 7.35 to 7.45.

22. **Q.** Given a patient's pH is 7.42, and both the bicarbonate and pCO_2 are abnormal, has the patient compensated?
    A. Yes, since the pH is in the normal range, the body has compensated.

23. **Q.** Given a pH of 7.57, a bicarbonate of 36 mmol/L, and a pCO_2 of 50 mm Hg, what is the main problem, what is trying to compensate or has compensated, and is the patient's main problem metabolic or respiratory?
    A. To solve this, first look at the pH. It is alkalotic. That tells you immediately that it is not fully compensated, since it is not in the normal range. Next, look at the bicarbonate value. Is it normal? No, it is slightly above normal. Does that fit the pattern that if the bicarbonate is elevated the pH is elevated? Yes. Now look at the pCO_2 range. Is it normal? No, the pCO_2 is elevated. Does that fit the pattern that if the pCO_2 is elevated the pH goes down? No. Now you know that the bicarbonate is the main problem and the lungs are trying to compensate. The more the lungs can retain the acid of the CO_2, the lower the pH can become. Therefore you have a partially compensated metabolic alkalosis.

24. **Q.** Given a pH of 7.39, a bicarbonate of 12 mmol/L, and a pCO_2 of 20 mm Hg, determine if it is a fully compensated, partially compensated, respiratory, or metabolic primary disorder.
    A. The pH is in the normal range of 7.35 to 7.45. This means that the condition is fully compensated. Now comes the fun part to determine whether it is respiratory or metabolic. The bicarbonate is low, which fits with a low pH; but the pCO_2 is also low, which does not fit with a low pH. Therefore the culprit is metabolic, and the lungs are trying to blow off acid to make the body more alkaline. Thus the main cause is metabolic acidosis that is fully compensated.

25. **Q.** Given a pH of 7.18, a bicarbonate of 24 mmol/L, and a pCO_2 of 65 mm Hg, determine if it is a fully compensated, partially compensated, respiratory, or metabolic primary disorder.
    A. The pH is acidotic, so it is not fully compensated. The bicarbonate is in the normal range, but the pCO_2 is very elevated. This is an example of an uncompensated respiratory acidosis.

26. **Q.** What is the anion gap of a sample with a $[Na^+]$ of 145 mmol/L, $[Cl^-]$ of 105 mmol/L, and $[HCO_3^-]$ of 30 mmol/L?
    A. The anion gap is a calculation used to detect changes in concentration of unmeasured anions and cations. In the body, the amount of cations should equal the amount of

anions. In some disease states and medical conditions, this balance may be altered. For example, in ketoacidosis, there is an increase in the concentration of ketoacids in the blood. These anions are not normally measured and so the anion gap will be increased. Using the data from the problem, the calculated anion gap is:

$$\text{Anion gap} = 145 \text{ mmol/L} - (105 \text{ mmol/L} + 30 \text{ mmol/L})$$
$$\text{Anion gap} = 145 \text{ mmol/L} - (135 \text{ mmol/L})$$
$$\text{Anion gap} = 10 \text{ mmol/L}$$

27. **Q.** Calculate the osmolal gap of a patient with a measured serum osmolality of 340 mOsm/kg, Na^+ of 141 mmol/L, K^+ of 3.5 mmol/L, glucose of 140 mg/dL, and BUN of 15 mg/dL.

   A. The osmolal gap is the difference between the calculated osmolality and the measured osmolality. The reference range for the osmol gap ranges from -6 to $+6$ mOsmol/kg H_2O. Theoretically, there should be no difference between the measured and calculated serum osmolality. The constituents of the calculation comprise the majority of dissolved solutes in the blood. When other nonmeasured solutes are present, such as ethanol, the measured serum osmolality value will differ from the calculated osmolality value. The formula to calculate osmolality is:

$$\text{Calculated osmolality} = 1.86\left[Na^+\right] + \frac{[\text{glucose}]}{18} + \frac{[\text{BUN}]}{2.8} \, (\text{mOsmol} / \text{kg } H_2O)$$

Substituting into the formula the values from the problem yields the following equation:

$$\text{Calculated osmolality} = 1.86(141 \text{ mmol} / L) + \frac{140 \text{ mg/dL}}{18} + \frac{15.0 \text{ mg/dL}}{2.8}$$
$$\text{Calculated osmolality (mOsm/kg } H_2O) = 262.3 + 7.8 + 5.4$$
$$\text{Calculated osmolality (mOsm/kg } H_2O) = 276$$

Next, the osmolal gap is calculated by determining the difference between the calculated osmolality and the measured osmolality.

$$\text{Osmolal gap} = \underset{(\text{calculated})}{276 \text{mOsm/kg } H_2O} - \underset{(\text{measured})}{340 \text{mOsm/kg } H_2O}$$
$$\text{Osmolal gap} = 64 \text{ mOsm/kg } H_2O$$

28. **Q.** What is the concentration of LDL cholesterol in a sample whose total cholesterol is 230 mg/dL, HDL cholesterol is 40 mg/dL, and triglyceride concentration is 150 mg/dL?

   A. At present, there are only a few methods that measure LDL cholesterol directly. Instead, the concentration of LDL cholesterol can be determined by a mathematical formula. This formula uses the triglyceride concentration. To measure an accurate triglyceride concentration in which dietary triglycerides do not interfere, a fasting specimen is required. Therefore a fasting specimen is also required for an accurate LDL cholesterol calculation. The mathematical formula to determine LDL cholesterol is:

$$\text{LDL cholesterol} = \text{Total cholesterol} - \left(\text{HDL cholesterol} + \frac{\text{Triglycerides}}{5}\right)$$

The fraction of triglycerides divided by 5 represents the VLDL fraction of cholesterol. This representation is only valid if the triglyceride concentration is below 400 mg/dL. Therefore the patient's LDL cholesterol is:

$$\text{LDL cholesterol} = 230 \text{ mg/dL} - \left(40 \text{ mg/dL} + \frac{150 \text{ mg/dL}}{5}\right)$$

$$\text{LDL cholesterol} = 230 \text{ mg/dL} - (40 \text{ mg/dL} + 30 \text{ mg/dL})$$

$$\text{LDL cholesterol} = 230 \text{ mg/dL} - 70 \text{ mg/dL}$$

$$\text{LDL cholesterol} = 160 \text{ mg/dL}$$

HOW PRACTICE PROBLEMS

Solve the following practice problems to further master the material. Answers and explanations to some problems can be found in the Answer Key.

Given the following % T values, calculate the absorbance values.

1. 25% T

2. 74% T

3. 32% T

Given the following absorbance values, calculate the % T values.

4. 0.188 absorbance

5. 1.625 absorbance

6. 0.730 absorbance

7. Calculate the concentration of a substance that has a molar absorptivity at 25°C of 45,000 M^{-1} cm^{-1} at 450 nm and a measured absorbance of 1.250. (Assume a 1 cm pathlength.)

8. Calculate the lactate dehydrogenase activity of a sample measured using NADH as the reaction indicator. The ΔAbs./min for the sample is 0.030. The molar extinction coefficient for NADH is 6.22×10^3 M^{-1} cm^{-1}. The sample volume is 100 mcL, and the reagent volume is 2.5 mL. Assume a pathlength of 1 cm.

9. Calculate the pH of 1.0 L of a buffer prepared by mixing equal volumes of a 0.80 M strong acid [HA] with its 0.50 M salt [A$^-$]. The pK_a of the acid is 3.6.

10. Calculate the pH of a patient's blood with a bicarbonate concentration of 31 mmol/L and a pCO_2 concentration of 45 mm Hg.

11. Calculate the bicarbonate of a whole blood sample with a pH of 7.4 and a pCO_2 concentration of 42 mm Hg.

12. Given a bicarbonate concentration of 20 mmol/L, a pCO_2 of 65 mm Hg, and a pH of 7.20, is the condition metabolic or respiratory; acidotic or alkalotic; partially compensated, compensated, or uncompensated?

13. Given a bicarbonate concentration of 16 mmol/L, a pCO_2 of 30 mm Hg, and a pH of 7.36, is the condition metabolic or respiratory; acidotic or alkalotic; partially compensated, compensated, or uncompensated?

14. Given a bicarbonate concentration of 40 mmol/L, a pCO_2 of 38 mm Hg, and a pH of 7.52, is the condition metabolic or respiratory; acidotic or alkalotic; partially compensated, compensated, or uncompensated?

15. Calculate the anion gap of a sample with the following concentrations:

$$Na^+ = 147 \text{ mmol/L}, \ Cl^- = 110 \text{ mmol/L}, \ HCO_3^- = 35 \text{ mmol/L}$$

16. Calculate the serum osmolality of a sample given the following data:

$$Na^+ = 147 \text{ mmol/L}, \ glucose = 410 \text{ mg/dL}, \ BUN = 20 \text{ mg/dL}$$

17. Calculate the osmolal gap of a sample given the following information:

$$Na^+ = 149 \text{ mmol/L}, \ glucose = 115 \text{ mg/dL}, \ BUN = 10 \text{ mg/dL, and}$$
$$\text{measured osmolality} = 290 \text{ mOsm/kg}$$

18. Calculate the LDL cholesterol concentration in a sample with a total cholesterol of 255 mg/dL, HDL cholesterol of 30 mg/dL, and triglycerides of 250 mg/dL.

Answer to Example 6-14

PROTEIN	%	G/DL
Albumin	61.8	4.39
Alpha-1	3.8	0.27
Alpha-2	9.4	0.67
Beta	15.2	1.08
Gamma	9.8	0.70
	Total Protein	7.1 g/DL

QUICK NOTES

- Abosrbance $= 2 - \log\% \text{ T}$.
- Beer's law: Absorbance = absorptivity coefficient × pathlenght × concentration, or A = abc. Since the absorptivity coefficient and the pathlenght are constant, then A is proportional to concentration.
- Absorbance is inversely proportional to percent transmittance (i.e., the higher the absorbance value, the lower the % transmittance value, or the lower the absorbance value, the higher the % transmittance value).

- Determining the concentrarion of an unknown value using the single point standard method uses ratio and proportion.
- When the absorbance value of an unknown (patient or control) is higher than the highest standard in a standard curve, or the absorbance value in a single point standard method, the sample has to be diluted and reanalyzed.
- Many modern analyzers use enzyme kinetics to determine the unknown value of analytes.
- No standard is used when performing an enzyme kinetic method. However, quality control samples are still analyzed per the laboratory's protocol.
- It is very uncommon in most clinical laboratories that the pH equation has to be manually calculated.
- If a patient's pH is outside the reference range, then the patient is uncompensated. To determine which analyte is the cause, the analyte that has a value opposite its normal effect on pH is the compensating analyte. Both bicarbonate and pCO_2 can have very abnormal values, but if the pH is now normal that is what the body works toward.
- The human body never overcompensates to get the pH value in the reference range.
- Doctors order osmolality to determine if there is another substance in the patient's blood (such as ethylene glycol). These patients will have an abnormal osmolality gap.
- When performing the LDL calculation, the triglyceride value cannot be more than 400 mg/dL.

BIBLIOGRAPHY

Bishop M, Fody E, Schoeff L, et al: *Clinical chemistry; principles, procedures, and correlations*, ed 8, Philadelphia, 2018, Lippincott Williams & Wilkins.

Burtis CA, Bruns DE, editors: *Tietz fundamentals of clinical chemistry and molecular diagnostics*, ed 7, St. Louis, 2015, Elsevier.

Friedewald WT, Levy RI, Frederickson DS: Estimation of the concentration of low density lipoprotein cholesterol in plasma without use of the preparative ultracentrifuge, *Clin Chem* 18:499, 1972.

Kaplan L, Pesce A: *Clinical chemistry: theory, analysis and correlation*, ed 5, St Louis, 2009, Mosby Company.

Report of the National Cholesterol Treatment Program expert panel on detection, evaluation, and treatment of high blood cholesterol in adults, *Arch Intern Med* 148:36–39, 1988.

Urinalysis Laboratory

OBJECTIVES

At the end of this chapter, the reader should be able to do the following:

1. Define the following terms: *clearance, glomerular filtration rate, intrinsic clearance,* and *extrinsic clearance.*
2. Correct refractometer readings due to increased glucose and protein concentration.
3. State the clearance formula.
4. Calculate uncorrected creatinine clearance rates.
5. Use a nomogram and calculate corrected creatinine clearance rates.
6. Define the estimated creatinine clearance formula.

WHAT URINE TESTS

At present, the routine urinalysis exam is one of the most common laboratory tests performed. Chemically impregnated strips allow the laboratory professional to screen the urine for chemical constituents. Microscopic evaluation of sediment helps to determine the cellular, crystals, microorganisms, and artifactual constituents of urine. Routine urinalysis is an excellent screening tool for many different diseases or conditions, such as diabetes, urinary tract infections, metabolic disorders, and liver disorders.

WHAT CORRECTIONS USED FOR THE REFRACTOMETER

Calibration

When a urinalysis is performed, the specific gravity of the urine is measured. The specific gravity is important because it is an indication of the quantity of dissolved solids in urine, such as urea and chloride.

The refractometer, or total solids (TS) meter (Figure 7-1), measures specific gravity indirectly by the refractive index of the urine. The refractive index is a ratio of the velocity of light in air to

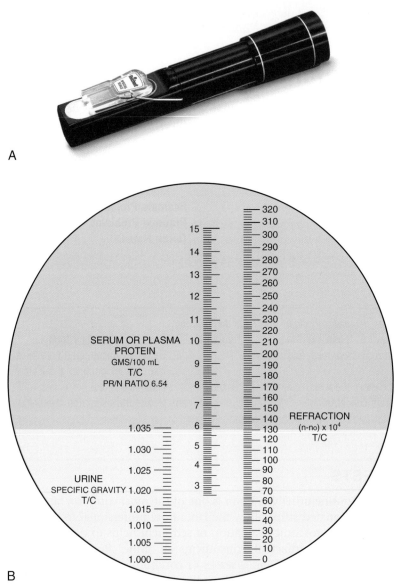

A

B

FIGURE 7-1 (A) and (B) Refractometer scale. (From Instructions for Use and Care of the Reichert TS Meter, Reichert Analytical Instruments Division, Buffalo, NY, with permission. Courtesy Reichert, Inc.)

the velocity of light in solution. The angle at which the light passes through the solution is mathematically converted into units of specific gravity. Only one drop of urine is required with a refractometer. The refractometer is calibrated with deionized water to read 1.000 and with 5.00%$^{(w/v)}$ NaCl to read 1.022.

HOW   *Example 7-1*

A refractometer used in a physician's office laboratory is checked with deionized water to determine if it is calibrated. The reading is 1.002. A quality control specimen also is measured using the refractometer with a specific gravity of 1.025. The refractometer is old and cannot be physically adjusted to a reading of 1.000 with deionized water. What adjustments or corrections must be made to the quality control result and all other control or patient results?

The specific gravity of deionized water as measured with a refractometer should measure 1.000. In this problem, the measurement is 1.002. All subsequent results (controls and patients) must be adjusted for the inaccuracy of +0.002 in the reading. The quality control specimen's specific gravity must be adjusted by subtracting 0.002 points from the measured reading. Therefore the corrected specific gravity for the quality control specimen is 1.023.

Example 7-1a   A refractometer in a hospital laboratory is checked with 5.00%$^{(w/v)}$ NaCl, and the reading is 1.021. What adjustments or corrections must be made to the quality control result and all other control or patient results?

The specific gravity should be checked with deionized water. If the result of the deionized water is 1.000, then the NaCl solution needs to be replaced. If, however, the deionized water did not have a value of 1.000, then the refractometer needs to be recalibrated.

WHAT   **Correction for Protein**

The refractometer must be corrected if large quantities of protein (1.0 g/dL or more) are present in the urine. Protein is a very-high-molecular-weight compound that will increase the density of urine by 0.003 for each 1.0 g/dL of protein. Protein is not normally found in urine because it is too large to pass through the glomerular membrane. When the integrity of the membrane is compromised due to injury or disease, protein molecules can pass through the glomerulus and will be present in urine. The purpose of performing the specific gravity analysis of the urine is to determine the concentrating ability of the kidney, which is primarily the work of the tubules. The presence of large amounts of protein (1.0 g/dL or more) in the urine can be an early indicator of renal disease and will falsely increase the specific gravity and result in erroneous assessment of the tubules.

HOW   *Example 7-2*

A urinalysis was performed on urine that contained 3 g/dL of protein. The specific gravity by refractometer was 1.026. What is the corrected specific gravity for this sample?

Each gram per deciliter of protein falsely elevates the specific gravity by 0.003. Because the urine contains 3 g/dL, the amount to be subtracted is $3 \times 0.003 = 0.009$.

$$\text{Corrected specific gravity} = 1.026 - 0.009 = 1.017$$

Therefore the specific gravity of the sample that accurately reflects the concentrating ability of the kidneys is 1.017.

Example 7-2a   A urinalysis was performed on a urine that contained 2 g/dL. The specific gravity by refractometer was 1.015. What is the corrected specific gravity?

Since each g/dL of protein falsely elevates the specific gravity by 0.003, then 0.006 must be subtracted from the obtained reading, giving a corrected specific gravity of 1.009.

WHAT   **Correction for Glucose**

The glucose molecule is a large molecular weight compound. When present in large quantities (1 g/dL or greater), the specific gravity of the urine will be increased by 0.004 for every 1 g/dL of glucose. As with increased protein, increased glucose levels do not accurately reflect the concentrating ability of the tubules but are a reflection of exceeding the renal threshold. The effect of 1 g/dL or higher of glucose must be subtracted from the specific gravity to obtain an accurate measurement.

HOW   *Example 7-3*

A urine specimen has a glucose concentration of 2 g/dL and a specific gravity of 1.018. What is the corrected specific gravity?

For each 1.0 g/dL of glucose, the specific gravity is elevated by 0.004. The corrected specific gravity would be as follows:

$$\text{Corrected specific gravity} = 1.018 - (0.004)(2)$$
$$= 1.018 - 0.008$$
$$= 1.010$$

Therefore the corrected specific gravity is 1.010.

Example 7-3a   A urine specimen has a glucose concentration of 1.0 g/dL and a specific gravity of 1.022. What is the corrected specific gravity?

Because every g/dL of glucose present in the urine raises the specific gravity by 0.004, the corrected specific gravity would be 1.018.

WHAT   # RENAL FUNCTION TESTS

Clearance Test

One of the most common renal function tests is the clearance test. This test provides information on the glomerular and tubular function of the kidneys. The kidney's main function is to excrete waste products while reabsorbing water and dissolved chemicals from the ultrafiltrate. By measuring the urine concentration per unit of time of a chemical that will be removed or "cleared" by the kidney tubules, the physiologic function of the tubules can be determined.

There are many variations on the clearance test. All variations measure three parameters: the plasma (or serum) concentration of the chemical to be cleared, the urine concentration of that same chemical, and the time interval of the clearance procedure. In this manner, the glomerular filtration rate (GFR) can be determined. This is the rate at which chemicals are filtered or "cleared" from the kidney. The clearance tests differ by the substance or chemical. Measurements of chemicals that are foreign to the body and completely cleared are known as extrinsic clearance tests. These chemicals include inulin and p-aminohippurate, among others. The extrinsic chemical is injected into the patient intravenously. After the chemical is injected, the plasma concentration is measured. All urine is collected during the clearance procedure and the volume is measured. After the time interval, which may be 6, 12, or 24 hours, the urine and plasma are analyzed for the chemical concentration. Intrinsic clearance tests measure chemicals that are intrinsic to the body, such as creatinine and urea. The urea clearance test was one of the first clearance tests performed. Because approximately 40% of urea is reabsorbed by the tubules, the urea clearance test does not provide an accurate clearance assessment.

Creatinine is a waste product of muscle metabolism, produced at a constant rate and proportional to muscle mass. Very little creatinine is secreted by the tubular cells; therefore the concentration of creatinine in urine is an excellent assessment of the tubular excretion function and the GFR. As with extrinsic clearance tests, the plasma levels of creatinine or urea are determined. Urine is collected for a fixed period ranging from 6, 12, or 24 hours. The 24-hour urine collection is the most commonly performed interval. The urine concentration of urea or creatinine is also determined.

All clearances are calculated by the following formula and reported in whole numbers:

$$\frac{UV}{P}$$

where:
U = urine concentration in mg/dL of the analyte that was cleared
V = volume of urine in mL/min
P = plasma concentration of analyte in mg/dL

HOW   **Example 7-4**

A 24-hour urine collection for a creatinine clearance was performed. The total volume of urine is 1500 mL. The plasma creatinine concentration is 1.4 mg/dL, and the urine creatinine concentration is 180 mg/dL. What is the creatinine clearance?

To solve this problem, first convert the volume of urine into milliliters per minute. Divide 1500 by 1440 to obtain the milliliters per minute because in 24 hours there are 1440 minutes (24 × 60).

$$mL/min = \frac{1500}{1440} = 1.04 \ mL/min$$

Next use the formula to obtain the creatinine clearance value.

$$\frac{UV}{P} = \frac{(180 \ mg/dL)1.04 \ mL/min}{1.4 \ mg/dL} = 133.71 \ mL/min$$

Therefore the creatinine clearance is equal to 134 mL/min.

Example 7-4a   Calculate the creatinine clearance of a 24-hour urine collection with a total volume of 2100 mL. The plasma creatinine concentration is 1.8 mg/dL and the urine creatinine concentration is 155 mg/dL.

To solve this problem, first convert the volume of urine into milliliters per minute. Divide 2100 by 1440 to obtain the milliliters per minute because in 24 hours there are 1440 minutes (24 × 60).

$$mL/min = \frac{2100}{1440} = 1.46 \ mL/minute$$

Next use the formula to obtain the creatinine clearance value.

$$\frac{UV}{P} = \frac{(155 \ mg/dL)1.46 \ mL/minute}{1.8 \ mg/dL} = 125.7 \ mL/min$$

Therefore the creatinine clearance is equal to 126 mL/min.

Example 7-4b   Calculate the creatinine clearance in a 24-hour urine collection with a total volume of 2200 mL, a blood urea nitrogen (BUN) of 17 mg/dL, a serum creatinine of 1.2 mg/dL, and a urine creatinine of 80 mg/dL.

Using the clearance formula, the result is 102 mL/min. Note that the BUN value is not part of the creatinine clearance calculation.

Example 7-4c   A 12-hour urine collection for a creatinine clearance was performed. The urine volume is 0.850 L, the plasma creatinine is 1.1 mg/dL, and the urine creatinine concentration is 117 mg/dL. What is the creatinine clearance?

To solve this problem, first determine the quantity of urine per milliliters per minute. In 12 hours there are 720 minutes (60 minutes × 12 hours). Divide 850 mL by 720 to determine the amount of urine produced in terms of milliliters per minute.

$$\frac{850}{720} = 1.181 \text{ mL/min volume of urine}$$

Using the clearance formula and substituting in the numbers:

$$\text{Clearance (mL/min)} = \frac{117 \text{ mg/dL} \times 1.181 \text{ mL/min}}{1.1 \text{ mg/dL}}$$

Creatinine clearance = 125.6 mL/min

Using the clearance formula, the result is 126 mL/min.

Example 7-4d   A 12-hour urine collection for a creatinine clearance was performed. The urine volume is 0.430 L, the plasma creatinine is 4.1 mg/dL, and the urine creatinine concentration is 130 mg/dL. What is the creatinine clearance?

To solve this problem, first determine the quantity of urine per milliliters per minute. In 12 hours there are 720 minutes (60 minutes × 12 hours). Divide 430 mL by 720 to determine the amount of urine produced in terms of milliliters per minute.

$$\frac{430}{720} = 0.597 \text{ mL/min volume of urine}$$

Using the clearance formula and substituting in the numbers:

$$\text{Clearance (mL/min)} = \frac{130 \text{ mg/dL} \times 0.597 \text{ mL/min}}{4.1 \text{ mg/dL}}$$

Creatinine clearance = 18.9 mL/min

Using the clearance formula, the result is 19 mL/min.

Example 7-4e   Calculate the creatinine clearance in a 12-hour urine sample with a total volume of 550 mL, a serum creatinine of 0.8 mg/dL, and a urine creatinine of 74 mg/dL.

Using the clearance formula, the clearance value is 71 mL/min.

WHAT **Clearance Formula Corrected for Body Size**

The clearance formula was developed to be used for patients with an adult "average" body size of 1.73 m². Patients with larger-than-average or smaller-than-average body dimensions would have inaccurate clearance values using this formula alone. In addition, this formula could not be used to accurately determine the clearance values of children because of their much smaller body size. Figure 7-2 is a nomogram that can be used to compensate for body sizes different from 1.73 m². To use the nomogram, the patient's height in centimeters or inches is required along with his or her weight in kilograms or pounds. Find the patient's height and weight on the nomogram. Using a ruler as a straightedge, line up the height and weight with the ruler. The surface area is the center scale, and the patient's body surface area is found at the intersection of the scale and the ruler.

Example 7-4f   A creatinine clearance was ordered for an obese patient with kidney disease. Her weight was 350 pounds and her height 5 foot 4 inches. The 24-hour urine volume was 650 mL, plasma creatinine 6.5 mg/dL, and urine creatinine 120 mg/dL. What is this patient's creatinine clearance?

To solve this problem, first determine the milliliters per minute quantity of urine creatinine.

$$\text{mL/minute} = \frac{650 \text{ mL/24 hr}}{(60 \text{ mL})(24 \text{ hr})} = \frac{650}{1440} = 0.45 \text{ mL/min}$$

Next, use **Figure 7-2** to determine the body surface area of the patient. The nomogram consists of three scales. The first on the left side of the nomogram is the height scale. Height can be measured both in feet/inches and in centimeters. The scale to the right is the weight scale. Weight can be measured both in pounds and in kilograms. The middle scale is the body surface area scale. To determine the patient's body surface area, first find the patient's height in feet and inches on the scale to the left. Next find the patient's weight on the scale to the right. Then, using a straightedge, draw a line through the body surface area scale connecting both measurements. The point of intersection through the body surface area will be the patient's body surface area. This patient has a body surface area of 2.30 m². Remember that the "average" person has a body surface area of 1.73 m². Finally, use the corrected clearance formula to determine the clearance value:

$$\text{Corrected creatinine clearance} = \frac{\text{UV}}{\text{P}} \times \frac{1.73 \text{ m}^2}{2.30 \text{ m}^2}$$

Using the values given, the formula becomes:

$$\left(\frac{120 \text{ mg/dL } (0.45 \text{ mL/min})}{6.5} \right) \times \frac{1.73 \text{ m}^2}{2.30 \text{ m}^2} =$$

8.3 mL/min × 0.752 = corrected creatinine clearance of 6.2 mL/min.

Notice that the corrected clearance value is lower than the uncorrected value because of the increased body size of the patient.

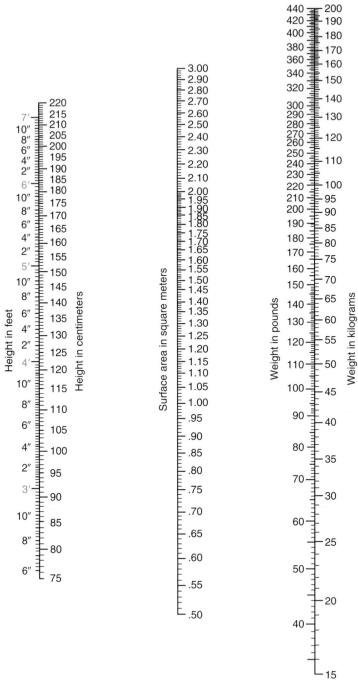

FIGURE 7-2 Nomogram for the determination of body surface areas.

Example 7-4g   A creatinine clearance is ordered for a patient who is 4 foot 11 inches and weighs 93 pounds. Her urine creatinine value is 75 mg/dL, the plasma creatinine is 1.5 mg/dL, and the urine volume on a 12-hour specimen was 750 mL. What is her corrected creatinine clearance?

To solve this problem, first determine the quantity of urine per minute.

$$\text{mL/min} = \frac{750}{(60)(12)} = 1.04 \text{ mL/min}$$

Because this patient does not have an average body size, the corrected version of the clearance formula will be used to obtain her creatinine clearance. Often, the height and weight of patients are unknown to the laboratory. Clearances are then reported as "uncorrected" for body size. To correct for body size, use the nomogram in **Figure 7-1** to determine the "corrected" body size. By drawing a line between the patient's height and weight, you find that this patient has a body surface area in square meters of 1.23. Next, use the modified creatinine clearance formula:

$$\frac{\text{UV}}{\text{P}} \times \frac{1.73 \text{ m}^2}{1.23 \text{ m}^2} = \frac{(75 \text{ mg/dL})(1.04 \text{ ml/min})}{1.5 \text{ mg/dL}} \times 1.41 =$$

$$\frac{78 \text{ mL/min}}{1.5} \times 1.41 = 73.3 \text{ mL/min corrected creatinine clearance}$$

What is this patient's uncorrected clearance?

To determine the uncorrected clearance, do not correct for body size. Use the unmodified clearance formula as in Examples 7-4 to 7-4d. Without the correction factor for her smaller-than-average body size of 1.23 m², this patient's uncorrected clearance is 52 mL/min.

Example 7-4h   A 24-hour urine sample was collected for a creatinine clearance test. The urine volume is 1800 mL, the plasma creatinine value is 2.4 mg/dL, and the urine creatinine result is 167 mg/dL. The patient is 6 feet 4 inches and 380 pounds. What is the patient's corrected creatinine clearance?

To solve, calculate the corrected creatinine clearance using the corrected clearance formula and substituting into it the values from this problem:

$$\text{Corrected creatinine clearance} = \frac{(167)(1.25)}{2.4} \times \frac{1.73 \text{ m}^2}{2.68 \text{ m}^2}$$

Using 2.68 the corrected creatinine clearance is 56.5 mL/min.

Example 7-4i   A 24-hour creatinine clearance was performed on a patient who is 4 feet 11 inches and 89 pounds. The patient's urine creatinine is 82 mg/dL, the serum creatinine is 0.8 mg/dL, and the total volume is 1455 mL. What is the corrected creatinine clearance?

The corrected clearance is 149 mL/min.

WHAT **Estimated GFR**

In 2002, the National Kidney Foundation Kidney Disease Outcomes Quality Initiative guidelines called for estimating GFR each time a serum creatinine test was performed. There are three equations in use for estimation of GFR, one of which is not commonly used. They are:

1. The Modification of Diet in Renal Disease (MDRD) (very cumbersome and not usually used)
2. The abbreviated or modified MDRD
3. The Crockroft-Gault equation

Modified MDRD Equation

$$\text{GFR}(\text{mL/min}/1.73 \text{ m}^2) = 175 \times (\text{Serum creatinine})^{-1.154} \times (\text{Age})^{-0.203} \times (0.742 \text{ if female})$$
$$\times (1.212 \text{ if African American})(\text{conventional units})$$

The modified MDRD equation may be used in laboratories with computer systems such as in hospitals. The equation is programmed into the computer, and as hospital laboratory computers are interfaced with the main hospital computers where the demographic information is stored, the calculation may be automatically generated once the creatinine level is known. However, many laboratory accreditation organizations require the laboratory to check on a monthly basis all calculations that are performed by the computer system to ensure that they are accurate.

Crockoft-Gault Equation

$$\text{Creatinine clearance (mL/min)} = \frac{(140 - \text{age}) \times \text{weight (kg)} \times (0.85 \text{ if female})}{72 \times \text{Serum creatinine (mg/dL)}}$$

This calculation is much simpler than the modified MDRD calculation and can be done on a simple calculator.

HOW **EXAMPLE PROBLEMS**

This section is designed to be useful to both the student and the laboratory professional. Students can use the additional problems to master the material. The laboratory professional can use the examples as templates for solving laboratory calculations. Find an example similar to the problem that you need to solve, and substitute the appropriate numbers into the equation.

1. Q. A urinalysis is performed on a urine specimen that contains 2 g/dL of protein. The specific gravity, performed by a refractometer, is 1.022. What is the correct specific gravity for this urine?

   A. Quantities of protein greater than 1 g/dL will falsely elevate the specific gravity reading by refractometer or urinometer. For every gram present, the specific gravity will be elevated by 0.003. Because the urine contains a protein concentration of 2 g/dL, the specific gravity is falsely elevated by 0.006. Subtracting 0.006 from the obtained specific gravity of 1.022 results in the correct specific gravity of the urine of 1.016.

2. Q. Urine from a diabetic patient has a glucose level of 3.0 g/dL. The specific gravity of the patient's urine by urinometer is 1.030. What is the patient's correct specific gravity?

A. For each gram per deciliter of glucose present in a urine specimen, the specific gravity is falsely elevated by 0.004. As the urine contains a glucose concentration of 3 g/dL, the effect is a false increase of 0.012 in specific gravity. By subtracting 0.012 from the obtained specific gravity of 1.030, the result of 1.018 is the correct specific gravity.

3. **Q.** A 24-hour urine sample was collected for a creatinine clearance test. The urine volume is 1800 mL, the plasma creatinine value is 2.0 mg/dL, and the urine creatinine result is 160 mg/dL. What is the patient's uncorrected creatinine clearance?

A. The formula for determining clearance is as follows:

$$\frac{UV}{P}$$

where:

U = urine concentration in milligrams per deciliter of the analyte that was cleared
V = volume of urine in milliliters per minute
P = plasma concentration of analyte in milligrams per deciliter
To determine the volume of urine in milliliters per minute, multiply the amount of hours of collection by 60 to determine the length of time in minutes:

$$24 \times 60 = 1440 \text{ minutes}$$

Next, divide the quantity of urine collected by the total minutes to obtain the milliliters per minute quantity:

$$\frac{1800 \text{ mL}}{1440 \text{ min}} = 1.25 \text{ mL/min}$$

Next, substitute into the clearance equation the data that are known:

$$\text{Clearance(mL/min)} = \frac{(160 \text{ mg/dL})(1.25 \text{ mL/min})}{2.0 \text{ mg/dL}}$$

$$\text{Clearance(mL/min)} = 100 \text{ mL/min}$$

4. **Q.** A 6-hour creatinine clearance was performed on a urine sample with a volume of 400 mL. The urine creatinine and plasma creatinine concentration are 50 mg/dL and 2.5 mg/dL, respectively. What is the patient's creatinine clearance?

A. To answer this question, first convert the amount of urine excreted in 6 hours to milliliters per minute excreted. In 6 hours there are 360 minutes. By dividing the volume of urine excreted, 400 mL, by 360, the amount of urine volume per milliliters per minute can be calculated. The milliliters per minute result is 1.11 mL/min. Using the clearance formula, the creatinine clearance can be calculated:

$$\text{Clearance (mL/min)} = \frac{(50 \text{ mg/dL})(1.11 \text{ mL/min})}{2.5 \text{ mg/dL}}$$

$$\text{Clearance (mL/min)} = 22$$

Therefore the creatinine clearance is 22 mL/min.

5. **Q.** A clearance test was performed on an 85-year-old woman who was 4 feet 10 inches and weighed 90 lb. The 24-hour urine specimen has a volume of 1250 mL and a urine creatinine of 115 mg/dL. The patient's plasma creatinine is 1.5 mg/dL. What is the patient's corrected creatinine clearance?

   A. The clearance formula was developed based on the average height and weight of men. Any person with a body size smaller or significantly larger should have the clearance formula adjusted for the difference in size. The nomogram **(Figure 7-2)** can be used to adjust the clearance formula for different body sizes. On the basis of the average male height and weight, the body surface area of the average man is 1.73 m². The clearance formula is slightly modified to correct for size differences. The corrected clearance formula is as follows:

$$\frac{UV}{P} \times \frac{1.73 \text{ m}^2}{\text{Body surface area of patient from nomogram}}$$

   Using the nomogram in **Figure 7-2**, determine the patient's body surface area by drawing a line from the point of 4 feet 10 inches on the height scale to 90 lb on the weight scale. The point of intersection on the body surface area scale is 1.20 m². Next, determine the patient's rate of urine flow in terms of milliliters per minute by dividing 1250 mL by the amount of minutes in 24 hours, or 1440 minutes. Next, use the clearance formula to determine the patient's clearance:

$$\text{Clearance} = \frac{(115 \text{ mg/dL})(0.87 \text{ mL/min})}{1.5 \text{ mg/dL}} \times \frac{1.73 \text{ m}^2}{1.20 \text{ m}^2}$$

$$\text{Clearance} = 66.7 \times 1.44$$

$$\text{Clearance (mL/min)} = 96 \text{ mL/min}$$

6. **Q.** A creatinine clearance is performed on a professional wrestler. The patient is 6 feet 6 inches and weighs 359 lb. A 24-hour urine sample was obtained with a total volume of 2200 mL. The urine creatinine result is 150 mg/dL, and the serum creatinine result is 1.5 mg/dL. What is the patient's corrected creatinine clearance?

   A. To solve this problem, first convert the total volume of urine collected into amount collected in terms of milliliters per minute. This is accomplished by dividing 2200 mL (amount collected) by 1440 (amount of minutes in 24 hours), yielding a milliliters per minute result of 1.53. Next, using the nomogram in **Figure 7-2**, determine the body surface area of the patient. Draw a line between the patient's height (6 feet 6 inches) and the patient's weight (359 lb). The line intersects the surface area scale at 2.68 m².

   Finally, substitute all data into the corrected clearance formula:

$$\text{Corrected creatinine clearance (mL/min)} =$$

$$\frac{(150 \text{ mg/dL})(1.53 \text{ mL/min})}{1.5 \text{ mg/dL}} \times \frac{1.73 \text{ m}^2}{2.68 \text{ m}^2} =$$

$$(153 \text{ mL/min})(0.645) =$$

$$\text{Corrected creatinine clearance} = 98.8 \text{ mL/min}$$

HOW **PRACTICE PROBLEMS**

Solve the following practice problems to further master the material. Answers and explanations to some problems are found in the Answer Key.

Correct the following specific gravity results obtained on a refractometer.

1. Specific gravity 1.020, urine protein concentration of 2.0 g/dL

2. Specific gravity 1.035, urine protein concentration of 4.0 g/dL

3. Specific gravity 1.042, urine glucose concentration of 4.0 g/dL

4. Specific gravity 1.027, urine glucose concentration of 2.0 g/dL

Calculate both the uncorrected and corrected creatinine clearance for practice problems 5 and 6.

Female patient: height 5 feet 8 inches, weight 225 pounds, urine creatinine 180 mg/dL, collection time 24 hours, plasma creatinine 1.7 mg/dL, urine volume 2400 mL.

5. Uncorrected creatinine clearance:

6. Corrected creatinine clearance:

Calculate both the uncorrected and corrected creatinine clearance for practice problems 7 and 8.

Male patient: height 5 feet 4 inches, weight 128 pounds, urine creatinine 150 mg/dL, collection time 24 hours, plasma creatinine 2.5 mg/dL, urine volume 1650 mL.

7. Uncorrected creatinine clearance:

8. Corrected creatinine clearance:

QUICK NOTES

- The refractometer has been replaced in many urinalysis laboratories as the automated urinalysis instruments perform specific gravity measurements.
- Many urine dipsticks have a test pad for the specific gravity of the urine, making the use of a refractometer unnecceessary.
- Insulin is the reference method for clearance tests but is never used in a clinical laboratory. Instead, creatinine clearance is commonly performed as the usual clearance method.
- The volume measurement in the creatinine clearance formula is the volume of the urine divided by the milliliters per minute. There are 1440 minutes in 24 hours.

BIBLIOGRAPHY

Burtis CA, Bruns DE, editors: *Tietz fundamentals of clinical chemistry and molecular diagnostics*, ed 7, St. Louis, 2015, Elsevier.
Strasinger K, Di Lorenzo MS: *Urinalysis and body fluids*, ed 6, Philadelphia, 2014, F.A. Davis Company.

Hematology Laboratory

OUTLINE

OBJECTIVES

At the end of this chapter, the reader should be able to do the following:

1. Estimate the hematocrit if given the hemoglobin using the rule of three and vice versa.
2. Estimate the hemoglobin if given the red blood cell count.
3. Calculate red blood cell indices (MCV, MCH, MCHC).
4. Correct the WBC count for the presence of nucleated red blood cells.
5. Calculate white blood cell, red blood cell, and platelet counts performed on a hemacytometer for blood and body fluids.
6. Calculate the sperm concentration per milliliter.
7. Calculate the sperm count per ejaculation.
8. Calculate the number of reticulocytes by both the slide and Miller disk method.
9. Correct the reticulocyte count for anemia using the reticulocyte index.
10. Correct the reticulocyte count when increased reticulocyte production is present.

WHAT **RULE OF THREE**

Hematology is the study of the cells within the blood. These include the white blood cells (WBCs), platelets, and the cells in the largest quantity, the red blood cells (RBCs). The RBCs carry oxygen from the lungs to the tissues and carbon dioxide from the tissues back to the lungs where it is exhaled. The oxygen is carried by hemoglobin molecules. The quantity of hemoglobin can be determined spectrophotometrically by automated hematology instruments. If the hemoglobin concentration is low, the oxygen-carrying capacity of the RBC is decreased as well. This will lead to the condition called anemia. The most common cause of anemia is iron deficiency. Iron is vital to the structure of the hemoglobin molecule, and if the iron concentration is low, the hemoglobin concentration will be adversely affected.

A second very common hematology test that is performed is the hematocrit. This is the ratio of the blood cells to the total volume of plasma expressed as a percent. The reference interval for hematocrit is 37% to 47% for adult women and 42% to 52% for adult men, meaning that approximately half of the whole blood in the body is made up of cellular components; the remainder is the liquid plasma portion. If the number of RBCs is decreased, the hematocrit will be decreased. If a person is anemic, the hemoglobin and hematocrit will both be decreased. The adult reference interval for hemoglobin is 14 to 18 g/dL for men and 12 to 16 g/dL for women.

There is a relationship between the hematocrit and the hemoglobin values that is useful as a quality assurance tool. The hematocrit is usually three times the hemoglobin value plus or minus 3. This is known as *the rule of three*. If the hematocrit is known, then the hemoglobin value can be estimated, and vice versa. This is a good rule of thumb to keep in mind even when the hemoglobin or hematocrit is either below or above the normal reference interval. When the rule of three is not found, it may indicate an error or an abnormality in the size of the RBC or the amount of hemoglobin in the RBC. This error may be an instrument malfunction of some sort, a mixup in patient identification, a problem in reporting the correct result, or a problem in the patient's RBCs.

HOW   *Example 8-1*

A finger stick was performed on a young boy in a pediatrician's office. The medical laboratory technician performed a spun hematocrit while the medical assistant performed the hemoglobin using a Clinial Laboratory Improvement Amendments (CLIA'88)-waived hemoglobin instrument. The hematocrit result was 45% and the hemoglobin was 11 g/dL. Are these results consistent with the rule of three?

No, these results do not follow the rule of three. The hemoglobin should be 15 g/dL if the hematocrit is accurate, or the hematocrit should be 33% if the hemoglobin is accurate. The medical laboratory technician should investigate the discrepancy.

Example 8-1a   If a hematocrit value is 36%, what would you estimate the hemoglobin value to be?

Using the rule of three, the hemoglobin would be estimated to be 12 g/dL.

Example 8-1b   If a hematocrit value is 45%, what would you estimate the hemoglobin value to be?

The hemoglobin would be estimated to be 15 g/dL.

WHAT   The rule of three can also be used to estimate the hemoglobin values using the RBC count. The RBC count × 3 should equal the hemoglobin value. The adult reference interval for RBC count is 4.5 to 5.5 (10^{12}/L) for men and 4.2 to 5.4 (10^{12}/L) for women. This additional relationship can also be used as part of the laboratory's quality assurance plan because errors may indicate preanalytical or analytical errors or a condition such as anemia in the patient.

HOW   *Example 8-2*

If a patient's RBC count is 4.7 (10^{12}/L), estimate the hemoglobin using the rule of three. The hemoglobin should be 14.1 g/dL if a normal weighted red blood cell is present.

Example 8-2a   If the RBC count is 3.7 (10^{12}/L), what would you estimate the hemoglobin to be?

The hemoglobin should be 11.1 g/dL if a normal weighted red blood cell is present.

Example 8-2b   If the RBC count is 4.3 (10^{12}/L), what would you estimate the hemoglobin to be?

The hemoglobin should be 12.9 g/dL if a normal weighted red blood cell is present.

WHAT   # RED BLOOD CELL INDICES

The size of the RBC is important in the treatment of anemias. Some anemias cause the RBC to be smaller than normal; others cause it to be larger. The relationship among size, hemoglobin, and hematocrit was mathematically determined by Wintrobe in the 1920s. Three formulas were developed to describe RBC morphology and to aid in the classification of anemia.

WHAT   ## Mean Corpuscular Volume

The first formula is the mean corpuscular volume (MCV). The MCV describes the average volume or size of the RBC in femtoliters (fL) and is calculated by the following formula:

$$\text{MCV (fL)} = \frac{\text{Hematocrit (\%)} \times 10}{\text{RBC count } (10^{12}/\text{L})}$$

The reference interval for MCV is 80 to 100 fL. MCV values less than 80 fL suggest RBCs that are smaller in size, whereas MCV values greater than 100 fL suggest RBCs that are larger than normal.

HOW   *Example 8-3*

Calculate the MCV of a sample if the hematocrit is 45% and the RBC count is 4.5 (10^{12}/L). Use the formula to calculate MCV:

$$\text{MCV} = \frac{\text{Hematocrit} \times 10}{\text{RBC count}} = \frac{45 \times 10}{4.5} = 100 \text{ fL}$$

The MCV of this sample is 100 fL.

Example 8-3a   Calculate the MCV of a sample if the hematocrit is 32% and the RBC count is 3.8 (10^{12}/L).

Use the MCV formula to solve:

$$\text{MCV} = \frac{\text{Hematocrit} \times 10}{\text{RBC count}} = \frac{32 \times 10}{3.8} = 84.2 \text{ fL}$$

Note: Sometimes in the clinical laboratory results are reported that do not adhere to the rules of significant figures. Notice that the MVC result is 84.2, not 84 fL.

Example 8-3b Calculate the MCV of a sample if the hematocrit is 48% and the RBC count is 5.3 (10^{12}/L).

Use the MCV formula to solve:

$$MCV = \frac{Hematocrit \times 10}{RBC\ count} = \frac{48 \times 10}{5.3} = 90.6\ fL$$

The MCV is 90.6 fL.

WHAT Mean Corpuscular Hemoglobin

The second formula is the mean corpuscular hemoglobin (MCH). As the name implies, it represents the average amount of hemoglobin present in the individual RBC in units of picograms (pg), significant only to the nearest tenth. It is calculated by the following formula:

$$MCH\ (picograms) = \frac{Hemoglobin\ (g/dL) \times 10}{RBC\ count\ (10^{12}/L)}$$

The adult reference interval for MCH is 27 to 31 pg.

HOW Example 8-4

Calculate the MCH of a patient with a hemoglobin concentration of 16 g/dL and a RBC count of 5.6 (10^{12}/L).
Use the formula to calculate MCH:

$$\frac{Hb \times 10}{RBC\ count} = \frac{16 \times 10}{5.6} = \frac{160}{5.6} = 28.6\ pg$$

The MCH is 28.6 pg.

Example 8-4a Calculate the MCH given a hemoglobin concentration of 14.0 g/dL and a RBC count of 5.1 (10^{12}/L).

Use the MCH formula to solve:

$$\frac{Hb \times 10}{RBC\ count} = \frac{14 \times 10}{5.1} = \frac{140}{5.1} = 27.4\ pg$$

The MCH is 27.4 pg.

Example 8-4b Calculate the MCH given a hemoglobin concentration of 11.5 g/dL and RBC count of 4.7 (10^{12}/L).

Use the MCH formula to solve:

$$\frac{Hb \times 10}{RBC\ count} = \frac{11.5 \times 10}{4.7} = \frac{115}{4.7} = 24.5\ pg$$

The MCH is 24.5 pg.

WHAT **Mean Corpuscular Hemoglobin Concentration**

The third calculation is the mean corpuscular hemoglobin concentration (MCHC). This calculation is a ratio of the hemoglobin to the hematocrit and is expressed in terms of grams per deciliter or grams per liter if using SI units. The MCHC is significant only to the nearest tenth. The MCHC represents the average hemoglobin content in the patient's RBC population.

$$MCHC = \frac{\text{Hemoglobin (g/dL)} \times 100}{\text{Hematocrit (\%)}}$$

The adult reference interval for MCHC is 32 to 36 g/dL.

HOW **Example 8-5**

Calculate the MCHC of a patient with a hemoglobin concentration of 10 g/dL and a hematocrit of 30%.
    Use the formula to calculate MCHC:

$$\frac{\text{Hb g/dL} \times 100}{30\%} = \frac{10 \times 100}{30} = \frac{1000}{30} = 33.3 \text{ g/dL}$$

The MCHC is 33.3 g/dL.

Example 8-5a   Calculate the MCHC of a patient with a hemoglobin of 15 g/dL and a hematocrit of 40%.

Use the MCHC formula to calculate:

$$\frac{\text{Hb g/dL} \times 100}{40\%} = \frac{15 \times 100}{40} = \frac{1500}{40} = 37.5 \text{ g/dL}$$

The MCHC is 37.5 g/dL.

Example 8-5b   Calculate the MCHC of a patient with a hemoglobin of 18 g/dL and a hematocrit of 45%.

Use the MCHC formula to calculate:

$$\frac{\text{Hb g/dL} \times 100}{45\%} = \frac{18 \times 100}{45} = \frac{1800}{45} = 40 \text{ g/dL}$$

The MCHC is 40.0 g/dL.

WHAT **Red Cell Distribution Width**

Red cell distribution width (RDW) is a measurement of the degree of anisocytosis present, or the degree of variability in RBC size, in a blood specimen.

$$\text{RDW-SD (\%)} = \frac{\text{Standard deviation (SD) of MCV}}{\text{Mean of MCV}} \times 100$$

Reference interval is 11.5% to 14.5%.
    This calculation is usually performed by the automated hematology analyzers but is presented here, as it is very commonly used in the hematology laboratory.

WHAT **CORRECTION OF THE WBC COUNT FOR NUCLEATED RBCS**

Nucleated RBCs (NRBCs) are immature RBCs that have not lost their nucleus. They are also called orthochromic normoblasts or metarubricytes. They are the last immature RBC that contains a nucleus, and when they further mature, they become reticulocytes. An even earlier nucleated red blood cell, the polychromatophilic nucleated red blood cell, may be seen too. Normally the NRBCs are found only in the bone marrow. In times of severe anemic stress they may be found in the peripheral blood, and they are also normally found in the peripheral blood of healthy newborns but disappear after a few days. Premature infants will have NRBCs present at birth and they may be present longer than a week.

Since NRBCs contain a nucleus, the WBC automated cell count should be adjusted downward, as the instrument may count the NRBC nucleus as a WBC. A correction calculation is usually performed when greater than 5 NRBCs per 100 WBCs are seen on a peripheral smear.

The formula to correct for NRBCs is:

$$\frac{\text{Automated WBC count} \times 100}{(\text{NRBC per 100 WBCs}) + 100}$$

HOW **_Example 8-6_**

A CBC with manual differential was ordered for a premature newborn born at 36 weeks of gestation. Twenty-six NRBCs were counted in the differential. The baby's WBC count was 27.5 (10^9/L). What is the corrected WBC count?

To solve this problem, use the previous formula:

$$\frac{(27.5)(100)}{(26) + 100} = 21.8\,(10^9/L)\,\text{WBC count}$$

Therefore the corrected WBC count is 21.8 (10^9/L).

WHAT **CELL COUNTING BY THE HEMACYTOMETER METHOD**

The majority of RBC, WBC, and platelet counts are performed by automated hematology analyzers. Occasionally, the count may be too low for the instrument to count the cells accurately. WBCs in body fluids are often counted manually. In these instances, cells are counted with the aid of a microscope using a counting chamber called a hemacytometer (Figure 8-1). The most common hemacytometer used in clinical hematology is the Neubauer hemacytometer. This hemacytometer consists of two identical counting chambers. Each chamber contains an etched grid constructed to have a total surface area of 9 mm². The chambers are identical, so that a sample can be counted in duplicate using the same hemacytometer. The count from each chamber should be within 10% of each other to ensure an accurate count. A dilution of whole blood is used, and a small amount of diluted sample is allowed to flow between the coverslip and hemacytometer chamber. The distance between the coverslip and the surface of the hemacytometer is 0.1 mm.

Figure 8-1 is a schematic of a Neubauer hemacytometer grid in which each of the large squares is numbered 1 to 9. WBCs are counted in the four corner squares (Nos. 1, 3, 7, and 9), whereas platelets and RBCs are counted in the central square (No. 5). Each large square is 1 mm² in area. The large squares are further divided into 16 smaller squares to facilitate ease of counting the

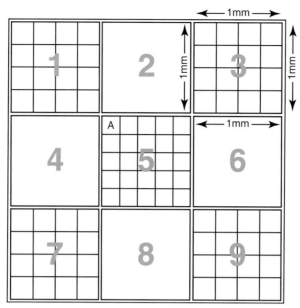

FIGURE 8-1 Neubauer hemacytometer.

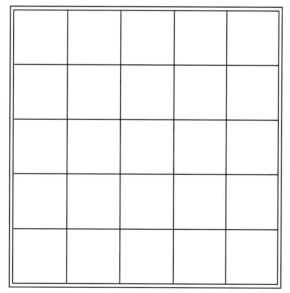

FIGURE 8-2 Enlargement of square A in Neubauer hemacytometer.

WBCs. The center square is divided into 25 small squares. Each of the 25 small squares is further divided into 16 smaller squares for RBC and platelet counting. The small square A is shown enlarged in Figure 8-2.

WHAT **White Blood Cell Count**

When the WBC count is abnormally elevated or decreased or the quantity of WBCs in fluid is requested, the hemacytometer method may be used to quantify the total WBC count. Using a micropipette, a $1/20$ dilution is usually used when counting the total WBC count. Occasionally, a

$^1/_{10}$ dilution is performed if the WBC count is abnormally decreased, and a $^1/_{100}$ dilution may be used if the WBC count is abnormally increased. WBCs are counted using high-power or $400\times$ magnification in each of the 16 smaller squares contained in each of the four corner squares. The area of each large square is 1 mm^2, and the depth is 0.1 mm. Therefore the volume in each large square is 0.1 mm^3 (volume = area × depth). Both sides of the hemocytometer are charged with the dilution and both sides are counted.

The mathematical formula to calculate the number of cells per cubic millimeter is as follows:

$$\text{No. cells/mm}^3 = \frac{\text{No. cells counted} \times \text{depth factor} \times \text{dilution factor}}{\text{Total area counted}}$$

where:
Area counted = number of large squares counted
Depth factor = reciprocal of depth $[1/(1/10)] = 10$
Dilution factor = reciprocal of dilution

The WBC count reference interval in adults is 4-11 (10^9/L)
Note: The number of WBCs counted *per side* should be within 20% of each other.
There are two ways to use this formula: The first is to add the number of WBCs counted on *both* sides of the hemocytometer and use the sum. The area counted would be 8 for the total area counted (4 squares per side). The second is to take the average of the number of WBCs counted on *each* side of the hemocytomter and average them. If the average of both sides is taken, then the total area counted should be 4, not 8.

HOW   **Example 8-7**

A WBC count was performed on a sample that was abnormally decreased below the linearity of the automated cell counter. A $^1/_{10}$ dilution was performed, and all WBCs in each of the four corner squares of both grids of the hemacytometer were counted. The sum of 75 WBCs was counted. What is the total WBC count?
In this problem, all eight squares were counted; therefore the area counted would be 8. The dilution factor would be 10, as a $^1/_{10}$ dilution was performed. Substituting into the basic formula for cell counting, the following equation is derived:

$$\text{\# WBC } (10^9/\text{L}) = \frac{75 \text{ WBCs counted} \times 10(\text{depth factor}) \times 10(\text{dilution factor})}{8(\text{total area counted})}$$

$$\text{\# WBC } (10^9/\text{L}) = 938$$

Example 8-7a   A manual WBC count was performed using a $^1/_{100}$ dilution; 145 cells were counted on one side and 149 cells were counted on the other side using the four large squares of the hemocytometer on each side. The average was calculated and determined to be 147 cells. The following equation is used to calculate the WBC count:

$$\text{\# WBC } (10^9/\text{L}) = \frac{147 \text{ WBCs counted} \times 10(\text{depth factor}) \times 100(\text{dilution factor})}{4(\text{total area counted})}$$

$$\text{\# WBC } (10^9/\text{L}) = 36,750$$

WHAT   *Factor Method*

For many WBC counts, the dilution performed is $^1/_{20}$, and all WBCs within the four corner squares are counted. Therefore within the volume in one large square is the amount of WBCs per $^1/_{200}$ 10^9/L (or mm^3) of blood (0.1 mm^3 × $^1/_{20}$). This amount is multiplied by the quantities of squares counted (four). Thus the typical WBC count quantifies the amount of WBCs per 50 (10^9/L) ($^1/_{200}$ × 4) of blood. The factor of 50 can be used to quickly calculate the WBC count using a hemacytometer. Simply multiply the total number of cells counted in the four large squares times 50 to yield the total WBC count (10^9/L).

> **NOTE:** This "factor" of 50 can only be used if the dilution performed is $^1/_{20}$ and all WBCs in the four large corner squares are counted.

The mathematical formula to calculate the factor is as follows:

Factor = 1/area × depth factor × dilution factor

Area counted = number of large squares counted

Depth factor = reciprocal of depth $[1/(1/10)]$ = 10

Dilution factor = reciprocal of dilution = $[1/(1/20)]$ = 20

$$\text{Therefore the factor} = \frac{1}{4} \times 10 \times 20 = 50$$

HOW   *Example 8-8*

A WBC count was performed using a hemacytometer and a $^1/_{20}$ dilution. There were 140 WBCs counted in the four large squares. Using the factor method, what is the total WBC count?

$$\text{The factor} = \frac{1}{4} \times 10 \times 20 = 50$$

Multiply the amount of cells counted by the factor of 50:

$$50 \times 140 = 7.0 \times 10^9 /\text{L or } 7000/\text{mm}^3$$

Therefore the WBC count is 7.0 (10^9/L). There are three ways that WBCs might be reported. Using SI units, the WBC count is reported as 7.0 × 10^9/L. Conventional units are 7.0 × 10^3/mcL, and an older way is 7.0 × 10^3/mm^3. The units are all equal in value as 1 mm^3 is equal to 1 mcL.

Example 8-8a   A manual WBC count was performed by a medical laboratory technician/ clinical laboratory technician student in a student laboratory experiment. The four large squares of one side of a hemacytometer were used, and the dilution used was $^1/_{20}$. The student counted 82 cells. What is the WBC count using the factor method?

Since the four large squares were used, and the dilution was $^1/_{20}$, the factor method can be used.

$$82 \times 50 = 4100/\text{mm}^3 = 4100/\text{mcL} = 4.1 \text{ WBCs} \times 10^9/\text{L}$$

Example 8-8b   A manual WBC count was performed by a medical laboratory technologist/clinical laboratory scientist student in a student laboratory experiment. The four large squares of one side of a hemacytometer were used, and the dilution was $^1/_{20}$. The student counted 135 cells. What is the WBC count using the factor method?

Since the four large squares were used, and the dilution was $^1/_{20}$, the factor method can be used.

$$135 \times 50 = 6.75 \text{ WBCs} \times 10^9/\text{L}$$

WHAT **Platelet Count**

Platelets are small fragments of cells found in the bone marrow called megakaryocytes. Platelets function in the initial phase of the coagulation process. The reference interval for platelets is 150 to 400 ($10^9/\text{L}$). All 25 squares in the central square of the hemacytometer are used to count platelets. Remember that within each of the 25 squares, there are 16 smaller squares, so the total amount of squares counted for platelets will be 400. As each of the 25 squares has an area of 0.04 mm^2, and all 25 squares are counted, the total area counted is 1 mm^2 (0.04 × 25). A $^1/_{100}$ dilution is performed on the whole blood for platelet counting. Just as for WBC and RBC counts, platelet counts can also have a calculated factor.

The mathematical formula for the factor for platelets is as follows:

Factor = 1/area × depth factor × dilution factor
Area counted = area of small squares counted (sum of five squares on *each* side of hemocytometer for a total of 10 squares)
Depth factor = reciprocal of depth [1/(1/10)] = 10
Dilution factor = reciprocal of dilution = [1/(1/100)] = 100

$$\text{Therefore the factor} = \frac{1}{1.0} \times 10 \times 100 = 1000$$

HOW   ***Example 8-9***

A platelet count was performed using a $^1/_{100}$ dilution and counting all platelets found in the 400 smallest squares of the central square in the hemacytometer; 150 platelets were counted. Using the factor method, what is the platelet count?

The factor for platelets is 1000. As 150 platelets were counted, the total platelet count is as follows:

$$150 \times 1000 = 150,000/\text{mm}^3$$

Example 8-9a   A platelet count was performed using a $^1/_{100}$ dilution and counting all platelets found in the 400 smallest squares of the central square of the hemacytometer; 85 platelets were counted. Using the factor method, what is the platelet count?

The factor for platelets is 1000. Therefore the platelet count is 1000 × 85 or 85,000/mm^3.

Example 8-9b   A platelet count was performed using a $^1/_{100}$ dilution and counting all of the platelets found in the 400 smallest squares of the central square of the hemacytometer by a medical technologist/clinical laboratory scientist student in a student laboratory. There were 274 platelets counted. Using the factor method, what is the platelet count?

The platelet count is 1000×274 or $274,000/mm^3$.

WHAT BODY FLUIDS

RBC, WBC, and platelet counts are not the only cell counts performed in the hematology laboratory. Cells from cerebrospinal fluid (CSF), transudates, and exudates, along with semen analysis, may be performed. The hemacytometer is used to count both RBCs and WBCs in the different types of fluids and to provide both qualitative and quantitative sperm counts.

Cell Counts for CSF Specimens

When a spinal tap is performed, three sterile tubes are collected and labeled 1, 2, and 3 in the order they are drawn. The first tube (Tube 1) will be sent to the chemistry laboratory for glucose and total protein analysis, and/or serology laboratory; Tube 2 will be sent to the microbiology laboratory for culture; and Tube 3 will be sent to the hematology laboratory for WBC and RBC counts. CSF cell counts should be performed within 1 hour of collection for the most accurate results. If that is not possible, the CSF tubes for hematology should be refrigerated. Some hematology analyzers, but not all, can perform cell counts on CSF and other body fluid specimens, which eliminates the need for manual cell counts.

WHAT Cell Counts for Synovial, Pleural, Pericardial, and Peritoneal Fluid

Samples for these fluids are usually collected in a heparinized or an EDTA tube. Table 8-1 contains the body fluid normal results.

TABLE 8-1 Normal Body Fluid Results

	Cerebrospinal Fluid		Serous (Pleural, Pericardial, Peritoneal)	Synovial
	Adult	**Neonate**		
Appearance	Clear and colorless	Clear and colorless	Pale yellow and clear	Pale yellow and clear
Red blood cell	$0–1/mm^3$	$0–3/mm^3$	$0–1/mm^3$	$0–1/mm^3$
White blood cell	$0–5/mm^3$	$0–30/mm^3$	$0–200/mm^3$	$0–200/mm^3$
Neutrophils (includes bands)	2%–6%	0%–8%	<25%	<25%
Lymphs	40%–80%	5%–35%	<25%	<25%
Monocytes	5%–45%	50%–90%	Included with others	Included with others
Others	Rare	Rare	Monocytes and macrophages 65%–75%	Monocytes and macrophages 65%–75%

From Ciesla B: *Hematology in practice*, ed 2, Philadelphia, 2011, FA Davis, p. 317, with permission.

Dilutions Associated With Body Fluids

Some fluid specimens may be clear enough that no dilution is necessary. Other fluid specimens must be diluted before analysis. The amount of dilution will depend on the appearance of the fluid. Unlike WBC dilutions, no acetic acid is used. Saline is used instead to dilute the fluids for analysis, and some laboratories use a small amount of methylene blue, or crystal violet is added to stain the nuclei of the WBCs for easier counting. Synovial fluid may have hyaluronidase added to it to reduce the viscosity of this fluid. Once diluted, the fluid is added to a hemacytometer chamber. How many squares to count may depend on the type and condition of the fluid and the policy of the laboratory. Table 8-2 and the dilution directions that follow present a unique method and calculation reference for performing fluid counts. Table 8-3 is an example of a completed worksheet.

To determine which dilution method to use, follow these directions:

Based on the gross appearance of the fluid, dilute the specimen by one of the following methods. Volumetric pipettes and hematocrit tubes are used by this unique method.

Method A: (Clear or Slightly Cloudy Fluid)

1. Dilute 1 to 2 with crystal violet (0.2 mL specimen and 0.2 mL crystal violet).

Method B: (Moderately Cloudy Fluid)

1. Dilute 1 to 11 with saline (0.1 mL specimen and 1.0 mL saline). Then dilute 1 to 2 with crystal violet (0.2 mL of a 1 to 11 dilution + 0.2 mL crystal violet).

Method C: (Very Cloudy or Bloody Fluid)

1. Dilute 1 to 101 with saline (0.1 mL specimen with 10.0 mL saline. Then dilute 1 to 2 with crystal violet (0.2 mL of a 1 to 101 dilution + 0.2 crystal violet).

TABLE 8-2 Reference Factors for Fluid Calculations

	Multiplication Factors		
Total No. of Squares Counted	**Method A**	**Method B**	**Method C**
1	×20	×220	×2020
2	×10	×110	×1010
3	×6.7	×73.3	×673.3
4	×5.0	×55	×505
5	×4.0	×44	×404
6	×3.3	×36.7	×336.7
7	×2.9	×31.4	×288.6
8	×2.5	×27.5	×252.5
9	×2.2	×24.4	×224.4
10 Small center	×100	×1100	×10,100
11 Small center	×50	×550	×5050

From Ciesla B: *Hematology in practice*, ed 2, Philadelphia, 2011, FA Davis, p. 315, with permission.

TABLE 8-3 **Body Fluid Worksheet**

	Dilution A, B, or C	No. of Squares Counted	No. of Cells		Average No. of Cells	Calculation	Result/ mcL
			Count 1	Count 2			
WBC							
RBC							

2. Fill each side of a hemacytometer chamber with the dilution. Place the hemacytometer in a premoistened petri dish. Allow the cells to settle for 3 to 5 minutes in the petri dish.
3. Place the hemacytometer on the microscope stage. Determining the number of squares to count depends on the initial viewing of the fluid on the hemacytometer under the microscope. This is the judgment of the technologist/technician.
4. Using the 20× or 40× objective, count the WBCs and RBCs on each side. Now enter the WBC and RBC of each dilution in the body fluid worksheet (see Table 8-3).
5. The WBC and RBC count of each side must agree within 10%. If not, reload the chamber and recount the fluid.
6. The average of the two WBC counts and the average of the two RBC counts is determined.

NOTE: If the RBCs are too numerous to count, record them as TNTC.

7. Use **Table 8-3** to calculate the WBC and RBC count. This final result will depend on the amount of squares counted and the method used.

HOW **Example 8-10**

A WBC count was performed on cloudy pleural fluid with a patient with pneumonia. The sample was diluted using method C; 40 WBCs were counted in the four corner squares on one side of the hemacytometer, and 48 WBCs were counted in the four corner squares on the other side of the hemacytometer. What is this patient's pleural fluid WBC count?

When performing a fluid count, each side of the hemacytometer is counted and the results must match within 10%. If they do not match, the count should be repeated by reloading the hemacytometer. If they do match within 10%, then they are averaged and that result is multiplied by the factor that is dependent on the method of dilution, and the number of squares counted shown in **Table 8-2**. In this example, the WBCs average 44, and the factor used is 505. Therefore the WBC count is 22,220 mcL. The following table shows how **Table 8-3** can be used as a worksheet to determine the cell count.

	Dilution A, B, or C	No. of Squares Counted	No. of Cells		Average No. of Cells	Calculation	Result/ mcL
			Count 1	Count 2			
WBC	C	4	40	48	44	44 × 505	22,220 mcL

Example 8-10a The RBC count on the pleural fluid from the same patient used in Example 8-10 was performed. Nine squares were counted on each side of the hemacytometer. There were 22 RBCs seen on one side and 26 RBCs seen on the other side. What is the patient's RBC pleural fluid count?

Using **Table 8-3**:

| | | | No. of Cells | | | | |
	Dilution A, B, or C	No. of Squares Counted	Count 1	Count 2	Average No. of Cells	Calculation	Result/ mcL
RBC	C	9	22	26	24	24 × 224.4	5386 mcL

The patient's pleural fluid RBC count is **5386/mcL**.

Example 8-10b Calculate a patient's WBC and RBC count in a clear CSF specimen to complete the following chart:

| | | | No. of Cells | | | | |
	Dilution A, B, or C	No. of Squares Counted	Count 1	Count 2	Average No. of Cells	Calculation	Result/ mcL
WBC	A	9	12	16			
RBC	A	9	06	09			

The results are:

| | | | No. of Cells | | | | |
	Dilution A, B, or C	No. of Squares Counted	Count 1	Count 2	Average No. of Cells	Calculation	Result/ mcL
WBC	A	9	12	16	14	14 × 2.2	31/mcL
RBC	A	9	06	09	7.5	7.5 × 2.2	16/mcL

Therefore the WBC count is 31/mcL and the RBC count is 16/mcL.

WHAT Correction for Contamination in CSF Cell Counts

Sometimes when a spinal tap is performed, a capillary may be nicked in the process. This will result in a bloody tap, and the CSF will appear bloody to some degree. Some laboratories will correct the WBC and CSF protein count depending on the degree of the contaminating bleed. The ratio of WBC to RBC in whole blood is compared with the ratio of the RBCs and WBCs in the spinal fluid. To correct for the added WBCs, use the following formula:

$$\text{WBCs (added)} = \text{WBC (blood)} \times \frac{\text{RBC (CSF)}}{\text{RBC (blood)}}$$

HOW   *Example 8-11*

A bloody tap was performed and a CSF RBC count of 3000/mm^3 was obtained (10^9/L is the SI unit). The peripheral blood RBC count was 4.2×10^{12}/L. The peripheral blood WBC count was 5.1×10^9/L. How many WBCs were added due to the bloody tap?

Using the formula:

$$\text{WBCs (added)} = 5100/\text{mm}^3 \times \frac{3000/\text{mm}^3}{4.2 \times 10^{12}/\text{L}}$$

$$\text{WBCs added} = 3.6 \times 10^9/\text{L} \left(\text{or } 3600 \text{ mm}^3\right)$$

Now, in this example, the peripheral blood WBC count was 5.1×10^9/L. The true CSF WBC count is 5.1×10^9/L $- 3.6 \times 10^9$/L or 1.6×10^9/L or 1.6×10^9/L.

WHAT **Semen Analysis**

Sperm counts are performed in the hematology laboratory to determine male fertility. Sperm are the male reproductive cells that are in semen. In an average ejaculation, there are more than 40 million sperm, and the average semen volume per ejaculate is 2 to 5 mL. There are two main counts that are performed: (1) the sperm concentration per milliliter, and (2) the sperm count per ejaculate. Fresh semen samples must liquefy within 1 hour of collection for an accurate sperm count to be performed.

Sperm Concentration per Milliliter

The liquefied semen sample is counted by diluting it $^1/_{20}$ in a diluting fluid that contains formalin and sodium bicarbonate. It is counted similarly to RBC in whole blood using a Neubauer hemacytometer; that is, within the large center square, the four corner squares and the center square are used. Both sides of the chamber are counted and the results must match within 10%. By counting the sperm in the five small squares on each side, averaging the result, and using a $^1/_{20}$ dilution, a factor of 1 million can be used to determine the amount of sperm per milliliter.

HOW   *Example 8-12*

A sperm count was performed using a $^1/_{20}$ dilution, with the five small squares used for each side. The average count was 72 sperm. What is the sperm count per milliliter?

The sperm count per milliliter $= 72 \times 1,000,000 = 72,000,000$/mL or 7.2×10^7/mL.

Example 8-12a   A sperm count was performed using a $^1/_{20}$ dilution, with the five small squares used for each side. The average count was 112 sperm. What is the sperm count per milliliter?

The sperm count per milliliter $= 112 \times 1,000,000 = 112,000,000$/mL or 1.12×10^8/mL.

Example 8-12b   A sperm count was performed using a $^1/_{20}$ dilution, with the five small squares used for each side. The average count was 94 sperm. What is the sperm count per milliliter?

The sperm count per milliliter $= 94 \times 1,000,000 = 94,000,000$/mL or 9.4×10^7/mL.

WHAT **Sperm Count per Ejaculation**

The sperm count per ejaculation is calculated by multiplying the sperm count by the semen volume.

HOW **Example 8-13**

Calculate the sperm count per ejaculation using the sperm count determined in Example 8-12 if the semen volume is 3 mL.
    To calculate:

$$\text{Sperm count} \times \text{semen volume} = \text{sperm count per ejaculate}$$
$$7.2 \times 10^7/\text{mL} \times 3 \text{ mL} = 2.16 \times 10^8 \text{ sperm/ejaculate}$$

Therefore, there are 2.16×10^8 sperm per ejaculate.

Example 8-13a Calculate the sperm count per ejaculation if the sperm count is $3.44 \times 10^7/$mL and the semen volume is 2.5 mL.

The sperm count per ejaculate would be $3.44 \times 10^7/\text{mL} \times 2.5 = 8.6 \times 10^7/\text{mL}$.

Example 8-13b Calculate the sperm count per ejaculation if the sperm count is $6.88 \times 10^7/$mL and the semen volume is 2.7 mL.

The sperm count per ejaculation is $6.88 \times 10^7/\text{mL} \times 2.7 = 1.86 \times 10^8/\text{mL}$.

WHAT **RETICULOCYTE COUNT**

Slide Method

Reticulocytes are slightly immature RBCs that usually cannot be distinguished from mature RBCs (erythrocytes) on a Wright-stained smear. Unlike mature RBCs, reticulocytes contain small clumps of ribosomal ribonucleic acid (RNA). The ribosomal RNA can be stained with a supravital stain, such as brilliant cresyl blue or new methylene blue, so that the reticulocytes can be distinguished from mature RBCs. When stained with the supravital stains, the ribosomal RNA looks like blue strands or granules in the RBC. To perform a reticulocyte count, equal amounts of blood and stain are mixed and incubated at room temperature for 10 minutes. A smear is made of the mixture and allowed to air dry. Using the oil immersion lens, 1000 mature RBCs are consecutively counted, and the number of reticulocytes found among the 1000 mature cells is noted. A reticulocyte count is a percentage count of the amount of reticulocytes per 1000 mature RBCs. It is calculated using the following formula:

$$\text{Reticulocytes} = \frac{\text{Number of reticulocytes counted per 1000 erythrocytes}}{1000} \times 100$$

The reference interval for reticulocytes in newborns in 2.0% to 6.0%, and in adults it is 0.5% to 2.0%.

HOW   *Example 8-14*

A reticulocyte count was performed and 38 reticulocytes were counted per 1000 erythrocytes. What is the reticulocyte percentage?

$$\text{No. reticulocytes} = \frac{\text{No. reticulocytes counted per 1000 erythrocytes}}{1000} \times 100$$

$$= \frac{38}{1000} \times 100 = 3.8\%$$

The reticulocyte count is 3.8%.

Example 8-14a   A reticulocyte count was performed and 45 reticulocytes were counted per 1000 erythrocytes. What is the reticulocyte count?

The reticulocyte count can be calculated using the formula:

$$\text{No. reticulocytes} = \frac{\text{No. reticulocytes counted per 1000 erythrocytes}}{1000} \times 100$$

$$= \frac{45}{1000} \times 100 = 4.5\%$$

The reticulocyte count is 4.5%.

Example 8-14b   A reticulocyte count was performed and 22 reticulocytes were counted per 1000 erythrocytes. What is the reticulocyte count?

The reticulocyte count can be calculated using the formula:

$$\text{No. reticulocytes} = \frac{\text{No. reticulocytes counted per 1000 erythrocytes}}{1000} \times 100$$

$$= \frac{22}{1000} \times 100 = 2.2\%$$

The reticulocyte count is 2.2%.

WHAT   **Miller Disk Method**

Another method of counting reticulocytes is the use of a special glass insert for the eyepiece lens of a microscope. The glass insert fits into one of the eyepiece lenses and has a central large square (B) within which is a smaller square (A) in the lower corner (Figure 8-3). The smaller square comprises $1/9$ the area of the larger square. Using random fields where the RBCs are evenly distributed, the reticulocytes found in both the large and small square are quantitated, whereas the amount of RBCs counted in the small square reaches at least 200 cells. The quantity of reticulocytes is determined using the following formula:

$$\% \text{ reticulocytes} = \frac{\text{No. reticulocytes in square Nos. 1 and 2}}{(\text{No. RBCs in square No. 2})(9)} \times 100$$

The factor of 9 is used in the denominator because the ratio of the area in which the RBCs are counted to the total square is 1:9.

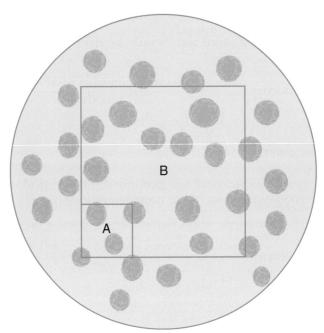

FIGURE 8-3 Miller disk.

Example 8-15

A reticulocyte count was performed on a patient using the Miller disk method. Thirty-five reticulocytes were counted along with 240 red blood cells. What is the patient's reticulocyte count?

Using the formula for calculating reticulocytes using the Miller disk, and substituting into it the data from the problem, the following equation is derived:

$$\% \text{ reticulocytes} = \frac{\text{No. reticulocytes in square Nos. 1 and 2}(35)}{(\text{No. RBCs in square No. 2}[240])(9)} \times 100$$

$$\% \text{ reticulocytes} = \frac{35}{2160} \times 100$$

$$\% \text{ reticulocytes} = 0.016 \times 100$$

$$\% \text{ reticulocytes} = 1.6\%$$

The reticulocyte count is 1.6%.

Example 8-15a A reticulocyte count was performed on a patient using the Miller disk method. There were 42 reticulocytes counted along with 180 RBCs. What is the patient's reticulocyte count?

To solve, use the Miller disk formula:

$$\% \text{ reticulocytes} = \frac{\text{No. reticulocytes in square Nos. 1 and 2}(42)}{(\text{No. RBCs in square No. 2}[180])(9)} \times 100$$

$$\% \text{ reticulocytes} = \frac{42}{1620} \times 100$$

$$\% \text{ reticulocytes} = 0.0259 \times 100$$

$$\% \text{ reticulocytes} = 2.6\%$$

Therefore the reticulocyte count is 2.6%.

Example 8-15b   A reticulocyte count was performed using the Miller disk method. There were 40 reticulocytes counted along with 198 RBCs. What is the patient's reticulocyte count?

Using the Miller disk formula, the result is 2.2%.

WHAT **Reticulocyte Count Correction for Anemia: Reticulocyte Index**

The bone marrow produces RBCs to replace those in the circulation that are damaged at a rate of about 1% per day. This is reflected by the normal reticulocyte count of approximately 0.5% to 1%. In cases of anemia, the total number of mature RBCs is decreased. This is reflected in a decreased hematocrit in patients with anemia. Because the reticulocyte count is based on the assumption that the RBC count is normal, a falsely elevated reticulocyte count may result in cases of anemia. A mathematical factor, the reticulocyte index, can correct the reticulocyte count in cases with abnormally low hematocrits by dividing the patient's hematocrit by 45 (the average normal hematocrit). The patient's reticulocyte count is multiplied by the reticulocyte index to correct for the decreased hematocrit.

HOW ***Example 8-16***

A patient with a hematocrit of 30% had a reticulocyte count of 6%. Using the reticulocyte index, what is the patient's corrected hematocrit?

$$\text{Corrected reticulocyte count} = \text{Patient's relative reticulocyte count} \times \frac{\text{patient's Hct}}{45}$$

$$\text{Corrected reticulocyte count} = 6\% \times \frac{30}{45}$$

$$\text{Corrected reticulocyte count} = 6\% \times 0.67$$

$$\text{Corrected reticulocyte count} = 4\%$$

Example 8-16a   A patient with a hematocrit of 27% had a reticulocyte count of 4.5%. Using the reticulocyte index, what is the patient's corrected reticulocyte count?

$$\text{Corrected reticulocyte count} = \text{Patient's reticulocyte count} \times \frac{\text{patient's Hct}}{45}$$

$$\text{Corrected reticulocyte count} = 4.5\% \times \frac{27}{45}$$

$$\text{Corrected reticulocyte count} = 4.5\% \times 0.60$$

$$\text{Corrected reticulocyte count} = 2.7\%$$

The patient's corrected reticulocyte count is 2.7%.

Example 8-16b   A patient had a hematocrit of 18% and a reticulocyte count of 2.1%. Using the reticulocyte index, what is the patient's corrected reticulocyte count?

The patient's corrected reticulocyte count is 0.8%.

TABLE 8-4 Red Blood Cell Production Index

Hematocrit (%)	Maturation Time (days)
40–45	1
35–39	1.5
25–34	2.0
15–24	2.5
<15	3

From Rodak BF, Fritsma GA, Doig K: *Hematology, clinical principles and applications,* ed 3, St. Louis, 2007, WB Saunders, p. 171.

WHAT   **Reticulocyte Correction for Increased Reticulocyte Production**

In many cases of anemia, the bone marrow tries to compensate by releasing young reticulocytes into the circulation earlier than usual. These young reticulocytes are called shift reticulocytes because the bone marrow has "shifted" toward prematurely releasing reticulocytes in an effort to correct the effects of the anemia. These shifted reticulocytes are larger than older reticulocytes and mature RBCs. They may have a slight bluish tinge to them in a Wright-stained smear. The reticulocyte count must be corrected for these shift reticulocytes because they are in the circulation longer than more mature reticulocytes. In addition, when shift reticulocytes are present, the patient usually has a decreased hematocrit, and the reticulocyte count must be corrected for the hematocrit as well. Table 8-4 shows the length of time in the peripheral blood the shift reticulocytes are present based on the hematocrit.

Using Table 8-4, the reticulocyte production index (RPI) can be calculated. This index is a good indication of the effective RBC production. The index formula combines both the reticulocyte index calculation with the factor for maturation. The following is the formula for the RPI:

$$\text{RPI} = \frac{\text{Reticulocyte count} \times \text{ reticulocyte index}}{\text{Maturation factor (from Table 8-4)}}$$

HOW   ***Example 8-17***

A patient had a reticulocyte count of 6% and a hematocrit of 25%. Shift reticulocytes were found when the cell differential was performed. Calculate the RPI for this patient.

$$\text{RPI} = \frac{\text{Reticulocyte count (6\%)} \times \text{ reticulocyte index (25\% \div 45\%)}}{\text{Maturation time correction (2.0)}}$$

$$\text{RPI} = \frac{3.33}{2}$$

$$\text{RPI} = 1.7\%$$

The initial reticulocyte count was 6%. However, when corrected for the patient's low hematocrit and increased production of reticulocytes, the RBC production index gives a clearer indication of the patient's true reticulocyte count of **1.7%**.

Example 8-17a   Using Example 8-17 as a guide, calculate the RPI for a patient with a reticulocyte count of 4.0% and a hematocrit of 20%.

The RPI for this patient is 0.71%.

Example 8-17b   Calculate the RPI for a patient with a reticulocyte count of 4.5% and a hematocrit of 26%.

The RPI for this patient is 1.3%.

WHAT # INTERNATIONAL NORMALIZED RATIO

In the coagulation laboratory, the prothrombin time (PT) is one of the most commonly performed tests. The prothrombin test uses thromboplastin as a reagent, and the thromboplastin comes from a variety of sources. What this means is that each lot of thromboplastin will have slightly different concentrations, and therefore the prothrombin times in the laboratory will reflect the slight difference. The thromboplastin is calibrated against a World Health Organization standard and given an International Standardization Index (ISI).

The difference in the thromboplastin can be a problem if a patient has a prothrombin test performed in different laboratories where each laboratory uses different thromboplastin, especially if that patient is on anticoagulant therapy. The physician cannot be sure, if there is a difference in the PT time, whether it is due to an actual change in the patient or due to the inherent difference between the laboratories. By using the International Normalized Ratio (INR), the difference between laboratories is smoothed out or "normalized." The INR is calculated by the coagulation instruments; it is not a calculation that is commonly performed by the clinical laboratory personnel and is used primarily for patients on warfarin (Coumadin). The formula for the INR is:

$$\left(\frac{\text{Patient's PT value}}{\text{Laboratory's mean PT value}}\right)^{\text{ISI}}$$

The recommended INR for a patient on warfarin is 2 to 3.

HOW *Example 8-18*

A patient on warfarin had a prothrombin time of 25.2 seconds. The laboratory's mean PT value is 12.7, and the ISI value for the thromboplastin used in the prothrombin assay is 1.287. Calculate the INR value for this patient.

Using the formula, or the numerous online INR calculators, the patient's INR is 2.4.

HOW # EXAMPLE PROBLEMS

This section is designed to be useful to both the student and the laboratory professional. Students can use the additional problems to master the material. The laboratory professional can use the examples as templates for solving laboratory calculations. By finding an example similar to the problem that you need to solve, substitute into the equation the numbers appropriate to your calculation.

1. **Q.** Calculate the mean corpuscular volume (MCV) of a sample if the hematocrit (Hct) is 25% and the RBC count is 4.6 (10^{12}/L).
   A. The MCV is calculated from the following formula:

$$\text{MCV (fL)} = \frac{\text{Hct} \times 10}{\text{RBC count}}$$

Substituting into the formula, the data from the problem yields the following:

$$\text{MCV (fL)} = \frac{25 \times 10}{4.6}$$

$$\text{MCV (fL)} = 54.3 \text{ fL}$$

2. **Q.** Calculate the MCV of a sample with a hematocrit of 46% and an RBC count of 4.5 $(10^{12}/\text{L})$.

   A. Using the formula for MCV, the following equation is derived:

$$\text{MCV (fL)} = \frac{46\% \times 10}{4.5(10^{12}/\text{L})}$$

$$\text{MCV (fL)} = 102.2 \text{ fL}$$

3. **Q.** Calculate the MCV of a sample with a hematocrit of 32% and an RBC count of 3.8 $(10^{12}/\text{L})$.

   A. The MCV is 84.2 fL.

4. **Q.** Calculate the mean corpuscular hemoglobin (MCH) of a sample with a hemoglobin of 16 g/dL and an RBC count of 4.2 $(10^{12}/\text{L})$.

   A. The MCH is calculated by the following formula:

$$\text{MCH (pg)} = \frac{\text{Hemoglobin (g/dL)} \times 10}{\text{RBC count }(10^{12}/\text{L})}$$

$$\text{MCH (pg)} = \frac{16 \times 10}{4.2}$$

$$\text{MCH (pg)} = 38.1 \text{ pg}$$

5. **Q.** Calculate the MCH of a sample with a hemoglobin (Hb) of 20 g/dL and an RBC count of 5.0 $(10^{12}/\text{L})$.

   A. Using the formula:

$$\text{MCH (pg)} = \frac{20 \text{ g/dL} \times 10}{5.0(10^{12}/\text{L})}$$

$$\text{MCH (pg)} = 40.0 \text{ pg}$$

6. **Q.** Calculate the MCH of a sample with a hemoglobin of 27 g/dL and an RBC count of 4.4 $(10^{12}/\text{L})$.

   A. The MCH is 61.4 pg.

7. **Q.** Calculate the MCHC of a sample with a hemoglobin concentration of 15 g/dL and a hematocrit of 45%.

   A. The MCHC is calculated by the following formula:

$$\text{MCHC (\%)} = \frac{\text{Hb (g/dL)} \times 100}{\text{Hematocrit (\%)}}$$

Substituting into the formula the data from the problem:

$$MCHC\ (\%) = \frac{15 \times 100}{45\%}$$

$$MCHC\ (\%) = 33.3\ g/dL$$

8. Q. Calculate the MCHC of a sample with a hemoglobin of 18 g/dL and a hematocrit of 52%.
   A. 34.6 g/dL

9. Q. A WBC count was performed on a $^1/20$ dilution using the four corner squares of the hemacytometer. The number of WBCs counted was 185. What is the total number of WBCs?
   A. As the WBC count was performed using the standard dilution and counting technique, the total WBC count is the sum of 185×50 or $9250/mm^3$ or $9.250 \times 10^9/L$.

10. Q. A manual WBC count was performed on a sample from a patient with a history of low WBC counts. A $^1/10$ dilution was performed and the number of WBCs found in all nine squares was counted; 58 WBCs were counted. What is the patient's total WBC count?
    A. The factor method cannot be used to calculate this patient's WBC count because the standard parameters were not used. The formula for calculating cells/mm^3 is as follows:

$$No.\ cells \times 10^9/L = \frac{No.\ cells\ counted \times depth\ factor \times dilution\ factor}{Area\ counted}$$

In this case, the number of cells counted is 58; the depth factor is still 10; the dilution factor is 10, not 20; and the total area counted is 9, not 4. Therefore, by substituting into the formula the data known, the total WBC count can be calculated:

$$No.\ WBCs \times 10^9/L = 644$$

11. Q. A WBC count was performed using a hemacytometer and a $^1/20$ dilution. There were 172 WBCs counted in the four large corner squares of the hemacytometer. Using the factor method, what is the total WBC count?
    A. The mathematical formula to calculate the factor is as follows:
    Factor = 1/area × depth factor × dilution factor
    Area counted = number of large squares counted
    Depth factor = reciprocal of depth [1/(1/10)] = 10
    Dilution factor = reciprocal of dilution = [1/(1/20)] = 20

$$Therefore\ the\ factor = \left(\frac{1}{4}\right)(10)(20) = 50$$

Therefore the number of cells counted (172) times the factor (50) is equal to the total WBC count: $172 \times 50 = 8600/mm^3$ or $8.6 \times 10^9/L$.

NOTE: The factor method can only be used to count WBCs if the dilution performed is $^1/20$ and all WBCs in the four large corner squares are counted.

12. **Q.** A WBC count was performed using a $^1/_{20}$ dilution. All WBCs in the four large corner squares of the hemacytometer were counted, resulting in a count of 294 WBCs. What is the total WBC count?

    A. Because the dilution performed was $^1/_{20}$ and all WBCs within the four large corner squares of the hemacytometer were counted, the factor method can be used. The total WBC count is equal to the factor of 50 multiplied by the number of WBCs counted. Therefore the total WBC count is 14,700/mm^3 or the equivalent units of 14.7 × 10^9/L.

13. **Q.** A platelet count was performed using a $^1/_{100}$ dilution and counting all platelets found in the 400 smallest squares of the central square in the hemacytometer. There were 375 platelets counted. What is the platelet count?

    A. A factor can also be used to calculate platelets. However, the dilution performed must be a $^1/_{100}$ dilution, and all platelets must be counted that are found in the 25 smallest squares within the central square. Each of the 25 squares is further divided into 16 squares. Therefore the total number of squares counted is 400 (16 × 25). The mathematical formula for the factor for platelets is as follows:

Factor = 1/area × depth factor × dilution factor
Area counted = area of small squares counted (0.04 × 25 = 1 mm^2)
Depth factor = reciprocal of depth [1/(1/10)] = 10
Dilution factor = reciprocal of dilution = [1/(1/100)] = 100

$$\text{Therefore the factor} = \left(\frac{1}{1.0}\right)(10)(100) = 1000$$

The number of platelets counted is multiplied by the factor to calculate the total platelet count

$$375 \times 1000 = 375,000/\text{mm}^3 \text{ or } 375 \times 10^3/\text{mcL or } 375 \times 10^9/\text{L}$$

14. **Q.** A platelet count was performed using a $^1/_{100}$ dilution. There were 150 platelets counted in the platelet counting area of the hemacytometer. What is the total platelet count?

    A. The factor method can be used for this problem because all standard parameters were used. The number of platelets counted (150) multiplied by the factor of 1000 is equal to a platelet count of 150,000/mm^3 or 150 ×10^3/mcL or 150 × 10^9/L.

15. **Q.** A platelet count was performed on a patient on chemotherapy. A $^1/_{50}$ dilution was performed. All 400 small squares within the central square were counted for a total of 13 platelets. What is the total platelet count?

    A. The factor method cannot be used to solve this problem because a $^1/_{50}$ dilution, not $^1/_{100}$, was performed. Instead, use the following formula:

$$\text{No. cells} \times 10^9/\text{L} = \frac{\text{No. cells counted} \times \text{depth factor} \times \text{dilution factor}}{\text{Area counted}}$$

$$\text{No. cells} \times 10^9/\text{L} = \frac{13 \times 10 \times 50}{1 \text{ mm}^2}$$

$$\text{No. cells} \times 10^9/\text{L} = 6.5 \times 10^9/\text{L}$$

16. **Q.** A WBC count was performed on a clear CSF specimen. Method A was used to perform the dilution, and an average of 18 cells were counted in a total of eight large squares. The factor was determined to be 2.5. What is the CSF WBC count?
    A. The WBC fluid count can be determined by multiplying the number of WBCs by a factor that is determined by both the method of dilution and the amount of squares counted. Since method A was used, and eight squares were counted, the factor is 2.5. Therefore $2.5 \times 18 = 45/\text{mcL}$ WBCs in the CSF specimen.

17. **Q.** Calculate the sperm count per milliliter in a sample that was diluted $1/20$ and counted in the five small RBC squares in a Neubauer hemacytometer. Both sides of the hemacytometer were counted, and the average was 62 sperm. What is the sperm count per milliliter?
    A. As with WBC, RBC, and platelet counts, a factor can be used to calculate the concentration of sperm per milliliter. Since the dilution was $1/20$ and the five small squares were used, and the concentration is in milliliters, the factor is 1 million. Therefore the sperm concentration per milliliter is 62 million/mL or $6.2 \times 10^7/\text{mL}$.

18. **Q.** Calculate the sperm concentration per milliliter in a semen specimen that was diluted $1/20$. There were 51 sperm counted in the five small squares used for RBC counts. What is the sperm concentration?
    A. The sperm concentration is 51 million/mL or $5.1 \times 10^7/\text{mL}$.

19. **Q.** Calculate the sperm count per ejaculate using the sperm concentration in Example Problem 17 and a semen volume of 2.5 mL.
    A. The sperm count per ejaculate is calculated by multiplying the sperm count per milliliter by the semen volume. Therefore the sperm count per ejaculate is 62 million/mL × 2.5 mL, or $1.55 \times 10^8/\text{mL}$.

20. **Q.** Calculate the sperm count per ejaculate using the information from Example Problem 18 if there was a semen volume of 3.0 mL.
    A. The sperm count per ejaculate is $1.5 \times 10^8/\text{mL}$.

21. **Q.** A reticulocyte count was performed, and 17 reticulocytes were counted per 1000 RBCs. What is the reticulocyte percentage?
    A. The formula to calculate reticulocytes is as follows:

$$\frac{\text{Number of reticulocytes counted per 1000 erythrocytes}}{1000} \times 100$$

Using the formula, and substituting the data from the problem:

$$\frac{17}{1000} \times 100 = 1.7\%$$

Therefore the reticulocyte count is 1.7%.

22. **Q.** A reticulocyte count is performed, and 24 reticulocytes are found among 1000 mature RBCs. What is the reticulocyte percentage?
    A. Using the formula for reticulocytes:

$$\frac{24}{1000} \times 100 = 2.4\%$$

Therefore the reticulocyte percentage is 2.4%.

23. **Q.** A reticulocyte count was performed using the Miller disk method. Twenty-six reticulocytes were counted along with 210 RBCs. What is the patient's reticulocyte count?

A. The Miller disk is a calibrated glass insert for the eyepiece lens of the microscope. The glass insert has a large center square (No. 1) within which is a smaller square (No. 2) in the lower corner. The reticulocytes within both the large and small squares are counted, until the number of RBCs counted only in the small corner square (No. 2) reaches at least 200 cells. The following formula is used to determine the percent of reticulocytes with a Miller disk:

$$\frac{\text{No. reticulocytes in square Nos. 1 and 2(or small and large squares)}}{(\text{No. RBCs in square No. 2})(9)} \times 100$$

Substituting into the equation the values from the problem:

$$\frac{\text{No. reticulocytes in small and large squares (26)}}{\text{No. RBCs in square No. 2}(210) \times 9} \times 100$$

$$\% \text{ reticulocytes} = \frac{26}{1890} \times 100$$

$$\% \text{ reticulocytes} = 0.014 \times 100$$

$$\% \text{ reticulocytes} = 1.4\%$$

24. **Q.** A reticulocyte count was performed using the Miller disk method, and 55 reticulocytes were counted among 230 RBCs. What is the reticulocyte percentage?

A. Using the formula for the Miller disk method, the following equation is derived:

$$\frac{\text{No. reticulocytes in small and large squares (55)}}{\text{No. RBCs in square No. 2}(230) \times 9} \times 100$$

$$\% \text{ reticulocytes} = \frac{55}{2070} \times 100$$

$$\% \text{ reticulocytes} = 0.027 \times 100$$

$$\% \text{ reticulocytes} = 2.7\%$$

25. **Q.** A patient with a low hematocrit of 21% had a reticulocyte count of 4.5%. Using the reticulocyte index, what is the patient's corrected reticulocyte count?

A. The reticulocyte index is used when a patient has an abnormally low hematocrit. The reticulocyte count is based on the assumption that the RBC count is normal; if this is not true, as in the case of anemia, then the reticulocyte count may be falsely elevated. The reticulocyte index corrects the reticulocyte count by the following formula:

$$\text{Corrected reticulocyte count} = \text{Patient's reticulocyte count} \times \frac{\text{Patient's Hct}}{45}$$

The factor of 45 is used because the average hematocrit is 45%. Using the formula, the patient's correct reticulocyte count is as follows:

$$\text{Corrected reticulocyte count} = 4.5\% \times \frac{21}{45}$$

$$\text{Corrected reticulocyte count} = 2.1\%$$

26. **Q.** An anemic patient with a hematocrit of 32% has a reticulocyte count of 3.7%. What is the patient's corrected reticulocyte count?

    A. The corrected reticulocyte count is calculated as follows:

$$\text{Corrected reticulocyte count} = 3.7\% \times \frac{32}{45}$$

$$\text{Corrected reticulocyte count} = 2.6\%$$

27. **Q.** A patient has a reticulocyte count of 6.5% and a hematocrit of 21%. Shift reticulocytes were found during the cell differential. What is the reticulocyte production index (RPI) for this patient?

    A. The RPI is an indicator of effective RBC cell production. When shift reticulocytes are found in the differential, the bone marrow is releasing reticulocytes earlier than normal. The RPI includes a factor accounting for the maturation rate of RBCs. The RPI is calculated as follows:

$$\text{RPI} = \frac{\text{Reticulocytecount} \times \text{reticulocyte index}}{\text{Maturation factor (from Table 8-4)}}$$

Table 8-4 shows that if a patient has a hematocrit of 21%, the RBC has a maturation time of approximately 2.5 days. Substituting the data from the problem into the formula yields:

$$\frac{6.5\% \text{ Reticulocyte count} \times \text{reticulocyte index } (21\% \div 45)}{\text{Maturation time correction } (2.5)} = 1.2\%$$

Therefore the corrected reticulocyte count for a low hematocrit and increased maturation time is 1.2%.

28. **Q.** An anemic patient has a reticulocyte count of 3.5% and a hematocrit of 25%. Shift reticulocytes were noted on the differential. What is the patient's reticulocyte count after correction for low hematocrit and increased maturation time?

    A. Using the formula for the RPI, the false increase in reticulocyte percentage due to both the low hematocrit and increased maturation time can be corrected.

$$\frac{3.5\% \text{ Reticulocyte count} \times \text{reticulocyte index } (25\% \div 45)}{\text{Maturation time correction } (2.0)} = 1.0\%$$

Thus the corrected reticulocyte percentage is 1.0%.

HOW **PRACTICE PROBLEMS**

Solve the following practice problems to further master the material. Answers and explanations to some problems can be found in the Answer Key.

Calculate the MCV, given the following information.

1. Hematocrit = 40.0%, RBC count = 4.4 $(10^{12}/\text{L})$

2. Hematocrit = 47%, RBC count = 5.2 $(10^{12}/\text{L})$

3. Hematocrit = 25%, RBC count = 2.8 $(10^{12}/L)$

Calculate the MCH, given the following information.

4. Hemoglobin = 6 g/dL, RBC count = 4.1 $(10^{12}/L)$

5. Hemoglobin = 10 g/dL, RBC count = 3.4 $(10^{12}/L)$

6. Hemoglobin = 15 g/dL, RBC count = 4.5 $(10^{12}/L)$

Calculate the MCHC, given the following information.

7. Hemoglobin = 11 g/dL, hematocrit = 33%

8. Hemoglobin = 7 g/dL, hematocrit = 21%

9. Hemoglobin = 16 g/dL, hematocrit = 48%

For the following WBC counts performed on a $1/20$ dilution and counting all WBCs in the four large corner squares of the hemacytometer, use the factor method to calculate the WBC count $\times 10^9/L$. WBCs counted:

10. 40

11. 148

12. 90

For the following platelet counts performed on a $1/100$ dilution and counting all platelets within the center square of the hemacytometer, use the factor method to calculate the platelet count $\times 10^9/L$. Platelets counted:

13. 380

14. 63

15. 180

Calculate the following cell counts without using the factor method.

16. WBC count: $1/10$ dilution performed, 65 WBCs counted in four corner squares

17. WBC count: $1/20$ dilution performed, 135 WBCs counted in eight large squares

18. Platelet count: $1/50$ dilution, 93 platelets counted within the large center square

Use **Table 8-2** to determine the factor necessary to calculate the fluid WBC and RBC counts for the following fluids.

19. Moderately cloudy CSF, diluted by method B, total of nine squares counted, factor is 24.4 and an average of 39 WBCs and 25 RBCs counted

20. Very cloudy peritoneal fluid, diluted by method C, total of nine squares counted, factor is 224.4, average of 162 WBCs and 74 RBCs counted

Calculate the sperm count per milliliter and the sperm count per ejaculate given the following data.

21. 88 sperm counted in the five center RBC squares in the Neubauer hemacytometer, a $1/20$ dilution performed. The total semen volume is 3.4 mL.

22. 134 sperm counted in the five center RBC squares in the Neubauer hemacytometer, a $^1/_{20}$ dilution performed. The total semen volume was 2.8 mL.

Calculate the percent reticulocytes given the following data.

23. 52 reticulocytes counted per 1000 RBCs

24. 15 reticulocytes counted per 1000 RBCs

25. 48 reticulocytes counted in large and small squares of Miller disk, 254 RBCs counted in square No. 2 of Miller disk

26. 22 reticulocytes counted in large and small squares in Miller disk, 180 RBCs counted in small square No. 2 of Miller disk

Correct the following reticulocyte percentages in questions 27 and 28 using the correction formula.

27. 5.9% reticulocytes, 28% hematocrit

28. 8.5% reticulocytes, 22% hematocrit

Correct the following reticulocyte percentages in questions 29 and 30 using the red blood cell production index (see **Table 8-4**).

29. 4.6% reticulocytes, 25% hematocrit

30. 2.9% reticulocytes, 14% hematocrit

QUICK NOTES

- A good rule to remember is the rule of three, where the Hb × 3 will equal the hematocrit, and the Hb ÷ 3 or the Hct ÷ 9 will equal the RBC count.
- The mean corpuscular volume (MCV) is calculated by multiplying the Hct × 10 and dividing that result by the RBC count. The MCV is an indicator of RBC size.
- Microcytic RBCs have MCV levels below 80 fL.
- Macrocytic RBCs have MCV levels above 100 fL.
- The mean corpuscular hemoglobin (MCH) is calculated by multiplying the hemoglobin value by 10 and dividing that value by the RBC count. The MCH is an indicator of how much hemoglobin is inside the RBCs. Low MCH levels infer hypochromia.
- The mean corpuscular hemoglobin concentration (MCHC) is a calculation of the ratio of the hemoglobin and hematocrit. The formula for MCHC is Hb × 100 in the numerator divided by the hematocrit in the denominator.
- Babies and very young children may have nucleated red blood cells in their peripheral blood, and these may be counted by some instruments as lymphocytes. Therefore some laboratories perform corrections to the WBC count to obtain an accurate count.
- The hemocytometer is not as frequently used for WBC counts or platelet counts as it once was. Platelets are counted within the center square, and many laboratory procedures call for WBCs to be counted in the four large corner squares.
- If a 1/20 dilution is performed for a WBC count, and all WBCs in the four large corner squares are counted, then the factor of 50 can be used to multiply the number of WBCs to arrive at the number of WBCs/mm^3.

- A factor of 1000 can be used if a platelet count is performed, and all platelets within the 25 small squares within the middle square are counted and a 1/100 dilution is performed.
- Many laboratories no longer perform a manual reticulocyte count as many hematology instruments can now perform a reticulocyte count.
- Every time a new lot number of thromboplastin is going to be used in the coagulation laboratory, a new reference INR must be performed.

BIBLIOGRAPHY

Ciesla B: *Hematology in practice*, ed 3, Philadelphia, 2019, FA Davis.

Rodak BF, Fritsma GA, Keohane E: *Hematology, clinical principles and applications*, ed 5, St. Louis, 2016, Elsevier-Saunders.

Immunohematology Laboratory

OBJECTIVES

At the end of this chapter, the reader should be able to do the following:

1. Determine the approximate increase in hematocrit and hemoglobin in patients receiving packed red blood cells.
2. Calculate the expected decrease in prothrombin and partial thromboplastin time in patients receiving fresh frozen plasma.
3. Calculate the approximate increase in platelet count in patients receiving pooled platelet concentrate or a platelet pheresis pack.
4. Calculate the appropriate dose of Rh-immune globulin to be given to Rh-negative patients.
5. Determine the percentage of compatible (or incompatible) units of blood in 100 random donors when patients have multiple antibodies.

WHAT **CALCULATIONS ASSOCIATED WITH THE MEDICAL EFFECTS OF TRANSFUSION SERVICES**

Immunohematology is the science of blood group serology and transfusion medicine. A more common name for the immunohematology laboratory is the blood bank. The primary function of the immunohematology laboratory is to supply the safest and most suitable blood and blood products to patients as quickly as possible. Surgical, trauma, maternity, and orthopedic patients are only a few of the types of patients that may require transfusion services. Routine blood products provided by the laboratory include packed red blood cells (RBCs), fresh frozen plasma, and platelet concentrates. When individuals donate a pint (or approximately 450 mL) of whole blood, that blood is referred to as a unit. The average adult body's total blood volume is between 7 and 10 pints or units of blood. The whole blood unit may be processed to provide three or more components, including packed RBCs, plasma, and platelets. The whole blood is centrifuged, and the plasma is expressed into an attached satellite bag. The RBCs left behind are referred to as a unit of packed RBCs. The plasma may be further centrifuged, and the platelets are expressed into a second satellite bag. In this manner, both a unit of fresh plasma and a unit of platelet concentrate are formed. The immunohematology laboratory performs tests to determine the compatibility between the patient's (recipient) blood and donor blood. Only when a unit has been extensively tested for compatibility with the patient is it transfused into the patient.

WHAT   ## Estimating Therapeutic Effects of Transfusions

In this era of HIV and other bloodborne pathogens, the decision to transfuse blood into a patient is not made lightly. In most cases, the patients are severely anemic, profusely bleeding, or undergoing major surgery. Patients who are severely anemic may require an infusion of packed RBCs to increase the oxygen-carrying capacity of the blood. Plasma may be given to patients who require an infusion of coagulation factors, whereas platelets may be given to patients with decreased platelet quantity or function. Patients on chemotherapy frequently require the transfusion of platelets. Determining the actual therapeutic effect of a unit of packed RBCs, plasma, or platelet concentrate on the patient can assist the physician in determining the number of units of blood or components to be transfused.

Determining Hemoglobin Increments

Because a unit of packed RBCs is highly concentrated with RBCs, for each unit of packed cells that is transfused into a patient who is not bleeding, the patient's hemoglobin concentration can be expected to increase by 1 g/dL. This ratio does not hold true if the patient is actively bleeding.

HOW   ### *Example 9-1*

An 87-year-old patient was admitted to the medical unit of a hospital while suffering from chronic renal failure. The patient was severely anemic, with a hematocrit of 12% and hemoglobin of 4.0 g/dL, and received five units of packed RBCs. What would be the patient's expected hemoglobin concentration posttransfusion?

    The hemoglobin concentration is expected to rise 1 g/dL for every unit of packed RBCs in nonbleeding patients. As this patient received five units of packed RBCs, it is expected that the posttransfusion hemoglobin concentration should be approximately 9.0 g/dL.

    Example 9-1a   Calculate the expected hemoglobin concentration if a patient had a hematocrit of 15%, a pretransfusion hemoglobin of 5 g/dL, and was given three units of packed RBCs.

    The expected hemoglobin would be 8 g/dL.

    Example 9-1b   Calculate the expected hemoglobin concentration if a patient had a hematocrit of 18%, a pretransfusion hemoglobin of 6 g/dL, and was given one unit of packed RBCs.

    The expected hemoglobin would be 7 g/dL.

Example 9-1c Calculate the expected hemoglobin concentration if a patient had a hematocrit of 20%, a pretransfusion hemoglobin of 7 g/dL, and was given three units of packed RBCs.

The expected hemoglobin would be 10 g/dL.

WHAT Determining Hematocrit Increments

One unit of packed RBCs has a hematocrit of approximately 79%. For every unit of packed RBCs, the hematocrit can be expected to rise 2 to 3 percentage points in a patient who is not bleeding. As with hemoglobin, this ratio does not apply if the patient is actively bleeding.

HOW *Example 9-2*

A woman delivered a child by cesarean section, during which she bled quite heavily. Three days after delivery, the hematocrit was 18%. Her physician ordered three units of packed RBCs to be administered. How will this affect the hematocrit?

For every unit of packed RBCs transfused, the hematocrit is expected to increase by 2 to 3 percentage points. As this patient received three units of packed RBCs, her hematocrit should rise to between **24% and 27%**.

Example 9-2a Calculate the expected hematocrit in a patient with a pretransfusion hematocrit of 15% and pretransfusion hemoglobin of 5 g/dL if given four units of packed RBCs.

The expected hematocrit would range from 23% to 27%.

Example 9-2b Calculate the expected hematocrit in a patient with a pretransfusion hematocrit of 16% and pretransfusion hemoglobin of 6 g/dL if given three units of packed RBCs.

The expected hematocrit would range from 22% to 25%.

Example 9-2c Calculate the expected hematocrit in a patient with a pretransfusion hematocrit of 24% and pretransfusion hemoglobin of 8 g/dL if given two units of packed RBCs.

The expected hematocrit would range from 28% to 30%.

WHAT Determining Fresh Frozen Plasma Increments

The plasma that is expressed from a unit of packed RBCs is further centrifuged to remove the platelets into a separate unit. The units of plasma are frozen within 8 hours of collection to preserve all coagulation factors. Before they are used, the fresh frozen units are thawed in a 37°C water bath or Food and Drug Administration (FDA)–approved microwave or other approved device specifically designed to thaw plasma. The fresh frozen plasma units contain all coagulation factors, and two units are usually sufficient to increase clotting factor activity by 15% to 20% in a patient with diminished clotting capacity.

HOW   *Example 9-3*

A patient with a history of spontaneous bleeding and bruising had an increased prothrombin time. Two units of fresh frozen plasma were transfused. What effect will this have on the prothrombin time?

For every 2 units of fresh frozen plasma, the clotting factors are elevated by 15% to 20%. By transfusing two units, the prothrombin time should be decreased approximately 15% to 20%.

Example 9-3a   A patient hemorrhaged after surgery, which elevated the prothrombin time to 40 seconds. If the patient was given two units of fresh frozen plasma post-operatively, estimate the effect on the prothrombin time.

The prothrombin time would be lowered to between 32 and 34 seconds (15%–20% lower).

Example 9-3b   Calculate the effect on the prothrombin time if a patient was given four units of fresh frozen plasma if the prothrombin time was elevated to 60 seconds.

The prothrombin time would be decreased by 30% to 40%, since four units were given. Therefore the prothrombin time should be between 36 and 42 seconds.

WHAT   ## Determining Platelet Increments

The normal concentration of platelets in a healthy person is between 150,000 and 450,000/ mcL of whole blood. Patients with bone marrow abnormalities, such as leukemia, may have diminished platelet production and may develop life-threatening drops in their platelet counts. Platelet concentrates are formed when plasma components are further centrifuged at high speed. All but approximately 50 mL of plasma are expressed off to form the plasma concentrate. The remaining 50 mL is the newly formed platelet concentrate that contains at least 5.5 to 7.0 × 10^{10} platelets per unit. This unit is called a **random platelet** unit. Each unit will increase the platelet count by an increment of approximately 10,000/mcL, which is not sufficient to provide a significant platelet increment in the patient. Routine practice advocates the administration of 4 to 6 platelet concentrates that have been pooled. The expected increment will vary depending on the number of platelet concentrates pooled and the product transfused. A post-transfusion platelet count should be drawn 10 to 60 minutes posttransfusion.

Platelet donors are persons who donate their platelets to patients by the process of apheresis. The apheresis instrument separates the platelets from the blood. All other constituents of the blood, except approximately 200 to 400 mL of plasma and a small number of RBCs, are returned to the donor. In this manner, large quantities of platelets may be harvested without harm to the donor. The use of a pherisis pack from one donor is the preferred method, as it minimizes the risk to the recipient. One pherisis pack will, at minimum, raise the platelet count by 30,000 mcL, but more likely the increase is between 40,000 and 100,000 platelets per pack.

HOW   *Example 9-4*

A patient with acute lymphocytic leukemia had a platelet count of only 10,000/mcL and was at risk for the occurrence of uncontrolled bleeding. The platelet donor was notified, and a pheresis pack was transfused into the patient. What should be the approximate platelet count of the patient after transfusion?

Each pheresis pack contains enough platelets comparable to 4 to 10 random platelet units and a minimum of 30,000 platelets/mcL. As each unit of platelets is estimated to increase the platelet concentration by 10,000 mcL, the estimated platelet count would be between 50,000 and 110,000 platelets/mcL.

WHAT **RH INCOMPATIBILITY**

Approximately 15% of the population lack the red cell antigen D and are therefore considered to be Rh negative. An Rh-negative person does not have naturally circulating antibodies to the D antigen. Rh-negative mothers who are carrying Rh-positive fetuses may run the risk of antibody production. Fetal-maternal bleeds can occur with any pregnancy, and the mixing of maternal and fetal blood may occur at delivery. In most cases, an Rh-negative mother with an Rh-positive fetus may not become sensitized to the Rh factor unless a fetal-maternal bleed occurs. In the mid-1960s, it was discovered that if nonsensitized Rh-negative persons received intramuscular doses of Rh-immune globulin (RhIG), their immune systems failed to produce D antibodies even after exposure to the D antigen. This finding ultimately led to the current immunization of Rh-negative pregnant women during and immediately after delivery with RhIG.

Determining the Quantity of Rh-Immune Globulin to Administer

It has been estimated that the average fetal-maternal bleed contains approximately 30 mL of whole blood or 15 mL of packed RBCs. The RhIG is formulated to contain 300 mcg of RhIG, which is sufficient to protect against an average bleed. One unit of RhIG is generally sufficient to protect an Rh-negative pregnant woman during pregnancy, and a second dose is administered within 72 hours of delivery. However, there may be incidences of increased fetal-maternal bleeding. In those cases, the quantity of RhIG units must be calculated to prevent formation of antibodies.

Kleihauer-Betke Acid-Elution Test

The Kleihauer-Betke test measures the quantity of fetal cells in the maternal circulation by using a blood smear made from blood drawn from the mother. The smear is placed in an acid buffer and the hemoglobin in adult RBCs (HbA) will leach out of the cells into the buffer. Fetal hemoglobin (HbF) is resistant to the acid and will stay within the RBC. The smear is then washed, stained with counterstain, and examined under oil immersion (1000×). Adult RBCs will look ghostlike because only the cell membrane remains, while the fetal cells will stain pink. The amount of fetal cells counted per 1000 adult cells is quantitated similarly to a reticulocyte count:

$$\text{Percent fetal cells} = \frac{\text{No. fetal cells counted}}{2000 \text{ adult cells counted}} \times 100$$

Some laboratories are using the more exact method of flow cytometry to quantitate fetal cells.

WHAT *Number of Units or Vials of RhIG*

The number of units or vials of RhIG to be administered is calculated by the following formula:

$$\text{Vials of RhIG} = \frac{\% \text{ fetal cells} \times 50}{30}$$

where:
% fetal cells = number of fetal cells per 1000 maternal cells
50 = factor to account for average maternal blood volume
30 = dose of RhIg that suppresses alloimmunization of 30 mL fetal blood exposure

To err on the side of caution, the result is rounded to the nearest whole number and an additional unit is added.

HOW **Example 9-5**

A woman was rushed into the emergency room hemorrhaging as a result of a miscarriage. Her blood type was B Rh negative, and the father was A positive. A Kleihauer-Betke acid elution test determined the percentage of fetal cells in the mother's circulation to be 3.2%. How many units of RhIG should the woman be given to prevent the formation of D antibodies?
The formula to determine the units of RhIG is as follows:

$$\text{Vials of RhIG} = \frac{\% \text{ fetal cells} \times 50}{30}$$

where:

% fetal cells = number of fetal cells per 1000 maternal cells
50 = factor to account for average maternal blood volume
30 = dose of RhIG that suppresses alloimmunization of 30 mL fetal blood exposure

Substituting into the formula the data from the problem:

$$\text{Vials of RhIG} = \frac{3.2\% \times 50}{30}$$

$$\text{Vials of RhIG} = 5.3$$

The amount calculated (5.3) is rounded to 5.0, and an additional vial is added to err on the side of safety. Therefore the woman would receive six vials of RhIG.

Example 9-5a Calculate the number of vials of RhIG that a Rh-negative woman would receive if the percent of fetal cells were determined to be 2.1%.

Using the formula used in Example 9-5, the following equation is derived:

$$\text{Vials of RhIG} = \frac{2.1\% \times 50}{30}$$

$$\text{Vials of RhIG} = 3.5$$

The number calculated (3.5) is rounded up to 4.0, and an additional unit is given. For purposes of giving RhIG, if the amount calculated ends in the number 5 or above it is rounded up; if it is less than 5, as in the first example, it is rounded down. In each case an extra vial of RhIG is given.

Therefore the final number of vials of RhIG given to this woman is five.

Example 9-5b   Calculate the number of vials of RhIG given to a woman if the amount of fetal cells were determined to be 1.7%.

Using the formula to determine vials of RhIG:

$$\text{Vials of RhIG} = \frac{1.7\% \times 50}{30}$$

$$\text{Vials of RhIG} = 2.8$$

The number of vials of RhIG given to the woman is four.

WHAT MONITORING PREGNANT PATIENTS FOR HEMOLYTIC DISEASE OF THE FETUS AND NEWBORN (HDFN) USING ANTIBODY TITRATION

Pregnant women with a history of anti-D antibody production or any other IgG antibody capable of crossing the placenta will have a baseline antibody titer performed during the first trimester. It is recommended that aliquots of the serum or plasma drawn are frozen for use in future titers performed every 4 to 6 weeks for the duration of the pregnancy. An eightfold 1 to 2 dilution series of the patient's serum with saline is performed to a final dilution of 1 to 256 (8 tubes: $\frac{1}{2}$, $\frac{1}{4}$, $\frac{1}{8}$, $\frac{1}{16}$, $\frac{1}{32}$, $\frac{1}{64}$, $\frac{1}{128}$, $\frac{1}{256}$). The red cell chosen to be tested is usually homozygous and tested using the tube antiglobulin technique using anti-IgG. The titer value is the reciprocal of the highest dilution that gives a 1+ reaction. Refer to Chapter 4 for additional information on titers.

For each subsequent testing, an aliquot of the original first-trimester blood draw is tested alongside the new sample. An increase in the new titer by 2 dilutions or higher as compared to the original sample is considered significant.

WHAT SCREENING FOR PROBABLE COMPATIBLE UNITS

Determining the compatibility of donor blood to the patient is the fundamental responsibility of the immunohematology laboratory. All units of blood are grouped for ABO and Rh and screened for significant circulating antibodies. The frequency of the occurrence of blood groups is important when a patient develops antibodies to any blood group antigen and must receive blood that is negative for the corresponding antigen. By knowing the frequency of the antigen, the probability of finding a compatible unit that is negative for the antigen can be determined.

WHAT *Example 9-6*

A woman developed anti-Fy^a antibodies because of a previous transfusion. She was admitted for surgery, and the doctor requested two units of packed cells. What is the chance of finding a Fy^a-negative unit?

The frequency of the Fy^a or Duffy antigen is approximately 65%, or 0.65. Therefore the chance of finding a negative unit for the Duffy antigen is 100% − 65% = 35%. This means that roughly one of three units will be Duffy negative for Fy^a.

Example 9-6a   A man developed autoantibodies to anti-Fy^b and was phenotyped as Fy(a-b+). What is the chance of finding an Fy^b-negative unit?

The frequency of this phenotype is 23%. Therefore, there is a 77% chance of finding an Fy^b-negative unit.

Example 9-6b A woman developed anti-S antibodies. What is the chance of finding an S-negative unit?

The frequency of the S antigen is 55%. Therefore, there is a 45% chance of finding an S-negative unit.

Example 9-6c A patient has developed antibodies to two antigens. One has a frequency of occurrence of 9.0%, and the other has a frequency of 30%. What is the chance of finding a compatible unit that is negative for both antigens?

The frequency of occurrence for the first antigen is 9.0%, or a frequency of 0.9, meaning that 91% (100% − 9%) of the population is negative for the antigen. The frequency of the second antigen is 30%, or 0.30, which means that 70% (100% − 30%) of the population is negative for that antigen. The chance of finding a unit of blood that is negative for *both* antigens is the product of the frequency of both negative antigens multiplied together.

Combined negative antigen frequency = 0.91 Negative frequency antigen 1

$$\times\ 0.70 \text{ Negative frequency antigen 2}$$

$$=0.637 \text{ or } 63.7\%$$

Therefore the chance of finding a unit negative for both units is 63.7%.

Example 9-6d A man required four units of packed cells. An antibody identification panel revealed that he had developed antibodies to the JK^a and e antigens from a previous transfusion. The antigen frequency of JK^a in the patient's ethnic population is 77%, and the frequency of the e antigen is 98%. How many units out of 100 random donors will be compatible with the patient for transfusion?

The frequency of a unit negative for the JK^a antigen is 100% − 77% = 23% or 0.23. The frequency of a unit negative for the e antigen is 100% − 98% = 2% or 0.02.

The chance of finding a unit negative for both antigens is the product of their individual negative frequencies:

$$0.02 \times 0.23 = 0.0046 \text{ or } 0.46\%$$

Therefore the chance of finding a compatible unit is extremely small, and most likely a unit will only be found by consulting with the rare donor file from the local blood center.

HOW **EXAMPLE PROBLEMS**

This section is designed to be useful to both the student and the laboratory professional. Students can use the additional problems to master the material. The laboratory professional can use the examples as templates for solving laboratory calculations. By finding an example similar to the problem that you need to solve, substitute the numbers appropriate to your calculation into the equation.

1. **Q.** Calculate the expected posttransfusion hemoglobin concentration if three units of packed RBCs are transfused into a nonbleeding patient with a hemoglobin concentration of 6 g/dL.
   A. For every unit of packed RBCs, the hemoglobin concentration should rise by 1 g/dL in nonbleeding patients. As this patient received three units, the posttransfusion hemoglobin concentration should be 9 g/dL.

2. **Q.** Calculate the expected posttransfusion hemoglobin concentration if six units of packed RBCs are transfused into a nonbleeding patient with a hemoglobin concentration of 4 g/dL.
   A. The patient's posttransfusion hemoglobin concentration can be expected to be 10 g/dL.

3. **Q.** Calculate the expected posttransfusion hemoglobin concentration if five units of packed RBCs are transfused into a nonbleeding patient with a hemoglobin of 10 g/dL.
   A. The patient's posttransfusion hemoglobin concentration can be expected to be 15 g/dL.

4. **Q.** Calculate the expected posttransfusion hematocrit percentage in a patient with a hematocrit of 15% who is given four units of packed RBCs. The patient is not an active bleeder.
   A. For every unit of packed RBCs, the hematocrit percentage will rise 2 to 3 percentage points. Because the patient received four units of packed RBCs, the hematocrit can be expected to increase between 8 and 12 percentage points, resulting in an expected posttransfusion hematocrit of between 23% and 27%.

5. **Q.** Calculate the expected posttransfusion hematocrit percentage in a patient with a hematocrit of 7% who is given six units of packed RBCs. The patient is not an active bleeder.
   A. The patient's posttransfusion hematocrit can be expected to be between 19% and 25%.

6. **Q.** Calculate the expected posttransfusion hematocrit percentage in a patient with a hematocrit of 20% who is given two units of packed RBCs.
   A. The patient's posttransfusion hematocrit can be expected to be between 24% and 26%.

7. **Q.** A patient with thrombocytopenia has an increased prothrombin time and requires an infusion of four units of fresh frozen plasma. What effect will the transfused plasma have on the patient's prothrombin time?
   A. Two units of fresh frozen plasma contain enough clotting factors to decrease the prothrombin time by 15% to 20%. As the patient received four units of plasma, the prothrombin time should decrease by 30% to 40%.

8. **Q.** A patient with a history of spontaneous bleeding and bruising has an increased partial thromboplastin time. The patient receives two units of fresh frozen plasma. What effect will the transfusion have on his clotting ability?
   A. As two units of fresh frozen plasma contain sufficient clotting factors to raise the clotting activity by 15% to 20%, the patient's clotting factor ability should be increased by 15% to 20%, and therefore the partial thromboplastin time should be decreased by approximately the same amount.

9. **Q.** A patient with a platelet count of 90,000/mcL received six pooled random platelet concentrates. What effect will this have on the patient's platelet count?
   A. Each random platelet concentrate contains at least 5.5×10^{10} platelets and will increase the platelet concentration by 10,000/mcL. As six concentrates are pooled, the platelet

count should be elevated by approximately 60,000/mcL platelets to elevate the platelet count to approximately 150,000/mcL.

10. **Q.** A patient on chemotherapy required a pheresis pack of platelets because her platelet count had fallen to 20,000/mcL. What effect will the transfusion of the pheresis pack have on the patient's platelet count?

A. A pheresis pack is formed when a donor undergoes apheresis, and a large quantity of platelets is harvested from the donor. Each pheresis pack contains enough platelets equivalent to 4 to 10 platelet concentrates. As each platelet concentrate will increase the platelet concentration by approximately 10,000 platelets/mcL, the overall increase in platelets should be between 40,000 and 100,000/mcL. Therefore the patient's platelet count should increase to between 60,000 and 120,000/mcL.

11. **Q.** A pregnant woman has premature rupture of the membranes. The woman's blood type was group B Rh negative, and the father was group B Rh positive. A Kleihauer-Betke acid elution test determined the percentage of fetal cells in the mother's circulation to be 3.5%. How many vials of RhIG should the woman be given to prevent the formation of D antibodies?

A. It is estimated that the average fetal-maternal bleed contains approximately 30 mL of whole blood or 15 mL of packed RBCs. Each vial of RhIG is formulated to contain 300 mcg of immune globulin, which is sufficient to protect against exposure to 30 mL of fetal blood. When a pregnant woman has increased bleeding, the following formula is used to determine the quantity of vials of RhIG necessary to prevent the formation of antibodies:

$$\text{Vials of RhIG} = \frac{\% \text{ fetal cells} \times 50}{30}$$

where:
% fetal cells = number of fetal cells per 1000 maternal cells
50 = factor to account for average maternal blood volume
30 = dose of RhIg that suppresses alloimmunization of 30 mL fetal blood exposure
Substituting into the formula the data from the problem:

$$\text{Vials of RhIG} = \frac{3.5 \times 50}{30}$$
$$\text{Vials of RhIG} = 5.8$$

The amount calculated (5.8) is rounded to 6.0, and an additional vial added to err on the side of safety. Therefore the woman would receive seven vials of RhIG.

12. **Q.** An Rh-negative pregnant woman carrying an Rh-positive fetus was a passenger in an automobile that crashed. The woman received blunt trauma to the lower abdominal area. An ultrasound revealed damage to the placenta. The percentage of fetal cells within the mother's circulation was calculated by the Kleihauer-Betke acid elution test to be 2.5%. How many vials of RhIG should the woman receive to prevent the formation of D antibodies?

A. Substituting the data from the problem into the formula used to determine the number of vials of RhIG to administer, the following equation is derived:

$$\text{Vials of RhIG} = \frac{2.5\% \text{ fetal cells} \times 50}{30}$$

$$\text{Vials of RhIG} = 4.2$$

Therefore five vials of RhIG will be administered to the patient.

13. **Q.** A woman developed anti-E antibodies because of a previous transfusion. She was admitted for surgery, and the doctor requested three units of packed RBCs. What is the chance of finding an E-negative unit?

   A. The prevalence of the E antigen is 30%. Therefore the chance of finding a unit negative for the E antigen is 100% − 30%, or 70%.

14. **Q.** A man with antibodies to M and Le^a requires four units of packed RBCs. The frequency of the M antigen is 70% and of the Le^a antigen is 23%. How many units out of 100 random donors will be compatible with the patient for transfusion?

   A. The frequency of a unit negative for the M antigen is 100% − 70% = 30%, or 0.30. The frequency of a unit negative for the Le^a unit is 100% − 23% = 77%, or 0.77. The frequency of finding a unit negative for both antigens is the product of their individual negative frequencies:

$$0.30 \times 0.77 = 0.23 \text{ or } 23\%$$

Therefore the chance of finding a compatible unit is 23%.

HOW   **PRACTICE PROBLEMS**

Solve the following practice problems to further master the material. Answers and explanations to some problems can be found in the Answer Key.

Determine the expected increase in hemoglobin concentration for the following patients. Note: None of the patients are active bleeders.

1. A patient with a hemoglobin of 5 g/dL receives seven units of packed RBCs.

2. A patient with a hemoglobin of 7 g/dL receives three units of packed RBCs.

3. A patient with a hemoglobin of 9 g/dL receives two units of packed RBCs.

Determine the expected increase in hematocrit percentage for the following patients who are not actively bleeding.

4. A patient with a hematocrit of 14% receives three units of packed RBCs.

5. A patient with a hematocrit of 10% receives four units of packed RBCs.

6. A patient with a hematocrit of 8% receives three units of packed RBCs.

Determine the expected increase in clotting factor activity for the following patients.

7. A patient receives five units of fresh frozen plasma.

8. A patient receives eight units of fresh frozen plasma.

Determine the expected increase in platelet concentration for the following patients.

9. A patient with a platelet count of 30,000/mcL receives nine units of platelet concentrate.

10. A patient with a platelet count of 4500/mcL receives a pheresis pack of platelets.

Determine the number of vials of RhIG necessary to prevent formation of the D antibody in the following women.

11. Percentage of fetal cells in maternal circulation = 4.1%

12. Percentage of fetal cells in maternal circulation = 1.4%

Out of 100 donor units, determine the chance of finding a unit negative for the following antigen(s).

13. Jka+ b+, frequency of 50%

14. K-k+, frequency of 98%, and Le a-b-, frequency of 22%

QUICK NOTES

- The hemoglobin rises 1 g/dL for every unit transfused, assuming no active bleeding is occurring.
- For every unit of packed RBCs, the hematocrit can be expected to rise 2 to 3 percentage points, assuming no active bleeding is occurring.
- Two units of fresh frozen plasma will increase clotting factor activity, and therefore lower PT and aPTT times, by 15% to 20% in a patient with diminished clotting ability.
- The number of vials of RhIG given to Rh-negative women is calculated after performing the Keihauer-Betke test to determine the quantity of fetal cells in the maternal calculation.
- The number of vials of RhIG is calculated by dividing the number of fetal cells counted by 2000 adult cells that are counted to calculate the percent of fetal cells. The result is multiplied by 100. To determine the number of vials of RhIG, the percent of fetal cells is multiplied by 50 and then divided by 30. The answer is rounded up to its next number, and an additional vial of RhIG is added.
- The chance of finding a negative unit for a particular antibody is to subtract the frequency of this antibody from 100.
- To determine the chance of finding units negative for patients with more than one antibody, the frequencies of both are determined and that value is subtracted from 100 for each antibody. The chance that *both* will be negative is determined by multiplying each antibody's chance of finding a negative unit together.

BIBLIOGRAPHY

Ciesla B: *Hematology in practice*, ed 3, Philadelphia, 2019, FA Davis.
Harmening DM: *Modern blood banking and transfusion practices*, ed 7, Philadelphia, 2019, FA Davis.

Microbiology Laboratory

OBJECTIVES

At the end of this chapter, the reader should be able to do the following:

1. Calculate the colony-forming units or concentration of bacteria per milliliter of sample in a urine specimen when using a calibrated loop.

2. Correlate the quantity of colony-forming units from a urine culture with probability of urinary tract infection.

WHAT COLONY COUNTS

A colony count determines the amount of bacteria present in a sample. The colony count is often used in the microbiology laboratory to determine the amount of bacteria present in a urine sample. Urine is a sterile fluid formed by the kidney and stored in the bladder until voided. As urine passes from the bladder into the urethra, it may become contaminated with the normal flora found in the urethra. Bacteria that is on the skin in the genital area may also contaminate the urine specimen.

The total amount of bacteria present as a result of contamination is less than 10,000 organisms per milliliter of urine or less than 10,000 or 10^3 colony-forming units (CFUs). Urinary tract infections are primarily caused by single strains of bacteria. Urinary tract infections that are caused by more than one strain of organism are not very common. If three strains of organisms are detected, then contamination of the specimen has most likely occurred. The most common organism responsible for urinary tract infections is *Escherichia coli*, a gram-negative rod.

When a physician suspects that a patient has a urinary tract infection, a clean-catch urine sample is collected by the patient. When the concentration of organisms is greater than 100,000 organisms per milliliter (10^5 CFUs/mL), a urinary tract infection is indicated. If a urine sample is to be used for both microbiologic studies and urinalysis, the microbiologic studies are performed first to avoid contamination of the sample with reagent strips, pipettes, and so forth.

Although there are other methods to perform a colony count, the streak method will be discussed in this chapter. In the streak method, a calibrated loop is used to inoculate a culture plate. Two different calibrated loops can be used. One calibrated loop will hold 0.01 mL of sample. The other loop will hold 0.001 mL of sample. The urine is streaked first with a primary streak down the middle of the plate. The plate is then turned 90 degrees and streaked across the primary streak the length of the plate. In some labs, the plate is again turned 90 degrees (or 180 degrees from the original orientation) and streaked across the secondary streaks. In this manner, the entire plate is streaked with urine, and isolation of any organisms can be achieved.

The plate is incubated aerobically at 37°C for 24 hours, and the number of colonies or CFUs/mL are counted. Each CFU/mL represents a single organism from the original sample. The total number of CFUs/mL are calculated by multiplying the amount of colonies by the dilution factor of the calibrated loop. If a 0.01 mL calibrated loop is used, the number of colonies is multiplied by 100. If a 0.001 mL calibrated loop is used, the number of colonies counted is multiplied by 1000. In this manner, the total number of CFUs/mL of urine can be obtained. Clean-catch urine specimens that contain less than 10^3 CFUs of bacteria are not indicative of a urinary tract infection. Clean-catch urine specimens that contain between 10^3 and 10^5 CFUs may indicate possible infection.

When a possible infection is indicated, the organism is identified, and antibiotic susceptibility testing is performed. Clean-catch urine specimens that contain more than 10^5 CFUs/mL indicate probable infection. As with a possible infection, the organism is identified and antibiotic susceptibility testing is performed.

Urine may also be collected from an indwelling catheter. Patients with indwelling catheters are at high risk for acquiring urinary tract infections; therefore sterile technique should be carefully followed. Urine is never collected for culture from the collection bag. Significant bacteriuria is indicated if greater than 10^5 CFUs/mL are counted.

Urine may also be collected by suprapubic aspiration. In this surgical procedure, urine is taken directly from the bladder and cultured. Any amount of CFUs/mL should be reported, the organism identified, and antibiotic susceptibility testing performed.

HOW   *Example 10-1*

A clean-catch urine specimen is obtained from a 17-year-old girl with a possible urinary tract infection. The urine is cultured using a 0.01 mL calibrated loop. After appropriate incubation, 350 colonies are counted. What is the patient's CFU/mL, and is it indicative of a urinary tract infection?

A 0.01 mL calibrated loop was used to inoculate this urine. Therefore the quantity of colonies (350) is multiplied by the conversion factor of 100, yielding 35,000 CFUs/mL.

A CFU count of at least 10^5 colonies is necessary to indicate probable infection. The patient's CFU/mL count was 3.5×10^4, indicating possible, but not probable, infection.

Example 10-1a   A clean-catch urine specimen was obtained from a 42-year-old woman with a possible urinary tract infection. The urine was cultured using a 0.01 mL calibrated loop. After appropriate incubation, eight colonies are counted. What is the patient's CFU/mL, and is it indicative of a urinary tract infection?

Since the 0.01 mL loop was used, the number of colonies (8) is multiplied by 100, yielding 800 CFUs/mL, or 8.0×10^2 CFUs/mL. Since this is less than 10^3 CFUs of bacteria, the result is not indicative of a urinary tract infection.

Example 10-1b   A clean-catch urine specimen was obtained from a 12-month-old boy with a possible urinary tract infection. The urine was cultured using a 0.01 mL calibrated loop. After appropriate incubation, 1245 colonies are counted. What is the patient's CFU/mL, and is it indicative of a urinary tract infection?

Since the 0.01 mL loop was used, the number of colonies (1245) is multiplied by 100, yielding 124,500 CFUs/mL, or 1.245×10^5 CFUs/mL. Since this is more than 10^5 CFUs of bacteria, the result is indicative of a probable urinary tract infection.

Example 10-1c   A urine specimen obtained by catheter on a 14-month-old boy is cultured for possible infection using a 0.001 mL calibrated loop. Following standard laboratory protocol, 120 organisms are counted. What is the baby's CFU/mL count, and is it indicative of an infection?

As a 0.001 mL calibrated loop was used to inoculate the specimen, the amount of colonies counted (120) is multiplied by 1000, yielding 1.2×10^5 CFUs/mL. This quantity of organisms indicates a probable infection.

Example 10-1d   A urine specimen obtained by a suprapubic aspiration is cultured for a possible infection using a 0.001 mL calibrated loop. After appropriate incubation, 45 colonies are counted. What is the patient's CFU/mL, and is it indicative of a urinary tract infection?

Because the 0.001 mL calibrated loop was used, the number of colonies (45) is multiplied by 1000, resulting in 45,000 or 4.5×10^4 CFUs/mL. Because this is a suprapubic aspiration, any amount of organisms indicates an infection and an antibiotic sensitivity workup.

Example 10-1e   A urine specimen obtained by a urinary catheter is cultured for a possible infection using a 0.001 mL calibrated loop. After appropriate incubation, one colony is counted. What is the patient's CFU/mL and is it indicative of a urinary tract infection?

The number of colonies counted (one) is multiplied by 1000, resulting in a 1.0×10^3 CFU/mL colony count. This quantity is not indicative of a urinary tract infection. Patients with urinary catheters are at a higher risk of developing a urinary tract infection.

WHAT ANTIMICROBIAL SUSCEPTIBILITY TESTING

Once an organism is identified as a possible pathogen, the microbiology laboratory must identify the possible antimicrobial agent(s) that can kill or inhibit the growth of the organism. An organism that is inhibited completely by a particular antimicrobial agent is said to be susceptible to that antimicrobial agent. On the other hand, if the organism continues to grow when exposed to the antimicrobial agent, the organism is considered to be resistant to that antimicrobial agent. The dose of antimicrobial agent to be given to the patient should be the lowest possible dose that will inhibit or kill the organism. This dose is termed the minimal inhibitory concentration (MIC) and is measured in micrograms per milliliter (mcg/mL). The MIC for a particular antimicrobial can be performed in either broth or agar. The broth method can be either by tube (macrotube) or by microtiter plate (microtube). There are automated instruments that are capable of reading the microtiter MIC plates, and most, if not all, clinical microbiology laboratories now use the microtiter method. Because the microtiter method is so prevalent, the dilutions necessary to perform the macrotube method will not be discussed but are placed in Appendix 10-A. Appendix 10-B contains information on the preparation of the 0.5 McFarland standard.

EXAMPLE PROBLEMS

This section is designed to be useful to both the student and the laboratory professional. Students can use the additional problems to master the material. The laboratory professional can use the examples as templates for solving laboratory calculations. By finding an example similar to the problem that you need to solve, substitute the numbers appropriate to your calculation into the equation.

1. **Q.** A urine specimen was obtained for a culture and sensitivity. A 0.01 mL calibrated loop was used to streak the plate. After appropriate incubation, 271 CFUs were counted. Is this indicative of a urinary tract infection?
   A. Because a 0.01 mL calibrated loop was used to inoculate the culture plate, the amount of CFUs found on the plate is multiplied by the conversion factor of 100. In this problem, there would be a quantity of 27,100 CFUs/mL, or 2.71×10^4 CFUs/mL. The patient's CFU count indicates a possible infection. However, a CFU of at least 10^5 is necessary to indicate probable infection.

   For questions 2 through 4, state if the amount of colonies counted using a 0.01 mL calibrated loop indicates a possible or probable infection or does not indicate an infection.

2. **Q.** 789 colonies counted
   A. 7.89×10^4 CFUs/mL: possible infection

3. **Q.** 4 colonies counted
   A. 4.0×10^2 CFUs/mL: not indicative of an infection

4. **Q.** 1153 colonies counted
   A. 1.153×10^5 CFUs/mL: probable infection

5. **Q.** A urine was cultured using a 0.001 mL calibrated loop, and 590 CFUs were counted after appropriate incubation. Is this indicative of a urinary tract infection?
   A. When a 0.001 mL calibrated loop is used to inoculate a urine specimen, the amount of colonies counted are multiplied by the conversion factor of 1000. In this case, there are 590,000 CFUs/mL, or 5.9×10^5 CFUs/mL, which indicates a probable urinary tract infection.

   For questions 6 through 8, state if the amount of colonies counted using a 0.001 mL calibrated loop indicates a possible or probable infection or does not indicate an infection.

6. **Q.** 32 colonies counted
   A. 3.2×10^4 CFUs/mL: possible infection

7. **Q.** 13 colonies counted
   A. 1.3×10^4 CFUs/mL: possible infection

8. **Q.** 112 colonies counted
   A. 1.12×10^5 CFUs/mL: probable infection

9. **Q.** What is an MIC?
   A. The MIC is the minimal inhibitory concentration of an antimicrobial agent. MICs are used to assess the dosage of antimicrobial necessary to inhibit the growth of organisms.

10. **Q.** How is a MIC performed?

    A. MICs can be performed on broth or agar. In addition, they can be in tubes (macro method) or microtiter plates (micro method). The organisms are adjusted in broth to a density of a standard McFarland 0.5 suspension. In the macrotube method, an equal amount of Mueller Hinton (MH) broth is added to 12 tubes. Then, a serial dilution of the antimicrobial agent to be tested is performed in the 12 tubes containing the MH broth. An equal amount of the test organism is then added to each tube. The tubes are then incubated overnight. The MIC is the lowest concentration in which there is no visual growth of the organism.

HOW PRACTICE PROBLEMS

Solve the following practice problems to further master the material. Answers and explanations to some problems can be found in the Answer Key.

1. If 1750 CFUs were counted on a urine culture that was inoculated with a 0.01 mL calibrated loop, what is the concentration of CFUs/mL?

2. If 272 CFUs were counted on a urine culture that was inoculated with a 0.001 mL calibrated loop, what is the concentration of CFUs/mL?

3. At what concentration of bacteria in a suspective urinary tract infection not indicative of an infection if the sample was a clean-catch urine?

4. At what concentration of bacteria is a urinary tract infection probable if the sample was a clean-catch urine?

5. In a macrobroth MIC, which tube has a *final* antibiotic concentration of 0.25 mcg/mL?

QUICK NOTES

- Urine colony counts below 1000 CFUs/mL are not indicative of a urinary tract infection and are more likely due to contamination.
- Urine colony counts between 10^3 and 10^5 CFUs/mL indicate a possible infection in a clean-catch urine specimen.
- Urine colony counts above 10^5 CFUs/mL indicate a probable infection in a clean-catch urine specimen.
- If a 0.01 calibrated loop is used to inoculate the urine onto the agar plate, the number of colonies that are counted is multiplied by 100 to determine the amount of CFUs/mL.
- If a 0.001 calibrated loop is used to inoculate the urine onto the agar plate, the number of colonies that are counted is multiplied by 1000 to determine the amount of CFUs/mL.
- The minimum inhibitory concentration (MIC) of an antibiotic is the lowest possible dose of that antibiotic that will inhibit or kill the organism.

BIBLIOGRAPHY

Forbes BA, Sahm DF, Weissfeld AS: *Bailey & Scott's diagnostic microbiology*, ed 14., St. Louis, 2018, Mosby Elsevier.

Clinical and Standards Laboratory Institute: *Methods for dilution antimicrobial susceptibility tests for bacteria that grow aerobically*, M07-Ed11, Wayne, PA, 2019.

Clinical and Standards Laboratory Institute: *Performance standards for antimicrobial susceptibility testing: twentyninth informational supplement*, M100-Ed29, Wayne, PA, 2019.

Appendix 10-A Macrotube Broths

To perform a macrotube broth MIC, a standard suspension of the test organism is prepared. Four or five pure colonies are placed in a suitable broth (usually Mueller-Hinton broth [MHB] or TSB) and vortexed until the turbidity of the broth is that of a 0.5 McFarland standard. McFarland standards are solutions of varying concentrations of barium sulfate and sulfuric acid. By forming increasingly turbid samples, the standards represent increasing numbers of bacteria in suspension. A 0.5 McFarland standard represents a bacterial suspension containing 10^8 CFUs/mL of organism. Typically, the broth inoculum is diluted $^1/_{100}$ to yield a concentration of 10^6 CFUs/mL prior to the inoculation into the antibiotic. The standard MIC dilutional scheme will result in a final diluted inoculum concentration in each tube of 5×10^5 CFUs/mL.

The MIC dilutional scheme is as follows:

1. Add 1 mL of MHB that contains the test organism at a concentration of 10^6 CFUs/mL to 12 sterile test tubes. One of the test tubes is kept aside as it will be the control. The control test tube can be labeled 13.
2. Place 2 mL of the stock antimicrobial in a test tube and label as tube 1.
3. Perform a twofold serial dilution using 1 mL of the stock antimicrobial on the 11 remaining tubes (labeled 2 to 12). For the last tube (tube 12), after the tube is mixed, discard 1 mL so the total volume is still 1 mL.

Figure 10-1 is a schematic of a procedure using ampicillin as the antimicrobial agent to be tested up to this point.

Note that the antimicrobial is serially diluted in this dilutional scheme. In the next step, the antimicrobial agent will be further diluted.

4. Add 1 mL of the test organism at a concentration of 1×10^6 CFUs/mL to each tube, including the control tube 13. By adding 1 mL to the 1 mL already in the tube, a 1/2 dilution is made of the antimicrobial agent and the test organism. Therefore, in the 12 tubes, the concentration of the test organism is 5×10^5 CFUs/mL ($^1/_2$ of 1×10^6), and the concentrations of the antimicrobial range from 256 mcg/mL to 0.125 mcg/mL as demonstrated in Figure 10-2.

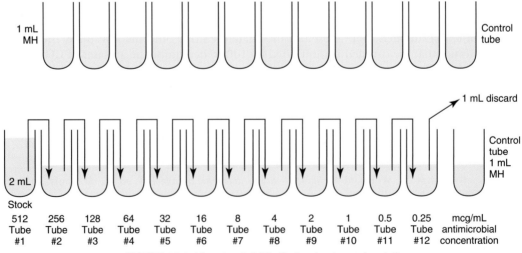

FIGURE 10-1 Macrobroth MIC dilutional scheme (partial).

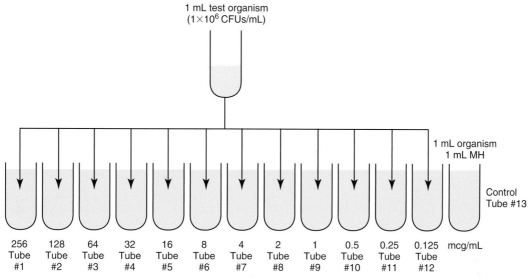

FIGURE 10-2 Macrobroth MIC dilutional scheme (completed).

5. Incubate the final 13 tubes overnight at 35°C. Check the tubes for the presence of turbidity, which represents growth of the organism in the antimicrobial agent. The MIC is the lowest concentration of antimicrobial in which there is no growth.

Appendix 10-B Preparing a 0.5 McFarland Standard

1. Add 0.5 mL of 0.048 M $BaCl_2$ (1.175% $BaCl_2 \cdot 2H_2O$ w/v) to 99.5 mL of 0.18 M H_2SO_4 (1% w/v).
2. Mix well with a magnetic stirrer.
3. Distribute 1 to 5 mL of the resulting standard into screw-cap tubes of the same size used in growing the broth culture inoculum. The amount placed in each tube should be the same volume as used in the tests.
4. Seal the tubes tightly with parafilm.
5. Store in the dark at room temperature.
6. Before use: Vigorously agitate the standard on a mechanical vortex.

Note: Cultures adjusted to this standard contain approximately 10^8 CFUs/mL.

Molecular Diagnostics Laboratory

OUTLINE

OBJECTIVES

At the end of this chapter, the reader should be able to do the following:

1. Convert between common metric units used in the clinical molecular laboratory.
2. Calculate common dilutions that are performed in the clinical molecular laboratory.
3. Calculate the concentration in micrograms per milliliter of single-stranded or double-stranded DNA, RNA, and oligonucleotides if given the optical density at 280 nm.
4. Correlate the absorbance 260/280 ratio to the purity of DNA samples.

WHAT COMMON UNITS OF MEASUREMENTS USED IN THE CLINICAL MOLECULAR LABORATORY

The clinical molecular laboratory has become an integral part of the diagnostic testing menu. Actual viral loads for the human immunodeficiency virus (HIV), or hepatitis B or C, have dramatically changed treatment options for patients. It no longer is adequate to be able to measure the presence of the HIV antibody in patients; now treatment protocols demand determination of the exact amount of virus present in the body. The recent COVID-19 outbreak showcases the vital role of the molecular laboratory professionals to respond to new viruses with new analytical techniques.

The work that is performed in a clinical molecular laboratory differs from that performed in a research molecular laboratory or in a biotechnology production laboratory. It is not the purpose of this chapter to go into detail on the many calculations that are associated with research protocols or biotechnology protocols that range from calculating bacterial growth to developing unique probes, to name just a few. There are many reference books on the subject; many reliable molecular biotechnology sources, blogs, and discussion forums that can be found on the Internet; and molecular and biotechnology professional organizations that

TABLE 11-1 Common Metric Units in the Clinical Laboratory

Prefix	Abbreviation	Compared to Base Unit	Metric Conversions
kilo	k	10^3 larger	There are 1000 k in a g
deci	d	10^{-1} smaller	There are 10 dg in a g
centi	c (lower case)	10^{-2} smaller	There are 100 cg in a g
milli	m (lower case)	10^{-3} smaller	There are 1000 mg in a g
micro	mc	10^{-5} smaller	There are 1,000,000 mcg in a g
nano	n	10^{-9} smaller	There are 1,000,000,000 mg in a g
pico	p	10^{-12} smaller	There are 1,000,000,000,000 pg in a g
femto	f	10^{-15} smaller	There are 1,000,000,000,000,000 fg in a g

provide a forum for discussion among members. A few of the professional societies are the American Society for Biochemistry and Molecular Biology, the American Society for Microbiology, the American Society for Cell Biology, and the European Laboratory for Molecular Biology. The University of Illinois's library has a comprehensive listing of molecular and cell biology weblinks. There is also an extensive molecular biology forum originally linked to the National Oceanic and Atmospheric Administration and the Northwest Fisheries Science Center **(http://molecularbiology.forums.biotechniques.com/index.php)**.

A list of organizations associated with molecular biology can be found at the end of the chapter.

The metric system was discussed in Chapter 3. However, in the molecular laboratory, much smaller quantities of materials and dilutions are performed versus what is performed in the core laboratory. For example, if a 1 to 10 dilution was to be performed in a clinical chemistry laboratory, the dilution might be performed with a 10 mcL sample to 90 mcL diluent. Compare that to the dilutions performed in the clinical molecular laboratory where a 1 to 10 dilution might be performed with 1 mcL sample in 9 mcL diluent.

Table 11-1 presents common metric units that are used in a clinical molecular laboratory.

WHAT Dilutions/Solutions Used in the Clinical Molecular Laboratory

Buffers are used in the clinical molecular laboratory for a variety of tests. For example, if samples are tested by electrophoresis, then buffers are integral in the electrophoresis technique. Common buffers used are Tris borate buffer, TE buffer, TAE or Tris acetate EDTA, STET buffer, and maleic acid buffer. The calculations used are generally C1V1 = C2V2 calculations to form a working buffer from a stock solution. What makes the difference between the molecular laboratory and the main laboratory is the volumes used. The clinical molecular laboratory, in general, uses much smaller quantities of patient sample and reagents than what is commonly used in the main clinical laboratory and also tends to use preassembled kits that contain premade reagents. Ethanol is also commonly used in many molecular techniques, many times at a $70\%^{v/v}$ concentration.

HOW Example 11-1

A medical laboratory scientist student needed to prepare a $70\%^{v/v}$ ETOH solution to be used in a hepatitis C molecular assay. The stock ETOH was at $100\%^{v/v}$ and 50 mL of the 70% ETOH solution was needed. How did the student prepare this solution?

The C1V1 = C2V2 formula is used to solve this problem.

C1 = stock concentration (100%)
V1 = volume of stock needed
C2 = 70%
V2 = 50 mL

Using C1V1 = C2V2 the following equation is derived:

$$(100\%)(X) = (70\%)(50 \text{ mL})$$

$$X = \frac{(70\%)(50 \text{ mL})}{100\%} = 35 \text{ mL}$$

Therefore 35 mL of the stock ETOH is added to a 100 mL volumetric flask, and 15 mL deionized water is added to form the 35%$^{v/v}$ ETOH solution.

WHAT CONVERSIONS COMMONLY PERFORMED IN A CLINICAL MOLECULAR LABORATORY

When double-stranded DNA (dsDNA), single-stranded DNA (ssDNA), or oligonucleotides are extracted, their quantity may be expressed in molar terms. Table 11-2 contains the molecular weight of DNA, RNA, and oligonucleotides in terms of picograms per picomole.

To convert dsDNA that is in terms of micrograms per milliliter to picomoles per microliters, use the following formula:

n = number of nucleotides
X = number of micrograms per milliliter of DNA that you have

$$\frac{X \text{ mcg dsDNA}}{\text{mL}} \times \frac{1 \text{ pmol}}{660 \text{ pg}} \times \frac{1 \text{ mL}}{1000 \text{ mcL}} \times \frac{10^6 \text{ pg}}{1 \text{ mcg}} \times \frac{1}{n} = X \text{ pmol/mcL DNA}$$

To convert from picomoles per microliter DNA to micrograms per milliliter DNA, use the following formula:

$$\frac{X \text{ pmol dsDNA}}{\text{mcL}} \times \frac{660 \text{ pg}}{\text{pmol}} \times \frac{1000 \text{ mcL}}{1 \text{ mL}} \times \frac{1 \text{ mcg}}{10^6 \text{ pg}} \times n = X \text{ mcg/mL dsDNA}$$

n = number of nucleotides
X = number of picomoles per microliter of double-stranded DNA.

To convert ssDNA or ssRNA, use 330 pg/pmol in the conversion formulas.

TABLE 11-2 Molecular Weights

Substance	Average Molecular Weight of a Base Pair
dsDNA	660 pg/pmol
ssDNA, RNA, and Nucleotides	330 pg/pmol

HOW   *Example 11-2*

A new employee in a large university hospital clinical molecular laboratory was being trained in the math associated with molecular techniques. She was told to convert a 12 mcg/mL concentration of a dsDNA sample consisting of 2500 base pairs into units of picomoles per microliter concentration. How much DNA in picomoles per microliter does this new employee have in this sample?

To solve, substitute the values given into the applicable formula:

$$\frac{12 \text{ mcg}}{\text{mL}} \times \frac{1 \text{ pmol}}{660 \text{ pg}} \times \frac{1 \text{ mL}}{1000 \text{ mcL}} \times \frac{10^6 \text{ pg}}{\text{mcg}} \times \frac{1}{2500}$$

$$X = 7.27 \times 10^{-3} \text{ pmol/mcL}$$

WHAT   ## ABSORBANCE TO CONCENTRATION CALCULATIONS

Sometimes the amount of DNA that has been produced is quantitated in a spectrophotometer by ultraviolet (UV) absorbance methods. As covered in Chapter 6, when a substance is turbid, it will block the light path of the spectrophotometer, leading to a decreased transmittance of light coming in contact with the detector. This decreased transmittance can be measured at two different wavelengths (260 and 280 nm) for DNA analysis. In research laboratories, these measurements are often taken for quantification of bacterial or viral growth cultures. In the clinical molecular laboratory the ratio of the measurements of the absorbance of 260/280 should be between 1.8 and 2.0 and indicate the purity of the DNA that was extracted. Values greater than this are an indication of contamination of the DNA.

There are conversion formulas that have been developed that will convert the absorbance at 260 nm to a micrograms per milliliter quantity of DNA or RNA. Table 11-3 contains the conversion formulas.

By using ratio and proportion, the micrograms per milliliter quantity of DNA or RNA can be calculated once the absorbance at 260 nm has been determined.

Example 11-3

A factor 2 assay was being performed. One step was to extract the dsDNA and determine the micrograms per milliliter quantity so that further calculations could be performed. The OD at 260 nm was measured as 1.425. What is the micrograms per milliliter quantity of the dsDNA?

By using the conversion factor in **Table 11-3** and ratio and proportion presented earlier, the following calculation can be performed:

$$\frac{1 \text{ Abs}}{\text{Conversion factor } 50 \text{ mcg/mL}} = \frac{1.425 \text{ OD}}{X}$$

$$X = (50)(1.425)$$

$$X = 71 \text{ mcg/mL}$$

Therefore, there are 71 mcg/mL dsDNA in this sample.

TABLE 11-3 **Relationship Between Absorbance 260 nm and Micrograms per Milliliter**

Absorbance at 260 nm	mcg/mL
1	50 mcg/mL dsDNA
1	40 mcg/mL RNA
1	33 mcg/mL ssDNA

EXAMPLE PROBLEMS

This section is designed to be useful to both the student and the laboratory professional. Students can use the additional problems to master the material. The laboratory professional can use the examples as templates for solving laboratory calculations. By finding an example similar to the problem that you need to solve, substitute the numbers appropriate to your calculation into the equation.

1. **Q.** Convert 5 mg to microgram units.
   A. A milligram is 1000 times smaller than a gram. (See **Table 11-1**). A microgram is 1 million times smaller than a gram and 1000 times smaller than a milligram. Therefore 5000 mcg are in 5 mg.

2. **Q.** Convert 80 picograms to nanograms.
   A. A nanogram is 1000 times larger than a picogram (1×10^{-9} vs. 1×10^{-12}). Another way of looking at it is that a picogram is 1000 times smaller than a nanogram. Therefore, by dividing 80 by a factor of 1000, the number of nanograms can be determined. Eighty picograms are equal to 0.08 or 8.0×10^{-2} nanograms.

3. **Q.** An assay needs 100 mL of a 10 mM TE buffer. The stock 20 mM TE buffer is available. How much of the stock buffer should be used to make the 10 mM buffer?
   A. This is a C1V1 = C2V2 problem. The calculation is 20 mM X = (10 mM)(100 mL); 20 X = 1000, X = 50 mL of the 20 mM TE buffer. Therefore 50 mL of the stock buffer would be added to 50 mL of deionized water to make 100 mL of a 10 mM TE buffer.

4. **Q.** What is the average molecular weight of a dsDNA?
   A. The average molecular weight of a dsDNA is 660 pg/pmol. See info in **Table 11-2.**

5. **Q.** What is the average molecular weight of a ssDNA?
   A. The average molecular weight of a ssDNA is 330 pg/pmol.

6. **Q.** How many picomoles per microliter of ssDNA are in a 250 mcg/mL sample with 600 base pairs?
   A. There are 1.26 pmol/mcL in this sample. Use the following conversion formula to convert mcg/mL to pmol/mcL:

$$\frac{X \text{ mcg ssDNA}}{mL} \times \frac{pmol}{330 \text{ pg}} \times \frac{1 \text{ mL}}{1000 \text{ mcL}} \times \frac{10^6 \text{ pg}}{1 \text{ mcg}} \times \frac{1}{n}$$

Substituting into the formula the values from this problem:

$$\frac{250 \text{ mcg ssDNA}}{mL} \times \frac{pmol}{330 \text{ pg}} \times \frac{1 \text{ mL}}{1000 \text{ mcL}} \times \frac{10^6 \text{ pg}}{1 \text{ mcg}} \times \frac{1}{600} = 1.26 \text{ pmol/mcL}$$

7. **Q.** Convert 1.60 pmol/mcL of a 725 nucleotide RNA sample to micrograms per milliliter.
   A. There are 383 mcg/mL in this sample. Use the following conversion formula:

$$\frac{\text{X pmol RNA}}{\text{mcL}} \times \frac{330 \text{ pg}}{\text{pmol}} \times \frac{1000 \text{ mcL}}{1 \text{ mL}} \times \frac{1 \text{ mcg}}{10^6 \text{ pg}} \times n = \text{mcg/mL RNA}$$

Substituting into the formula the values from the problem:

$$\frac{1.6 \text{ pmol RNA}}{\text{mcL}} \times \frac{330 \text{ pg}}{\text{pmol}} \times \frac{1000 \text{ mcL}}{1 \text{ mL}} \times \frac{1 \text{ mcg}}{10^6 \text{ pg}} \times 725 = 383 \text{ mcg/mL RNA}$$

8. **Q.** Given an absorbance ratio of 260/280 of 1.9 for a DNA sample, is this sample pure DNA?
   A. Yes, since the ratio is between 1.8 and 2.0.

9. **Q.** Given an absorbance of 1.444 for a ssDNA sample, what is its concentration in micrograms per milliliter?
   A. 47.65 mcg/mL

HOW   # PRACTICE PROBLEMS

Solve the following practice problems to further master the material. Answers and explanations to some problems can be found in the Answer Key.

For problems 1 through 4, convert the following:

1. 30 mcg/mL to picograms per milliliter

2. 120 fg to picograms

3. 62 mg to nanograms

4. 2.8 mcg to milligrams

5. How much diluent is needed to make 40 mL of a 70%$^{v/v}$ ETOH solution from a 95% ETOH stock?

6. Convert 0.45 pmol/mcL, 480 nucleotide ssDNA to micrograms per milliliter.

7. Convert 80 mcg/mL 1325 base pair dsDNA to picomoles per microliter.

8. Given an absorbance of 1.485 for an RNA sample at 260 nm, what is its concentration in micrograms per milliliter?

QUICK NOTES

• To convert dsDNA that is in terms of mcg/mL to pmol/mcg dsDNA, use the factor of 660 pg/mL in the formulas.
• To convert ssDNA or ssRNA, use 330 pg/pmol in the formulas.

MOLECULAR BIOLOGY RESOURCES
Professional Societies

Note: This is not a comprehensive list of all molecular biology organizations.

American Society for Biochemistry and Molecular Biology (ASBMB)
11200 Rockville Pike, Suite 302
Bethesda, MD 20814-3996
Ph: 240-283-6600
Fax: 301-881-2080
http://www.asbmb.org

American Society for Cell Biology
8120 Woodmont Avenue, Suite 750
Bethesda, MD 20814-2762
Ph: 301-347-9300
Fax: 301-347-9310
http://www.ascb.org

American Society for Microbiology
1752 N Street NW
Washington, DC 20036-2904
Ph: 202-737-3600
http://www.asm.org

American Society for Virology (ASV)
3000 Arlington Avenue, Mail Stop 1021
Toledo, OH 43614-2598
Ph: 419-383-5173
Fax: 419-383-2881
http://www.asv.org/

European Molecular Biology Laboratory (EMBL)
EMBL Heidelberg
Meyerhofstraße 1, 69117 Heidelberg, Germany
Ph: +49 (0) 6221 3870
Fax: +49 (0) 6221 3878306
http://www.embl.org

European Molecular Biology Organization (EMBO)
Postfach 1022.40
D-69012 Heidelberg, Germany
Ph: +49 6221 8891 0
Fax: +49 6221 8891 200
http://www.embo.org

Pan American Society for Clinical Virology
http://www.virology.org/

Internet Resources

Molecular Biology Resources (University of South Carolina)
https://sc.edu/study/colleges_schools/artsandsciences/biological_sciences/research/mcdb/index.php

The Bio-Web: Your Source for Molecular and Cell Biology-Bioinformatics-Technology News and Online Bio-Resources
http://www.cellbiol.com

Molecular Biology Core Facilities (Dana-Farber Cancer Institute)

http://mbcf.dfci.harvard.edu/
Computational Molecular Biology (National Institutes of Health)

https://www.nihlibrary.nih.gov/services/bioinformatics-support

Molecular Biology Resources on the Web (New York University)
http://sun-lab.med.nyu.edu/protocols-reagents/molecular-biology-resources-web

CHAPTER 12

Quality Assurance in the Clinical Laboratory: Basic Statistical Concepts

OBJECTIVES

At the end of this chapter, the reader should be able to do the following:

1. Define the following terms: *mean, median, mode, Gaussian distribution, variance, standard deviation,* and *coefficient of variation.*
2. Calculate the mean of a group of numbers.
3. Calculate the median of a group of numbers.
4. Calculate the mode of a group of numbers.
5. Calculate the variance and the standard deviation of a group of numbers.
6. Calculate the coefficient of variation for a group of numbers.
7. Compare two or more groups of numbers and determine the group with the highest precision.
8. Define confidence limits.
9. Calculate the confidence limits or standard deviation limits for a given set of data.

As laboratory professionals, we strive to produce accurate laboratory results. Statistical analysis of data is one tool we can use to help us accomplish this goal. To fully understand the analysis of data, we first must understand some basic statistical terms.

WHAT MEAN

The mean is the average of a group of numbers. In statistical analysis its symbol is $\overline{X}$. We sometimes use the mean value to perform other statistical tests on the group. The mean is one indicator of central tendency. Central tendency is the distribution of data around a central value.

HOW   *Example 12-1*

A student was performing a manual wet chemistry laboratory in which she obtained five replicate absorbance values for her unknown. What is the mean absorbance value for the unknown?

REPLICATE	ABSORBANCE VALUE
1	0.425
2	0.430
3	0.435
4	0.432
5	0.428

To calculate the mean, first add the five absorbance values.

$$0.425 + 0.430 + 0.435 + 0.432 + 0.428 = 2.15$$

The next step is to divide the sum by the total number of absorbance values, in this case, 5. The quantity of numbers included in a set is referred to as n.

$$\frac{2.15}{n \text{ or } 5} = 0.430$$

$$\text{Therefore, } \overline{X} = 0.430$$

The mean value for this group of absorbance values is 0.430.

In this case, the mean value also happened to be the same as one of the numbers of the group. This does not always occur.

Example 12-1a   What is the mean of the following group of magnesium values?

3.5 mg/dL, 5.4 mg/dL, 2.8 mg/dL, 4.1 mg/dL, 2.5 mg/dL, 3.6 mg/dL, 4.7 mg/dL

The mean value for this group of numbers is 3.8 mg/dL.

Example 12-1b   What is the mean of the following group of sodium values?

144 mEq/L, 137 mEq/L, 141 mEq/L, 143 mEq/L, 138 mEq/L, 140mEq/L, 141 mEq/L, 146 mEq/L, 147 mEq/L, 140 mEq/L

The mean value for this group of numbers is 142 mEq/L.

WHAT **MEDIAN**

Another indicator of central tendency is the median. The median is the central number in a set of numbers when the numbers are arranged in sequential order. In a set of numbers, an equal quantity of numbers is greater than the median value, and an equal quantity of numbers is less than the median value. The median value may or may not be the same as the mean value.

HOW   *Example 12-2*

Using the same group of absorbance values as in Example 12-1, find the median value.
    To find the median value, first rank the numbers from lowest to highest value.

Lowest value	0.425
	0.428
	0.430
	0.432
Highest value	0.435

Notice that the total number of values (five) in this set is an odd number. To determine the median of a set of values containing an odd number of values, first add 1 to the total number of values (five). Divide the total number of values (plus 1) by 2.
    In this example, there are five values.

$$5 + 1 = 6$$

$$\frac{6}{2} = 3$$

Next, go down the list to the third number on the list, which is 0.430. This number is the median value for this group of numbers.

Lowest value	0.425	
	0.428	
	0.430	←MEDIAN
	0.432	
Highest value	0.435	

Notice that there is an equal quantity of numbers above and below the median value.

Example 12-2a   Find the median of the following group of creatinine values:

1.2 mg/dL, 1.0 mg/dL, 1.3 mg/dL, 1.1 mg/dL, 1.4 mg/dL, 1.2 mg/dL, 1.1 mg/dL

To find the median value, first rank the group of numbers from lowest value to highest value: 1.0, 1.1, 1.1, 1.2, 1.2, 1.3, 1.4.

Since there are seven numbers, add 1 to the number 7 (8), divide by 2 (4). Find the fourth number: 1.2. Therefore the median value in this group of creatinine values is 1.2 mg/dL.

Example 12-2b   Find the median value in the following group of glucose values:

88 mg/dL, 75 mg/dL, 79 mg/dL, 81 mg/dL, 83 mg/dL

Since there are five values, after ranking the numbers from lowest to highest value, find the third value in the list of numbers [(5 + 1)/2 = 3].

75, 79, 81, 83, 88

Therefore the median value in this group of glucose values is 81 mg/dL.

Example 12-2c In Example 12-2b, the quantity of numbers in the group was an odd number (5). If the quantity of a group of numbers is an even number, the median must be calculated slightly differently. Given the following number set, determine the median value.

27, 24, 22, 25, 20, 21, 23, 26

The first step is to arrange the numbers in order from lowest to highest value.

Lowest	20
	21
	22
	23
	24
	25
	26
Highest	27

Next, divide the total quantity of numbers in this group by 2. There are eight numbers in this group.

$$\frac{8}{2} = 4$$

Next, add 1 to this value.

$$4 + 1 = 5$$

The median in this group of numbers is found to be the average of the fourth and fifth numbers in this group.

20
21
22
23   **Fourth number = Median = 23.5**
24   **Fifth number**
25
26
27

The median for this group of numbers is 23.5. Notice that there is an equal quantity of numbers above and below the median value.

Example 12-2d What is the median value for this set of chloride values?

107 mEq/L, 105 mEq/L, 110 mEq/L, 109 mEq/L

To calculate the median, first rank from lowest to highest value:

105, 107, 109, 110

Next, since there are four values (an even quantity), divide 4 by 2, yielding 2; then add 1, equaling 3. Therefore the median value will be the average of the second and third value, or 108 mEq/L.

Example 12-2e What is the median value for this set of blood urea nitrogen (BUN) values?

10.8 mg/dL, 10.2 mg/L, 10.7 mg/L, 10.2 mg/L, 10.3 mg/L, 10.4 mg/L

First, rank from lowest to highest value:

10.2, 10.2, 10.3, 10.4, 10.7, 10.8

Next, take the average of the third and fourth value (6 values/2 = 3, + 1 = 4). Therefore the median for this group of BUN values is 10.35, rounded to 10.4 mg/dL.

WHAT **MODE**

The third indicator of central tendency is the mode. The mode is the number that occurs most frequently in a group of numbers.

HOW ***Example 12-3***

What is the modal number for the following group of glucose values? All values are in milligrams/deciliter units.

75, 74, 72, 70, 76, 73, 72, 71

The first step is to arrange the data from the lowest value to the highest.

Lowest	70
	71
	72
	72
	73
	74
	75
Highest	76

Next, determine the number(s) that occurs most frequently.

NUMBER	FREQUENCY
70	1
71	1
72	2
73	1
74	1
75	1
76	1

From this chart, you can see that the number 72 occurs two times, so 72 mg/dL is the modal number for this group of glucose values.

Example 12-3a   Calculate the modal value of the following group of potassium values:

4.5 mEq/L, 4.6 mEq/L, 4.5 mEq/L, 4.7 mEq/L

To solve, rank the values from lowest to highest value:

4.5, 4.5, 4.6, 4.7

The modal value is 4.5 mEq/L.

Example 12-3b   Calculate the modal value of the following group of aspartate aminotransferase (AST) values:

36 IU/L, 22 IU/L, 25 IU/L, 21 IU/L, 22 IU/L

The modal value is 22 IU/L.

WHAT   GAUSSIAN DISTRIBUTION

Mean, median, and mode are all indicators of central tendency. When the mean, median, and mode are all the same number, we say that the group of numbers has a Gaussian distribution. Figure 12-1 is a Gaussian distribution. Another term for Gaussian distribution is normal distribution. A Gaussian distribution is bell shaped, with an equal amount of results above (right) and below (left) the highest point of the bell (center). In the laboratory, many times it is assumed that our data have a Gaussian distribution when we perform statistical analysis of the data. It is outside of the scope of this book to go into detail about the statistical analysis of data that do not have a Gaussian distribution. In a normal Gaussian distribution, as the mean, median, and mode are equal, a frequency distribution of the data has a bell shape.

WHAT   ACCURACY VERSUS PRECISION

In the laboratory, we strive to produce results that correctly assess the patient's condition. Two terms are used to describe the quality of the results that are produced. These are *accuracy* and *precision*. An accurate result correctly reflects the true value of the result. Imagine a target value that should be obtained for an analyte. If the results obtained reflect the target value, then we can say that the results are accurate. The mean value we obtained in our data should be very close to the target value. In the laboratory, by using quality assurance, we try to ensure that the tendency for the results to be centrally located or "hitting the target" can be achieved.

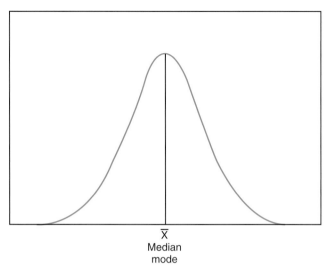

FIGURE 12-1 Gaussian distribution, or normal distribution where the mean = median = mode.

Precision occurs when, after repeated analysis, the same result is achieved. Precision is related to the amount of dispersion of the data around the target value. If there is a wide degree of dispersion, the results are not precise. However, precise results are those that are tightly clustered together. In the laboratory, we want results that are tightly clustered around the true value—that is, both accurate and precise. The statistical tools of variance, standard deviation, and coefficient of variation help assess the degree of dispersion of the data.

WHAT **VARIANCE**

The precision of a group of numbers is indicated by the variance. The symbol for variance is s^2. The variance indicates how close together, or how precise, the numbers are within a group. A group of numbers with a large variance would be expected to have a wide range of values. A group of numbers with a small variance would be expected to have numbers that are very close in value. The smaller the variance of a group of numbers, the more precise they are. Variance is calculated using the following formula:

$$s^2 = \frac{\sum (X_d - \overline{X})^2}{n - 1}$$

where:

s^2 = variance
Σ = the sum of the numbers within the parentheses
X_d = an individual data point within the group
$\overline{X}$ = the mean of the group of numbers
n = the total amount of numbers within the group

Most scientific calculators have a variance function. By using the statistical mode of the calculator, the variance can be easily obtained. The variance can also be calculated using computer software such as Microsoft Excel. Manually calculating the variance of a group of numbers may be time consuming but necessary if a scientific calculator or computer is not available.

To calculate the variance of a group of numbers, the mean of the group is first determined. Then the mean is subtracted from each individual number in the group. Sometimes a negative number will result if the mean is of a greater value than a particular number in the group. The differences will be individually squared. The next step is to determine the sum of the individually squared numbers. This value is the numerator of the formula and is divided by one less than the total amount of numbers in the group (n). The number obtained from this calculation is the variance of the group. The units associated with the variance value will also be squared (e.g., mg^2/dL^2) and will not be the same as the units of the group of numbers for which the variance was calculated.

HOW   *Example 12-4*

Calculate the variance of the following group of glucose values. All values have the unit of milligrams per deciliter.

$$94, 93, 92, 100, 101, 93, 105, 98, 99, 87$$

To calculate the variance, first rank the numbers from lowest to highest.

Lowest	87
	92
	93
	93
	94
	98
	99
	100
	101
Highest	105

Next, find the mean of the group of numbers by first determining the sum of the set of numbers:

$$87 + 92 + 93 + 93 + 94 + 98 + 99 + 100 + 101 + 105 = 962 \text{ mg/dL}$$

Therefore the sum, or Σ, of this set of numbers is 962 mg/dL.
Next, divide the sum by n:

$$\frac{962}{10 \text{ or } n} = 96.2 \text{ or } 96 \text{ mg/dL}$$

Now subtract the mean, 96 mg/dL, from each of the numbers in the set.

GLUCOSE RESULT (mg/dL)	$(X_d - \overline{X})$
87	$87 - 96 = -9$
92	$92 - 96 = -4$
93	$93 - 96 = -3$
93	$93 - 96 = -3$
94	$94 - 96 = -2$
98	$98 - 96 = +2$
99	$99 - 96 = +3$
100	$100 - 96 = +4$
101	$101 - 96 = +5$
105	$105 - 96 = +9$

Next, square the difference obtained in column 2.

GLUCOSE RESULT (mg/dL)	$(X_d - \overline{X})$	$(X_d - \overline{X})^2$
87	$87 - 96 = -9$	$(-9)^2 = 81$
92	$92 - 96 = -4$	$(-4)^2 = 16$
93	$93 - 96 = -3$	$(-3)^2 = 9$
93	$93 - 96 = -3$	$(-3)^2 = 9$
94	$94 - 96 = -2$	$(-2)^2 = 4$
98	$98 - 96 = +2$	$(+2)^2 = 4$
99	$99 - 96 = +3$	$(+3)^2 = 9$
100	$100 - 96 = +4$	$(+4)^2 = 16$
101	$101 - 96 = +5$	$(+5)^2 = 25$
105	$105 - 96 = +9$	$(+9)^2 = 81$

Now find the sum of the numbers obtained in column 3.

$$81 + 16 + 9 + 9 + 4 + 4 + 9 + 16 + 25 + 81 = 254$$

Using the variance formula, substitute into it the numbers that have been calculated so far.

$$s^2 = \frac{\sum (X_d - \overline{X})^2}{n - 1}$$

$$s^2 = \frac{254}{9} = 28.2 \text{ mg}^2/\text{dL}^2$$

The variance for this group of glucose values is $28.2 \text{ mg}^2/\text{dL}^2$.

WHAT STANDARD DEVIATION

In the clinical laboratory, the standard deviation is the most frequently used measure of precision. The symbol for standard deviation is **s**. The standard deviation is the square root of the variance. Notice that the units of measurement for the variance are also squared. By taking the square root of the variance, the units become expressed in the same terms as the mean, median, and mode.

HOW *Example 12-5*

Using the same group of glucose values in Example 12-4, calculate the standard deviation. The formula for the standard deviation is as follows:

$$s = \sqrt{\frac{\sum (X_d - \overline{X})^2}{n - 1}}$$

The variance calculated in Example 12-4 was $28.2 \text{ mg}^2/\text{dL}^2$.

$$s = \sqrt{28.2 \text{ mg}^2/\text{dL}^2}$$

$$s = 5.3 \text{ mg}/\text{dL}$$

This group of glucose values has a standard deviation of 5.3 mg/dL. This means that within this group of numbers, the numbers deviated from the central value or mean not more than 5.3 mg/dL. This deviation is referred to as "plus/minus 1 SD" or "+/− 1 SD." The smaller the standard deviation for a group of numbers, the closer the numbers are together in value and the higher the precision of the group of numbers. When the standard deviation is high for a group of numbers, there is a greater dispersion of value among the numbers.

Example 12-5a   Calculate the variance and standard deviation of the following group of sodium values:

144 IU/L, 145 IU/L, 143 IU/L, 139 IU/L, 147 IU/L, 140 IU/L, 144 IU/L, 142 IU/L, 145 IU/L, 147 IU/L

To solve, first rank the values and determine the mean.

$139 + 140 + 142 + 143 + 144 + 144 + 145 + 145 + 147 + 147 = 1436/10 = 144$ IU/L

Next, determine the variance of the group of numbers:

SODIUM RESULT (mEq/dL)	$(X_d - \overline{X})$	$(X_d - \overline{X})^2$
139	$139 - 144 = -5$	$(-5)^2 = 25$
140	$140 - 144 = -4$	$(-4)^2 = 16$
142	$142 - 144 = -2$	$(-2)^2 = 4$
143	$143 - 144 = -1$	$(-1)^2 = 1$
144	$144 - 144 = 0$	$(0)^2 = 0$
144	$144 - 144 = 0$	$(0)^2 = 0$
145	$145 - 144 = +1$	$(1)^2 = 1$
145	$145 - 144 = +1$	$(1)^2 = 1$
147	$147 - 144 = +3$	$(3)^2 = 9$
147	$147 - 144 = +3$	$(3)^2 = 9$

Next, determine the sum of the squared differences:

$$\sum (X_d - \overline{X})^2 = 66$$

Using the variance formula and substituting into it the appropriate calculated values yields:

$$s^2 = \frac{\sum (X_d - \overline{X})^2}{n - 1}$$

$$s^2 = \frac{66}{9} = 7.3 \text{ mg}^2/\text{dL}^2$$

The variance is 7.3 mg²/dL². By obtaining the square root of the variance, the standard deviation is determined to be 2.7 mg/dL.

Example 12-5b   Calculate the variance and standard deviation of the following group of hematocrit values:

45%, 42%, 44%, 41%, 44%, 43%, 41%, 40%, 48%, 43%

The variance of this group of hematocrit values is $5.4\%^2$, and the standard deviation is 2.3%.

WHAT   # PROBABILITIES ASSOCIATED WITH STANDARD DEVIATION

Statistically, if a sample is analyzed 30 times and the mean and standard deviation established for the results obtained, 68.2% of the time the results will fall within plus or minus $(+/-)$ 1 SD of the mean, 95.5% of the time the results will fall within $+/-$ 2 SD of the mean, and 99.7% of the time the results will fall within $+/-$ 3 SD of the mean. This concept is shown in Figure 12-2. These statistical probabilities are used when establishing the acceptable limits of our quality control (QC) results.

HOW   ### Example 12-6

If the mean for glucose in a quality control sample is 100 mg/dL, and 1 SD is 5 mg/dL, what is the probability that if the control sample is reanalyzed, the result will fall between 95 and 105 mg/dL $(+/-$ 1 SD)?

Statistically, it is known that 68.2% of the time a result will fall within $+/-$ 1 SD of an established value (mean). In this case, if the sample was analyzed 100 times, in 68 analyses the results will be between 95 and 105 mg/dL. However, 32 of the analyses will fall outside of this range.

Example 12-6a   What is the probability that a quality control value will fall outside of 2 SD?

Statistically, 95% of the time the quality control results will fall within $+/-$ 2 SD; therefore 5% of the time the result may fall outside of the $+/-$ 2 SD range.

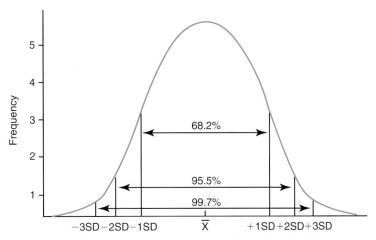

FIGURE 12-2 Probabilities associated with standard deviations.

Example 12-6b   If quality control material were analyzed 40 times, how many of the results could be expected to be outside of 2 SD?

Two of the 40 results would be expected to be outside of 2 SD, as 5% translates into 1 of 20, 2 of 40, 3 of 60, etc.

WHAT   **ESTABLISHING STANDARD DEVIATION LIMITS, STANDARD DEVIATION INTERVALS, OR CONFIDENCE INTERVALS**

When establishing acceptable limits for quality control, the standard deviation is not generally used by itself; instead, the standard deviation limit or interval is more useful. The terms *standard deviation range, standard deviation interval, standard deviation limits,* and *confidence intervals* have the same meaning. For the purposes of clarity, the term *standard deviation limits* will be used to explain the concept. The standard deviation limits are a measurement of dispersion. The limits are calculated by subtracting the standard deviation value from the mean value to establish the lowest number in the limit and adding the standard deviation value to the mean value to establish the highest number in the limit. In this manner, the standard deviation limits are the range of numbers from lowest to highest that are clustered or dispersed around the mean. Standard deviation limits are established for quality control material by the laboratory as a method of setting acceptable quality control limits. Frequently 1, 2, and 3 SD ranges are established.

HOW   **Example 12-7**

A single bottle of quality control was analyzed for sodium 20 times. The mean sodium value was 140 mEq/L. The standard deviation result was 3 mEq/L. Establish the 1, 2, and 3 SD ranges, or confidence intervals, for the quality control.

To establish the standard deviation range, the standard deviation value is subtracted from, and also added to, the mean value to establish the lower and upper limits. The 1 SD limits are established as follows:

$$1 \text{ standard deviation} = 3 \text{ mEq/L; mean} = 140 \text{ mEq/L}$$

$$140.0 - 3.0 = 137.0 \text{ mEq/L}$$

$$140.0 + 3.0 = 143.0 \text{ mEq/L}$$

The 1 SD limits are 137 to 143 mEq/L. This means that all numbers from 137 to 143 mEq/L are within 1 SD of the mean.

$$2 \text{ standard deviations} = 1 \text{ standard deviation} \times 2 = 3.0 \times 2 = 6 \text{ mEq/L}$$

$$140.0 - 6.0 = 134.0 \text{ mEq/L}$$

$$140.0 + 6.0 = 146.0 \text{ mEq/L}$$

The 2 SD limits are 134 to 146 mEq/L. Therefore all numbers from 134 to 146 mEq/L are within 2 SD from the mean.

$$3 \text{ standard deviations} = 1 \text{ standard deviation} \times 3 = 3.0 \times 3 = 9 \text{ mEq/L}$$

$$140.0 - 9.0 = 131.0 \text{ mEq/L}$$

$$140.0 + 9.0 = 149.0 \text{ mEq/L}$$

The 3 SD limits are 131 to 149 mEq/L. Therefore all numbers from 131 to 149 mEq/L are within 3 SD of the mean.

Example 12-7a   If the mean for 20 glucose QC results was 150 mg/dL, and 1 SD was 8 mg/dL, calculate the 1, 2, and 3 SD limits.

To calculate the 1 SD limits:

$$150 + 8 = 158\text{mg/dL}$$
$$150 - 8 = 142 \text{ mg/dL}$$

The 1 SD limits are 142 to 158 mg/dL.

To calculate the 2 SD range:

$$150 + 16 = 166 \text{ mg/dL}$$
$$150 - 16 = 134 \text{ mg/dL}$$

The 2 SD limits are 134 to 166 mg/dL.

To calculate the 3 SD range:

$$150 + 24 = 174 \text{ mg/dL}$$
$$150 - 24 = 126 \text{ mg/dL}$$

The 3 SD limits are 126 to 174 mg/dL.

Example 12-7b   Calculate the 1, 2, and 3 SD limit for QC Level 1 for hemoglobin if the mean was determined to be 8.0 mg/dL, and 1 SD was determined to be 1.2 mg/dL.

The 1 SD limits are 6.8 to 9.2 mg/dL.

The 2 SD limits are 5.6 to 10.4 mg/dL.

The 3 SD limits are 4.4 to 11.6 mg/dL.

Example 12-7c   If the +/− 2 SD limit for a glucose quality control level was 80 to 110 mg/dL, what is the mean, and what is 1 SD?

To solve, remember that the spread between 80 and 110 is 4 SD. Therefore, first take the average of 80 and 110, which is 95. This is the mean. Now you know that the −2 SD limit from the mean is from 80 to 95, and the + 2 SD limit from the mean is from 95 to 110. There is a 15 mg/dL difference for each 2 SD range, so a 1 SD would be half of 15, or 7.5. Therefore 1 SD is 7.5, and the mean is 95 mg/dL. You can prove this by adding and subtracting 7.5 from 95 to reach the +/− 1 SD range of 80 to 110:

$$95 - 7.5 = 87.5$$
$$95 + 7.5 = 102.5$$

Therefore, +/− 1 SD limits are 87.5 to 102.5 mg/dL.

$$87.5 - 7.5 = 80$$

$$102.5 + 7.5 = 110$$

Therefore, the $+/-$ 2 SD limits are 80 to 110 mg/dL.

WHAT **COEFFICIENT OF VARIATION**

The last statistical term to describe dispersion or precision is the coefficient of variation. The coefficient of variation (CV) is useful when comparing two or more groups of data to determine which has the greatest precision. The lower the coefficient of variation for a group of data, the more precise the data. In the laboratory, an instrument with a CV of 2% would be more precise than one with a CV of 5%. The coefficient of variation is calculated by the following formula:

$$\%CV = \frac{s}{X} \times 100$$

The coefficient of variation is expressed as a percentage.

HOW **Example 12-8**

Using the information from Examples 12-4 and 12-5, calculate the coefficient of variation for the group of glucose results.

From Example 12-4, the mean was determined to be 96 mg/dL. From Example 12-5, the standard deviation was determined to be 5.3 mg/dL. Using the coefficient of variation formula, the following calculation is derived:

$$\%CV = \frac{5.3 \text{ mg/dL}}{96 \text{ mg/dL}} \times 100 = 5.5\%$$

The coefficient of variation for the group of glucose values is 5.5%.

Example 12-8a   For a hematocrit method, given a standard deviation of 2.0%, and a mean of 45%, what is the coefficient of variation?

The coefficient of variation is calculated by dividing the standard deviation by the mean and multiplying that value by 100. Therefore the coefficient of variation for the hematocrit method is $(2/45) \times 100 = 4.4\%$.

Example 12-8b   Given a standard deviation of 1.5 mEq/L, and a mean of 141 mEq/L for a sodium method, what is the coefficient of variation?

The coefficient of variation is 1.1 mEq/L.

Example 12-8c   A technologist performed a glucose assay using the same specimens but two different methods. The CV for glucose method A was 2.7%, whereas the CV for glucose method B was 1.5%. Which method is more precise?

The lower the CV of a group of numbers, the higher the precision of the set of numbers. Therefore glucose method B is more precise than glucose method A.

EXAMPLE PROBLEMS

This section is designed to be useful to both the student and the laboratory professional. Students can use the additional problems to master the material. The laboratory professional can use the examples as templates for solving laboratory calculations. By finding an example similar to the problem that you need to solve, substitute the appropriate numbers appropriate to your calculation into the equation.

1. **Q.** What is the mean of the following set of BUN values? (All values are in mg/dL.)
   15, 20, 21, 24, 21, 19, 26, 20, 18, 23
   A. The mean of a set of numbers is calculated by adding the numbers and dividing the sum by the quantity of numbers in the number set. In this problem, there are 10 numbers, and the sum of the 10 numbers is equal to 207. The mean is calculated by dividing the number 207 by 10, resulting in a mean of 20.7, which is rounded to 21.

2. **Q.** What is the mean of the following set of numbers?
   135.7, 122.1, 132.2, 130.2, 129.1, 126.9
   A. The mean for this set of numbers is 129.4.

3. **Q.** What is the mean of the following set of sodium values? (All values are in units of mEq/L.)
   140, 144, 145, 138, 137, 144, 147, 150, 146, 145, 143, 140
   A. The mean for this set of numbers is 143.

4. **Q.** What is the median number of this set of serum creatinine values? (All values are in units of mg/dL.)
   1.43, 1.42, 1.49, 1.54, 1.40, 1.46, 1.41
   A. The median number is the number that is in the middle of a group of ranked numbers. An even number of digits is above and below the median number in a set of numbers. To calculate the median number, first rank the numbers in order from lowest to highest:
   1.40, 1.41, 1.42, 1.43, 1.46, 1.49, 1.54
   As the total quantity of numbers in the set is an odd number, 7, add 1 to the total quantity of numbers and divide the sum by 2. In this case, $7 + 1 = 8$. Eight divided by 2 equals 4. Finally, find the fourth number in the list of numbers. In this case it is 1.43.
   1.40, 1.41, 1.42, 1.43, 1.46, 1.49, 1.54
   Notice that the median number is the middle number in the group and that there is an equal quantity of values above and below the median value.

5. **Q.** What is the median number of this set of numbers?
   185, 177, 187, 178, 179, 180, 182
   A. The median number of this set of numbers is 180:
   177, 178, 179, 180, 182, 185, 187

6. **Q.** What is the median number of this set of glucose values? (All values are in units of mg/dL.)
   466, 471, 466, 473, 461, 470, 475, 472, 476, 469
   A. The first step is to rank the numbers in order from lowest to highest:
   461, 466, 466, 469, 470, 471, 472, 473, 475, 476
   This set of numbers is composed of 10 numbers, an even number.
   When the median must be found in a group of numbers in which the total quantity of numbers is an even number, the median is calculated by first dividing the total quantity

of the set of numbers, in this case 10, by 2, resulting in the number 5. Next, add 1 to the number 5: $5 + 1 = 6$. The median value for this set of numbers is the *average* of the fifth and sixth numbers.

461	
466	
466	
469	
470	Fifth number
471	Sixth number
472	
473	
475	
476	

The average of 470 and 471 is 470.5. The median number is not rounded. Therefore the median number for this set of numbers is 470.5. Notice that there is an equal quantity of values above and below the median value.

7. **Q.** What is the median value for this set of numbers?
   135, 128, 132, 134, 129, 131
   A. The median value for this set of numbers is 131.5, the average of the third and fourth numbers.

8. **Q.** Determine the modal number for this set of numbers:
   589, 580, 585, 579, 585, 577, 582, 585, 587, 590, 592, 591
   A. The modal number, or mode, is the number in a set of numbers that occurs the most frequently. In a Gaussian distribution, there will be only one modal number. Sometimes in other distribution patterns there may be more than one modal number. The modal number is calculated by first ranking the numbers from lowest to highest:
   577, 579, 580, 582, 585, 585, 585, 587, 589, 590, 591, 592
   Next, determine the frequency of occurrence for each number:

NUMBER	FREQUENCY
577	1
579	1
580	1
582	1
585	3
587	1
589	1
590	1
591	1
592	1

The modal number is the number that occurs most frequently. From the frequency chart, the number 585 occurs three times, whereas all other numbers occur only once. Therefore the modal number for this group of numbers is 585.

9. **Q.** What is the modal number for the following set of numbers?
55, 52, 57, 55, 52, 58, 57, 55, 56, 55
A. The modal number for this set of numbers is 55, which occurs four times. Other numbers within this set occur more than once, but none as many as four times.

10. **Q.** What is the modal number for the following set of serum magnesium values? (All values are in units of mg/dL.)
2.5, 2.8, 2.1, 2.0, 2.4, 2.1, 2.7
A. The modal number for this set of numbers is 2.1.

11. **Q.** Calculate the variance of the following set of serum chloride values. (All chloride values are in units of mEq/L.)
95, 90, 98, 88, 91, 101, 99, 100
A. The variance can be calculated by three methods. The first, and fastest, is with a scientific calculator using the statistical mode. Because scientific calculators may vary in specific keystrokes, consult the manufacturer's instructions on usage of this function. The second method is a computer program, and the third method is the manual calculation of variance. First, determine the total quantity of numbers, or n. In this example there are eight numbers, so n = 8. Next, determine the mean of the set of numbers. In this case, the mean value is 95. Next, rank the numbers in order from lowest to highest and subtract the mean (95) from each number. The term X_d denotes each digit in this set of numbers.

COLUMN 1	COLUMN 2
88	88 − 95 = −7
90	90 − 95 = −5
91	91 − 95 = −4
95	95 − 95 = 0
98	98 − 95 = +3
99	99 − 95 = +4
100	100 − 95 = +5
101	101 − 95 = +6

Next, square the difference in column 2, and determine the sum of the numbers in column 3:

COLUMN 1	COLUMN 2	COLUMN 3
X_d	$(X_d - \overline{X})$	$(X_d - \overline{X})^2$
88	88 − 95 = −7	49
90	90 − 95 = −5	25
91	91 − 95 = −4	16
95	95 − 95 = 0	0
98	98 − 95 = +3	9
99	99 − 95 = +4	16
100	100 − 95 = +5	25
101	101 − 95 = +6	36
		$\Sigma = 176$

Using the variance formula, substitute into it the numbers that have been calculated so far:

$$s^2 = \frac{\sum (X_d - \overline{X})^2}{n - 1} = \frac{176}{7}$$

$$s^2 = 25.1$$

12. **Q.** Using the data from Example Problem 11, calculate the standard deviation of the set of serum chloride values.
    A. The standard deviation is the square root of the variance. As the variance is 25.1, the square root of 25.1 is 5.0. Therefore the standard deviation, or average preciseness of this set of serum chloride values, is 5.0.

13. **Q.** Calculate the variance for the following group of glucose results. All results are in mg/dL.
    240, 238, 233, 247, 237, 240, 239, 240, 241, 242
    A. The variance is 12.9 mg^2/dL^2.

14. **Q.** Calculate the standard deviation for the group of numbers from Example Problem 13.
    A. The standard deviation is the square root of the variance. Since the variance was 12.9 mg^2/dL^2, the standard deviation is 3.6 mg/dL.

15. **Q.** Calculate the variance for the following group of creatinine results. All results are in mg/dL.
    1.2, 1.6, 1.4, 1.3, 1.7, 1.2, 1.5, 1.6
    A. The mean for this group of numbers is 1.4 mg/dL. The n is 8, as there are eight numbers in the group. The variance for this group of numbers is 0.037 mg^2/dL^2. Notice that the units are squared for the variance value.

16. **Q.** Given the variance value for Example Problem 15, what is the standard deviation of this group of creatinine values?
    A. The standard deviation is the square root of the variance. The square root of 0.037 is 0.19. The units will now become expressed in their original form. Therefore the standard deviation of this group of creatinine values is 0.19 mg/dL.

17. **Q.** What is the probability that a quality control result will fall within +/− 1 SD from the mean?
    A. The probability that a quality control result will fall within +/− 1 SD from the mean is 68.2%.

18. **Q.** What is the probability that a quality control result will fall outside of +/− 1 SD from the mean?
    A. Since the probability that a control result will fall within +/− 1 SD is 68.2%, the probability that the control result will fall outside of this limit is 100 − 68.2, or 31.8%.

19. **Q.** What is the probability that a quality control result will fall outside of +/− 2 SD from the mean?
    A. The probability that a quality control result will fall outside of +/− 2 SD from the mean is 4.5%, or approximately 5%.
    This is because the probability that a quality control result will fall within +/− 2 SD is 95.5%; that is, if a quality control sample was measured 100 times, approximately 95 results will fall within the +/− 2 SD limits, and 5% will fall outside of the limit.

20. **Q.** What is the probability that a quality control result will fall within the $+/-$ 3 SD interval?

    A. The probability that a result will fall within the $+/-$ 3 SD interval is 99.7%. Therefore, there is only a 0.3% chance that a result that falls outside of this interval is valid.

21. **Q.** Calculate the $+/-$ 2 SD limits for the creatinine results in Examples 15 and 16.

    A. The mean of the group of numbers was calculated to be 1.4 mg/dL. One SD was calculated to be 0.19 mg/dL. Therefore 2 SD would be twice the value of 1 SD, or 0.38 mg/dL (0.19×2). The $+/-$ (plus and minus) 2 SD limit from the mean is calculated by adding and also subtracting the 2 SD value from the mean. Therefore,

$$\text{Plus 2 SD} = 1.4 + 0.38 = 1.78 \text{ or } 1.8 \text{ mg/dL}$$
$$\text{Minus 2 SD} = 1.4 - 0.38 = 1.02 \text{ or } 1.0 \text{ mg/dL}$$

    Therefore the $+/-$ 2 SD limits for this group of creatinine values is from 1.0 mg/dL to 1.8 mg/dL.

22. **Q.** A new lot of the low-level QC material was assayed 30 times for cholesterol to establish the acceptable QC limits. The mean of the cholesterol values was 155 mg/dL. The standard deviation was calculated to be 4.5 mg/dL. Calculate the $+/-$ 3 SD limits for cholesterol performed on this lot of control material.

    A. The $+/-$ 3 SD limits are calculated by first determining the value of 3 SD. One standard deviation is equal to 4.5 mg/dL. Therefore 3 SD would be 3 times 4.5 mg/dL, or 13.5 mg/dL. Therefore the 3 SD limit would be calculated by adding 13.5 mg/dL to the mean (155 mg/dL) to determine the highest value in the limit and subtracting 13.5 mg/dL from the mean of 155 mg/dL to determine the lowest value in the limit:

$$\text{Plus 3 SD} = 155 + 13.5 = 168.5 \text{ mg/dL}$$
$$\text{Minus 3 SD} = 155 - 13.5 = 141.5 \text{ mg/dL}$$

    Therefore the plus and minus 3 SD limits for cholesterol analysis for this level of QC material includes all values including and between 141.5 and 168.5 mg/dL.

23. **Q.** If the $+/-$ 2 SD limit for a hematocrit control was 30% to 40%, what is the mean for this control?

    A. The mean is the average of the $+/-$ 2 SD range, or 35%.

24. **Q.** What is the standard deviation for the hematocrit control in Example Problem 23?

    A. The standard deviation can be determined by first calculating the spread between the mean and the $+$ 2 SD value, or 35 to 40, which has a spread of 5. This means that 2 SD is equal to 5, so 1 SD will be half of the 2 SD value, or 2.5%. You can prove this by multiplying 2.5 by 4, the total spread of the standard deviation between the $+/-$ 2 SD range of 30% to 40%. Thus $2.5 \times 4 = 10$, the spread between 30% and 40%.

25. **Q.** Calculate the coefficient of variation for a group of QC results assayed for sodium. The mean value was 142 mEq/L, and the standard deviation was calculated to be 1.8 mEq/L.

    A. The coefficient of variation is calculated by the following formula:

$$CV = \frac{s}{\overline{X}} \times 100$$

    The coefficient of variation is expressed as a percentage. By substituting into the equation the values from the problem, the following equation is derived:

$$CV = \frac{1.8 \text{ mEq/L}}{142 \text{ mEq/L}} \times 100$$

$$CV = 1.3\%$$

Therefore the coefficient of variation for this set of sodium results is 1.3%.

26. **Q.** A new supervisor performs 30 replicate hemoglobin determinations on the same tube of blood on two different hematology analyzers. The CV of the hemoglobin determinations on analyzer A was 1.4%, and the CV of the hemoglobin determinations on analyzer B was 2.0%. Which analyzer is more precise?

   A. The coefficient of variation is a measurement of the precision of a method. The smaller the CV, the more precise the method. Coefficients of variation measurements do not reveal anything about the accuracy of the method. When comparing two methods, the method with the smaller CV is more precise. Therefore, in this comparison, analyzer A has a smaller CV than analyzer B and yields more precise results.

HOW **PRACTICE PROBLEMS**

Solve the following practice problems to further master the material. Answers and explanations to some problems can be found in the Answer Key.

Given the following set of AST values, solve the following problems. (All values are in units of IU/L.)

538, 551, 542, 549, 562, 550, 543, 544, 538, 546, 541

1. Calculate the mean for the set of AST values.

2. Calculate the median number in this set.

3. Calculate the modal number in this set.

4. Calculate the variance for this set of AST levels.

5. Calculate the standard deviation of this set of AST values.

6. Calculate the coefficient of variation associated with this group of AST values.

Given the following group of glucose results, solve the following problems:

320 mg/dL, 330 mg/dL, 325 mg/dL, 330 mg/dL, 329 mg/dL, 336 mg/dL, 327 mg/dL, 322 mg/dL, 333 mg/dL, 328 mg/dL

7. Calculate the mean for the group of glucose values.

8. Calculate the median glucose value.

9. Calculate the modal glucose value.

10. Calculate the variance for this set of glucose values.

11. Calculate the standard deviation for the set of glucose values.

12. Calculate the coefficient of variation associated with this group of glucose values.

List the probabilities associated with each event.

13. A control result falls within +/− 1 SD of the mean.

14. A control result falls within + 2 SD of the mean. (Note that it is only asking for one side.)

15. A control result falls within +/− 3 SD of the mean.

16. A control result falls outside of +/− 2 SD of the mean.

17. A control result falls outside of +/− 3 SD of the mean.

18. If a group of data has a standard deviation of 5.0 and a mean value of 75, calculate the +/− 2 SD range for the data.

19. If a group of data has a standard deviation of 10.0 and a mean value of 250, calculate the +/− 3 SD range for the data.

20. If the +/− 2 SD range for a group of cholesterol control results was 140 to 200, what is the mean?

QUICK NOTES

- The mean is the average of a set of numbers.
- The median is the number that is in the middle of the set of numbers when they are ranked low to high or high to low.
- The mode is the most frequent number in a set of numbers.
- An accurate result reflects the true value of the result. The mean value is a measurement that we can use to determine accuracy.
- A precise result is related to the amount of dispersion of the data around the target value. The standard deviation is a measurement that we can use to determine precision.
- The standard deviation is the square root of the variance of a set of numbers.
- There is a 68.2% probability that a quality control value will fall within the +/− 1 SD and a 31.8% probability that a QC value will fall outside of this same range.
- There is a 95.5% (many labs use 95%) probability that a QC value will fall within the +/− 2 SD range and a 4.5% or 5% probability that a QC value will fall outside of this same range.
- There is a 99.7% probability that a QC value will fall within the +/− 3 SD range and a 0.3% probability that a QC value will fall outside of this same range.
- A 5% probability is the same as 1 in 20 replicates, 2 in 40, 3 in 60, etc.
- If you need to compute the probability that a QC value only falls in one direction, the probability numbers are cut in half (15.9%, 2.25% or 2.5%, and 0.15% for 1, 2, and 3 SD ranges).
- The coefficient of variation is an indicator of precision. The lower the CV the more precise the method.

BIBLIOGRAPHY

Bishop M, Fody E, Schoeff L, et al: *Clinical chemistry; principles, procedures, correlations,* ed 8, Philadelphia, 2018, Lippincott Williams & Wilkins.

Burtis CA, Bruns DE, editors: *Tietz fundamentals of clinical chemistry and molecular diagnostics,* ed 7, St Louis, 2015, Elsevier.

Kaplan L, Pesce A: *Clinical chemistry: theory, analysis and correlation,* ed 5, St Louis, 2009, Mosby.

CHAPTER 13

Quality Assurance and Quality Control in the Clinical Laboratory

OBJECTIVES

At the end of this chapter, the reader should be able to do the following:

1. Define the following terms: *quality control material, outlier, shift, trend, random error, systematic error.*
2. Plot quality control results on a Levey-Jennings chart.
3. Evaluate quality control results for shifts and trends.
4. Evaluate quality control results and determine, using Westgard rules, whether the results are acceptable.

WHAT   BASIC QUALITY ASSURANCE CONCEPTS

In the laboratory, the instruments and methodologies must be monitored to ensure accurate results. Quality assurance is the process in which this occurs. Quality assurance is the monitoring of any activity that is associated with a laboratory result. Activities that occur before the sample reaches the laboratory are called preanalytical activities, those that occur in the laboratory that directly deal with the analysis of the sample are called analytical activities, and those that occur after the analysis is performed are called postanalytical activities. The laboratory must monitor each of these activity phases for errors to ensure accurate results. For example, if the wrong patient's sample is drawn, that is a preanalytical error. If the sample is analyzed incorrectly, that is an analytical error. Similarly, if a diluted sample's result was not multiplied by the dilution factor correctly, that is a postanalytical error. One technique that laboratories can use to check the quality assurance procedures is to follow random samples as they proceed from collection to analysis to charting of the results.

WHAT **Quality Control Material**

Within the laboratory, one method that is used to ensure the quality of patient results is to use quality control material. Quality control material is analyzed along with patient specimens, and should be treated as patient specimens. Quality control material should be of the same matrix as the patient sample. The term matrix refers to the chemical and physical characteristics of the material that contains the analytes to be measured. If measurement of analytes in serum is being performed, a serum-based quality control material should be used. Likewise, if measuring analytes in urine specimens, a urine-based quality control material should be used. Quality control material is usually manufactured to contain many different analytes so that it can be used on multichannel analyzers. The concentration of the analytes will vary depending on the level of the quality control. When two or more levels of quality control material are included in an assay, one level may have the concentration of the analyte found in the normal population. The second level may have either the elevated or the low concentration of the analyte. Whether the second control has an elevated or decreased concentration of the analyte will depend on the medical usefulness of the particular concentration. Some analytes require three levels of control because both the decreased level of the analyte and the elevated level of the analyte are medically useful. For example, when analyzing therapeutic drugs such as theophylline, three levels of control (low, medium, and high or levels 1, 2, and 3) are used. Under the final rules of CLIA'88 published in the *Federal Register* on January 23, 2003, at least two levels of quality control material must be included for every assay at a minimum of at least once a day, unless specialty requirements apply or the method has met the criteria for the new Individualized Quality Control Plan (IQCP), which replaced equivalent quality control on January 1, 2016. The CLIA'88 final rules regarding quality control divided the laboratory tests into waived and nonwaived categories. For waived tests, the quality control rules are very simple: Laboratories should follow the manufacturer's instructions for performing quality control. IQCP and equivalent quality control will be discussed later in this chapter. The remainder of this chapter will focus on the quality control that must be performed for nonwaived tests.

The mean and standard deviation (SD) for each analyte is established for each level of quality control material. In this manner, the entire method can be monitored for errors because whatever occurs to the patient samples also occurs to the quality control samples. For example, if the wrong pipette is used in an analysis, and twice as much serum is used, the results for the quality control samples will be twice as high as they should be. Without quality control material to check the accuracy of the method, errors can occur. If the quality control results fall outside of the laboratory's established limits of acceptable results, the patient results should not be reported. Instead, the laboratory's troubleshooting policy for unacceptable quality control results should be followed.

Three forms of quality control are available:

- Lyophilized, or "freeze-dried," quality control material must be reconstituted with diluent before use. It is crucial to use the correct diluent and the proper quantity of diluent to ensure accurate quality control results. Before use, lyophilized controls must be fully reconstituted. Often, after the diluent is added, the control material is swirled gently to mix the diluent and lyophylized material. Then the control is undisturbed for a period of approximately 5 to 20 minutes, which allows for all of the lyophylized material to go into solution. If the quality control material is used immediately after the diluent is added, inaccurate results may occur.
- The second form of quality control material comes from the manufacturer prediluted and ready for use. Reconstitution is not necessary for this type of control.
- The third type of QC material is ethylene glycol-based controls. This type is prediluted in ethylene glycol. Ethylene glycol-based controls should not be used on analytes measured by ion-specific electrodes because the ethylene glycol may damage the electrodes. Ethylene glycol controls are stored in liquid form at $0°C$.

WHAT **Quality Control Analysis**

After quality control materials are used, their results must be analyzed before patient results are reported to the physician. There are many different methods of analysis of quality control results; however, it is beyond the scope of this book to list all of them. Statistical concepts discussed in Chapter 12 form the basis for quality control analysis.

- Recall that 68.2% of the time a control result will fall within +/−1 SD of the mean.
- 95.5% of the time the results will fall within +/−2 SD of the mean.
- 99.7% of the time the results will fall within +/−3 SD of the mean.
- Likewise, approximately 32% of the time results will fall outside of the +/−1 SD limit.
- 5% of the time QC results will fall outside of the +/−2 SD limit OR 2.5% of the time EITHER outside the +2 or − 2 SD limit.
- 0.3% of the time the result will fall outside of the +/−3 SD limit.
- These statistical probabilities are used to establish the acceptable limits of quality control results.

An important question for the laboratory professional to address is, "What is an acceptable quality control material result?" Remember, if the quality control result is outside of the acceptable limit established by the laboratory, the patient results should not be reported until the problem is solved. If a laboratory uses the 2 SD limits, 5 of 100 (or 1 of 20) quality control results will fall outside of the +/1 2 SD limit. In this case, if a result falls outside of 2 SD, there is a 95% chance that the result is invalid and only a 5% chance that the result is valid and fell outside of the limit by chance. Figure 13-1 shows a frequency distribution of 30 quality control results for glucose. The frequency of each SD limit is noted. If a result falls outside the laboratory's established quality control result limit, it is called an outlier. The method is termed **out of control**, and action must be taken to determine the problem. Patient results should not be reported until the method is "in control."

Whether or not outlier control values should be included in the laboratory's quality control statistics depends on each individual laboratory's quality assurance protocol. In general, if the outlier value can be directly traced back to a problem with the control itself—for example, an outdated control—the outlier value is not included in the statistics.

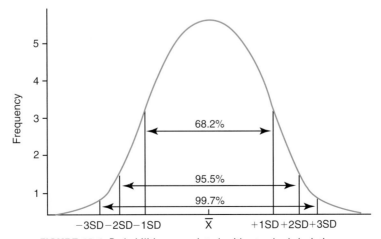

FIGURE 13-1 Probabilities associated with standard deviations.

In the hematology laboratory, the quality control technique of moving averages may be used on automated analyzers to establish the control limits for the erythrocyte indices. Erythrocyte indices tend to be stable within a given population. In the technique of moving averages, 20 consecutive patient samples are batched, and the mean is calculated by the instrument. An overall mean is established for every 20 batches of patient samples (400 different patients). This technique uses a complex mathematical formula to smooth the individual results within the batches, thereby allowing calculation of means and standard deviations for each index.

WHAT Errors That Cause a Method to Be Out of Control

A method may be out of control for two main reasons: random error and systematic error.
- Random error is error that occurs solely by chance. In the 2 SD limit, random error accounts for 5 of 100 (or 1 of 20) QC results outside of the limit, although there is really nothing wrong with the method. Laboratory professionals strive to keep the occurrence of random error as low as possible.
- An example of random error may be a 100 mcL pipette that delivers 100 mcL of sample in most samples for analysis but delivers only 90 mcL of sample in only a few samples. The 90 mcg/L samples will produce inaccurate results because insufficient sample was pipetted.
- Routine maintenance and calibration can reduce the occurrence of this type of random error.
- Random error is related to precision of the method.
- Other examples of random error include a bubble in the sample or reagent that results in inaccurate pipetting by the instrument, an electrical surge or transient power reduction, improperly mixed reagents, pipette tips that do not fit properly, or a clot in the sample that results in a so-called short sample being pipetted.
- Systematic error affects all samples. Systematic error may produce a bias in the method.
- One cause of systematic error may be a refrigerator that does not keep reagents at the proper temperature. Reagents containing enzymes may degrade in potency if not stored properly. Reagents not stored properly may cause falsely lowered and inaccurate results for all patient samples and QC material used.
- Another example of a systematic error is a method with improper calibration. All results will be adversely affected either in a positive or negative direction.
- Systematic error can be reduced with proper calibration and routine maintenance of all laboratory equipment and instruments.
- Systematic error is related to the accuracy of the method.
- Other causes of systematic errors include a change in the lot number of the reagents or calibrators, wrong calibrator or quality control values being used, incorrectly prepared reagents and controls, incorrect storage of reagents and controls, change in temperature of reaction blocks and incubators in the instruments, deterioration of the light source, and a change in procedure from one technologist to another.

WHAT Levey-Jennings Charts

CLIA'88 and good laboratory practice require the use of at least two quality control materials per day for each nonwaived method to ensure accurate and reliable patient results (assuming IQCP is not how the laboratory performs their quality control). The results of the quality control material must be analyzed to determine if the method is "in control" before patient results are reported. One mechanism for quickly analyzing each control value is to plot the value on an individual Levey-Jennings control chart. Figure 13-2 is a Levey-Jennings chart of Level 1

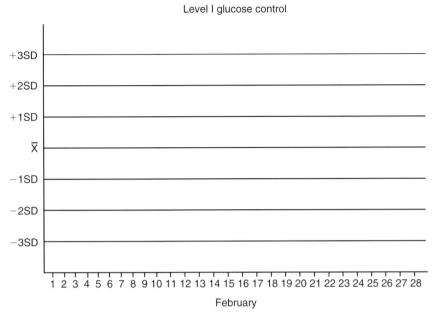

FIGURE 13-2 Levey-Jennings chart for Level 1 glucose control.

glucose control. It consists of a graph in which the mean and SD limits are plotted on the *y* axis, and the days of the month are plotted on the *x* axis. Each level of quality control material for a particular analyte has its own Levey-Jennings chart. For example, although CLIA'88 requires the use of two levels of quality control material for automated hematology analyzers each day, many laboratories use three levels instead and spread them out over the three shifts. This also satisfies the CLIA'88 requirement that the QC is rotated among all staff who perform the tests. If the analyte was hemoglobin, the hemoglobin results obtained from the three different levels of controls would be plotted on three different Levey-Jennings charts, one for each level of control.

HOW   *Example 13-1*

Three levels of control are run daily on an automated hematology analyzer in a physician's office laboratory. The mean for the normal level is 15 mg/dL with a SD of 1.5 mg/dL. What will the Levey-Jennings chart look like if a technician plotted hemoglobin results obtained from the normal level of quality control material over a 5-day period? The quality control hemoglobin results that were obtained are as follows:

Day 1 = 13 mg/dL, Day 2 = 12.5 mg/dL, Day 3 = 16.0 mg/dL,
Day 4 = 15.5 mg/dL, Day 5 = 14 mg/dL

The Levey-Jennings chart is labeled with the days of the week or times of the run on the *x* axis and the mean and SD intervals for the particular level of quality control material on the *y* axis. The 1, 2, and 3 SD intervals must be calculated first. The mean for the level to be plotted is 15 mg/dL, and the SD is 1.5 mg/dL. Therefore the +/−1 SD interval will be from 13.5 to 16.5. The +/−2 SD interval will be from 12 mg/dL to 18 mg/dL, whereas the +/−3 SD interval will be from 10.5 to 19.5 mg/dL. These interval values are plotted on the *y* axis of the chart. The days of the run are plotted on the *x* axis. Figure 13-3 illustrates the Levey-Jennings chart up to this point.

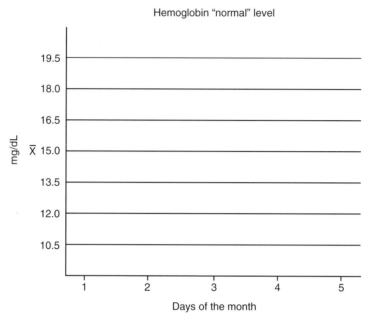

FIGURE 13-3 Constructing a Levey Jennings chart for hemoglobin "normal" levels.

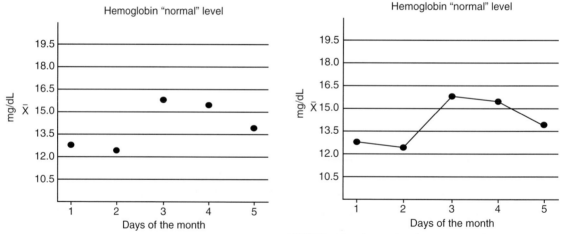

FIGURE 13-4 Plotting the 5 daily Hemoglobin "normal" levels.

FIGURE 13-5 Levey-Jennings chart for normal level hemoglobin control.

Next, the five values obtained are plotted on the chart by placing a dot or circle at the intersection of where the value is found on the *y* axis and the day analyzed on the *x* **axis**, as demonstrated by Figure 13-4.

Last, each result obtained from the same lot number is connected to the next by a line, as illustrated in Figure 13-5. When a new lot number is used, the mean and SD may be different and should be recalculated before use. Then, either a new Levey-Jennings chart is used or the same Levey-Jennings chart is used with a new labeled *y* axis reflecting the mean and SD of the new lot. The results from the two different lot numbers are not connected by a line. A notation should be placed on the chart where the results from the new lot number begin.

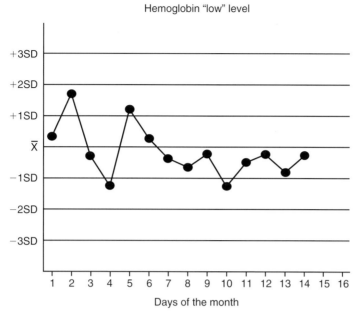

FIGURE 13-6 Levey-Jennings chart demonstrating a shift.

WHAT Shifts and Trends

By plotting quality control results on a Levey-Jennings chart, shifts and trends in the quality control results can be quickly discovered. A shift occurs when the quality control results are all distributed on one side of the mean or the other for 5 to 7 consecutive days. Shifts occur because of systematic error (e.g., a new lot of reagent might have inadvertently been used or a method has not been calibrated). Figure 13-6 demonstrates a shift on a Levey-Jennings chart of the low level of hemoglobin quality control material. When a shift occurs, the cause must be determined and corrected because the method is said to be "out of control."

HOW *Example 13-2*

The following quality control results obtained on days 6 through 11 for a normal level of control material for aspartate transaminase (AST) must be plotted on the following Levey-Jennings chart (Figure 13-7). Days 1 through 5 have already been plotted.

Day 6 = 60 IU/L, Day 7 = 65 IU/L, Day 8 = 62 IU/L, Day 9 = 61 IU/L,
Day 10 = 61 IU/L, Day 11 = 62 IU/L

Is there anything wrong with these quality control results? If there is, what are some of the predominant causes?

The quality control results demonstrate a shift. All the results fall on the same side of the mean, which is statistically unlikely, and there is an abrupt change in the pattern of the quality control results. The most likely cause of the shift is a new lot of reagent used without the assay being recalibrated, or another type of systematic error has occurred.

A trend occurs when the quality control results either decrease or increase consistently over a period of 5 to 7 days. A trend is also due to systematic error, but a trend tends to occur more slowly. For example, reagents may slowly deteriorate if stored in a refrigerator that does

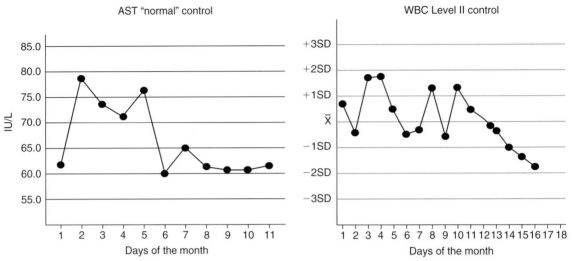

FIGURE 13-7 Levey-Jennings chart demonstrating a shift.   FIGURE 13-8 Levey-Jennings chart demonstrating a trend.

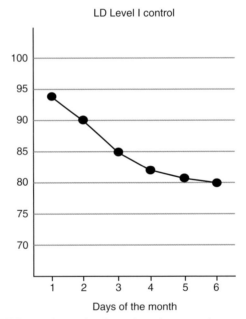

FIGURE 13-9 Levey-Jennings chart demonstrating a trend.

not maintain proper temperature. Another example is if a light source in an instrument slowly deteriorates. Figure 13-8 demonstrates a trend occurring in Level II of a quality control material for automated white blood cell counts. As with shifts, when trends occur, the cause must be determined and corrected.

Example 13-2a   The following Level 1 lactate dehydrogenase (LD) enzyme control results for days 1 through 6 have been plotted on a Levey-Jennings chart (Figure 13-9).

Is there anything wrong with these quality control results? If so, what could be the cause?

Day 1 = 94 IU/L, Day 2 = 90 IU/L, Day 3 = 85 IU/L, Day 4 = 83 IU/L,
Day 5 = 81 IU/L, Day 6 = 80 IU/L

The quality control results demonstrate a trend. Over the course of at least five runs, the results of the control show a consistent downward slide in value. This is not statistically likely to occur. Rather, it is most likely caused by a systematic error that is slowly decreasing the LD results. One cause could be a malfunctioning refrigerator that is slowly losing cooling function, thereby causing the LD reagent to deteriorate, resulting in decreased activity.

HOW   *Example 13-2b*   Evaluate the following Level I glucose QC results that were obtained over the first 10 days of the month. Do these values indicate a shift, trend, or normal distribution?

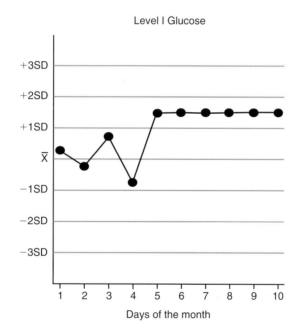

Level I Glucose

Days of the month

This is an example of a shift. From day 5 to day 10, all of the QC results are on the same side of the mean with little variation.

Example 13-2c   Evaluate the following group of QC values to determine if they show a shift, a trend, or a normal distribution. The mean is 150 mg/dL; 1 SD is 5 mg/dL.

Day 1: 145 mg/dL, Day 2: 142 mg/dL, Day 3: 146 mg/dL, Day 4: 155 mg/dL,
Day 5: 157 mg/dL, Day 6: 149 mg/dL, Day 7: 147 mg/dL, Day 8: 145 mg/dL,
Day 9: 143 mg/dL, Day 10: 141 mg/dL

These values show a trend: from day 6 through day 10 the values fall 2 mg/dL each day.

WHAT **QUALITY CONTROL ASSESSMENT**

Each laboratory is responsible for establishing its own criteria for acceptance or rejection of quality control results. For some laboratories, this may mean using the $+/-2$ SD limits as the cutoff point for accepting results. Any quality control results more than or less than 2 SD are rejected, and the method is considered out of control. For most laboratories, this criterion is too stringent. Remember that approximately 5% of the time, a perfectly valid result will fall outside of the 2 SD limit. Other laboratories may use a 2.5 SD limit as the cutoff. Today it is possible with many laboratory instruments to program the instrument with the laboratory's control criteria. When a control result is outside of the criteria, the result is flagged by the computer. Quality control assessments, including Levey-Jennings charts, can be recalled by the computer on a daily or monthly basis.

WHAT **Individualized Quality Control Plan**

CLIA'88 requires a minimum of two levels of controls to be used daily for most methods unless the new IQCP is used. The IQCP has three parts: (1) a risk assessment (RA), in which potential errors and failures in the testing process are identified and evaluated; (2) a quality control plan (QCP), which is the laboratory's standard operating procedure that describes how the laboratory is going to control the quality of a particular test method; and (3) a quality assessment plan (QA), which is the laboratory's written plan to ensure the quality of the laboratory results. Using IQCP is voluntary but gives the laboratory the ability to customize its quality control procedures. The laboratory quality control procedures must follow, at minimum, the instructions given by the manufacturer. If manufacturer's instructions are not given or are less stringent than what is listed in Appendix 13-A, the laboratory must follow either the current CLIA quality control regulations or customize its quality control procedures and develop its own IQCP procedures. Further information on IQCP can be found at www.cms.gov.

HOW **WESTGARD MULTIRULES**

In 1981, Westgard and colleagues developed a set of quality control rules for interpretation of quality control results in the clinical laboratory.

The rules pertaining to two levels of control will be discussed next. Westgard and colleagues have also developed computerized rules for interpreting control results.

The Westgard multirules are designed to be used in a schematic manner, as shown in Figure 13-10. The quality control result is first assessed against the first, or "warning," rule. If this is not broken, the next rule is assessed, and so on. If at any point a rule is violated, except for the warning rule, the result is rejected and the method may be out of control. Some rules are designed to be used with only one of the two control levels; other rules are designed to be interpreted with the results of both levels of controls. The large number (1, 2, 4, or 10) tells you the number of QC results that are out of control. The subscript numbers tell you the standard deviations that have been violated. For example, 1_{2S} means 1 QC value has violated 2 SD.

WHAT **The Warning Rule or 1_{2S} Rule**

The 1_{2S} rule is only a warning rule. This rule is violated if either of the two controls exceeds 2 SD from the mean in either a positive or negative direction. When this rule is violated, the other rules are applied. If the quality control results do not violate any other rule, even if one of the two results violates the 1_{2S} rule, the control results are accepted. This is why the 1_{2S} rule is referred to as the "warning" rule.

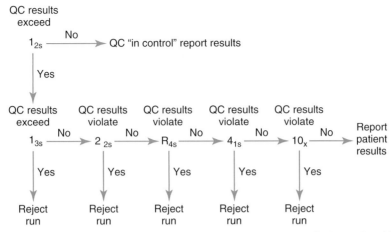

FIGURE 13-10 Quality control rule flow chart for two levels of controls. (Redrawn from Westgard JO, Barry PL, Hunt MR, et al: A multi-rule Shewhart chart for quality control in clinical chemistry, *Clin Chem* 27:493–501, 1981.)

HOW *Example 13-3*

The following are two Levey-Jennings charts for Level 1 (Figure 13-11A) and Level II (Figure 13-11B) glucose control. Notice the results obtained for both levels on day 5. Do the results violate any Westgard rules?

On day 5, the result for the Level 1 control exceeded +2 SD but was within +3 SD. However, the result for the Level 2 control was within 2 SD. Because only one of the two quality control results exceeded +2 SD, the 1_{2s} warning rule was violated. As no other rule was violated on that day, the run can be accepted.

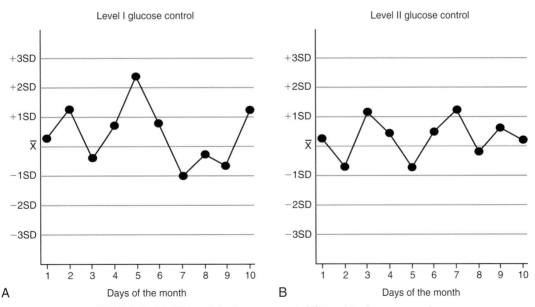

FIGURE 13-11 (A) Level 1 glucose control. (B) Level 2 glucose control.

HOW ***Example 13-3a*** A medical laboratory technician student was reviewing 12 days of Level II QC results for potassium as part of a student laboratory assignment to determine if any of the results violated the 1_{2S} rule. The mean was 6.0 mEq/L with a standard deviation of 0.7 mEq/L. The QC results were as follows:

Day 1: 5.5 mEq/L, Day 2: 6.7 mEq/L, Day 3: 4.5 mEq/L, Day 4: 5.9 mEq/L, Day 5: 6.8 mEq/L, Day 6: 6.1 mEq/L, Day 7: 6.0 mEq/L, Day 8: 5.7 mEq/L, Day 9: 7.7 mEq/L, Day 10: 5.4 mEq/L, Day 11: 6.1 mEq/L, Day 12: 6.5 mEq/L

Do any results violate the 1_{2S} rule?

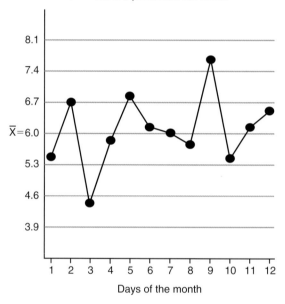

The 1_{2S} rule was violated on days 3 and 9. Since the mean was 6.0 mEq/L, and 1 SD was 0.7, the +/−2 SD limits are from 4.6 mEq/L to 7.4 mEq/L.

Example 13-3b A medical laboratory science student was given 10 days of a Level 1 glucose control to evaluate. The mean was 98 mg/dL, and 1 SD was 4 mg/dL. The control results are as follows:

Day 1: 95 mg/dL, Day 2: 97 mg/dL, Day 3: 101 mg/dL, Day 4: 99 mg/dL, Day 5: 98 mg/dL, Day 6: 94 mg/dL, Day 7: 103 mg/dL, Day 8: 109 mg/dL, Day 9: 103 mg/dL, Day 10: 97 mg/dL, Day 11: 96 mg/dL, Day 12: 100 mg/dL

Do any results violate the 1_{2S} rule?

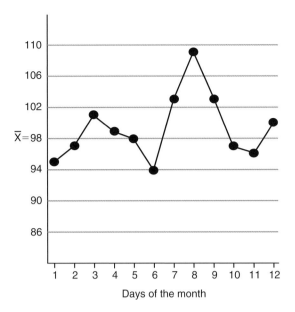

The 1_{2S} rule was violated on day 8 as the result of 109 mg/dL being higher than the +2 SD cutoff of 106 mg/dL.

WHAT   **The 1_{3S} Rule**

The 1_{3S} rule is violated when the result of one of the two quality control results is outside of 3 SD. Remember that, statistically, approximately 99% of all results should fall within +/−3 SD of the mean. Therefore, if a result is outside of 3 SD, there is less than a 1% chance that the result is accurate but a 99.7% chance that the result is an outlier. Because the chance of a QC result falling outside of 3 SD is so remote (<1%), when either of the quality control results violates this rule, the result is rejected, and the run is out of control and should not be accepted. The 1_{3S} rule is often violated due to random error. Causes of random error should be investigated and corrected if possible. For example, if a QC level violates the 1_{3S} rule, but an air bubble is seen in the sample cup, then the quality control level in question should be reanalyzed. If no rules are violated on the repeat analysis, the patient results can be released.

HOW   *Example 13-4*

The following are two Levey-Jennings charts for a Level 1 (Figure 13-12A) and Level 2 (Figure 13-12B) cholesterol control. Notice the result for day 7. What rule, if any, is violated?
    On day 7, the result for the level 2 cholesterol control was greater than 350 mg/dL, which exceeded the +3 SD limit for this cholesterol control. Notice that by default, if a result exceeds +/−3 SD, it will violate the 1_{2S} warning rule, thereby triggering the sequential chain of analysis of the other Westgard rules. According to Figure 13-10, the next rule to analyze after a result has broken the warning rule is the 1_{3S} rule. The Level 2 cholesterol control has violated this rule. The run should not be accepted, and the control should be repeated. Usually, when a control exceeds 3 SD, it is because of a random error and is unlikely to occur again. However, if, upon repeat analysis, the result is still more than 3 SD, an additional rule (discussed next) has been violated, and the cause is due to systematic error. Remember that

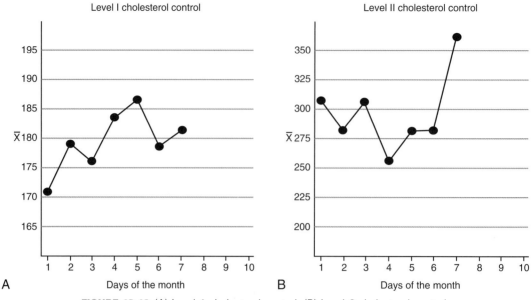

FIGURE 13-12 (A) Level 1 cholesterol control. (B) Level 2 cholesterol control.

systematic error may also be caused by an incorrect lot number of reagent or quality control being used. The medical laboratory scientist or technician should check for causes of systematic errors and correct them, if possible. Sometimes the cause is a bottle of control that, although in date, might have been in use for a while and deteriorated. By using a fresh bottle of control, the new QC result may be acceptable and the run can be accepted.

HOW

Example 13-4a   A new medical laboratory technician reviewed the quality control results obtained that day for a thyroid-stimulating hormone (TSH) assay. The mean for Level 1 was 1.5 mIU/L with a SD of 0.3. The mean for Level 2 was 4.0 mIU/L with a SD of 0.6. The control results were as follows; all units are in mIU/L, and the previous control values for both levels of control were acceptable and within 2 SD.

Level 1: 2.0
Level 2: 6.0

Are these results acceptable? What should the technician do next?

The results for Level 1 shown are acceptable: they are within 2 SD, so there is no 1_{2S} warning rule violation. The results for Level 2, however, violate the 1_{3S} rule as the value of 6.0 mIU/L is outside of the 3 SD upper level of 5.8 mIU/L. The technician should check for causes of random error, correct them if possible, and reanalyze the control (assuming the control itself is not the problem).

Example 13-4b   While pipetting the QC for a manual hexokinase glucose method in a student laboratory, the student noticed that the pipette tip was loose but did not stop and repipette the control. What Westgard rule might be violated because of the loose pipette tip?

A loose pipette tip may cause a random error because the volume of QC pipette will not be the correct amount. The Westgard rule most likely to be violated would be a 1_{3S} rule violation.

WHAT The 2_{2S} Rule

The 2_{2S} rule can be violated in two ways. The first is if both control results tested in a day exceed 2 SD from the mean. Both control results must be greater than 2 SD or less than 2 SD to violate this rule. The second way this rule can be violated is if one of the control results also exceeded 2 SD in the same manner in the previous run or day. For example, if one of the control results fell +2.2 SD from the mean for an assay, and the next time the assay was performed they again fell greater than +2 SD, the 2_{2S} rule would be violated.

HOW *Example 13-5*

The following are two quality control charts for Level 1 (Figure 13-13A) and Level 2 (Figure 13-13B) serum creatinine. Notice the quality control results for day 10. Is a Westgard rule violated on that day, and if so, which one?

On day 10, both the Level 1 and Level 2 creatinine quality control results are greater than 2 SD from the mean. Using the Westgard schematic, on day 10 it is noted that the 1_{2S} warning rule is violated for Level 1 (as well as Level 2). This triggers the evaluation of the other rules. The next rule to be evaluated is the 1_{3S} rule. Neither control value violates the 1_{3S} rule. The next rule is the 2_{2S} rule. When this rule is evaluated, it is noted that both control levels exceed +2 SD from the mean, therefore violating the 2_{2S} rule. No other rule is found to be violated. The 2_{2S} rule is violated because of a systematic error in the method. The cause of the error must be determined and corrected because the method is out of control. Patient results should not be reported until the error is corrected and the control results are acceptable.

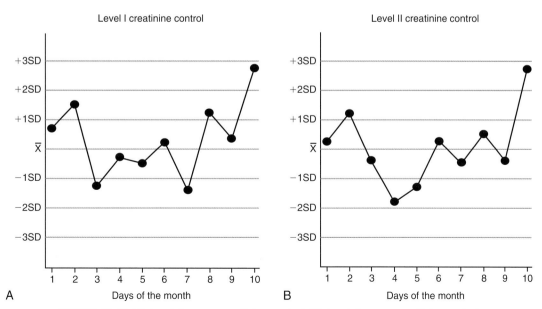

FIGURE 13-13 (A) Level 1 serum creatinine control. (B) Level 2 serum creatinine control.

HOW   ***Example 13-5a***   A medical laboratory scientist was evaluating the hemoglobin QC results at the beginning of the shift. The mean for the Level 2 QC was 13.0 mg/dL, and 1 SD was 0.8 mg/dL. The obtained QC result for Level 2 was 11.1 mg/dL. The mean for the Level 3 QC was 18 mg/dL with a standard deviation of 1.0 mg/dL. The value obtained for Level 3 was 15.5 mg/dL. What should the medical laboratory scientist do next?

The medical laboratory scientist should review the results for the Level 2 control first. The QC value of 11.1 mg/dL is, at minimum, a 1_{2S} warning rule violation because it exceeds the −2 SD value of 11.4 mg/dL. Next, the medical laboratory scientist should review the results of the Level 3 control. These results are also a 1_{2S} warning rule violation. Therefore, there is a 2_{2S} rule violation, and the medical laboratory scientist should troubleshoot for a systematic error.

Example 13-5b   The lead technologist in a hospital core laboratory showed the following QC results for two levels of control for a blood urea nitrogen (BUN) assay for the past week to a medical laboratory science student. Are any Westgard rules violated?

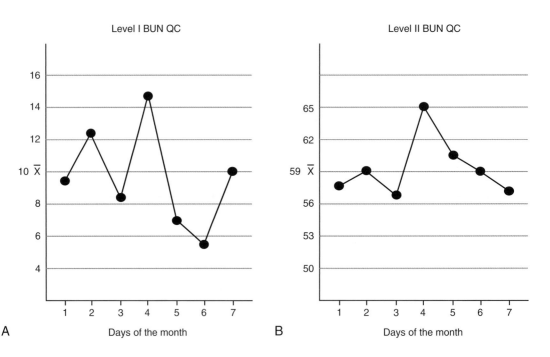

There was a 1_{2S} warning rule violation on both days 4 and 6 for the Level 1 control; however, although the result for day 4 of the Level 2 control is the same as the 2 SD value of 65 mg/dL, it did not *exceed* that level. Therefore no rule was violated. If that value had been higher than 65 mg/dL, the 2_{2S} rule would have been violated because the QC results for both Level 1 and Level 2 would each have been higher than 2 SD on the same side of the mean.

HOW   **Example 13-5c**   The following are two quality control charts for Level 1 (Figure 13-14A) and Level 2 (Figure 13-14B) sodium results. Notice the quality control result on day 4 for Level 2. Is the control result in violation of any rule? If so, which one?

On day 4, the Level 2 control exceeded the -2 SD from the mean control interval. Thus the control violated the 1_{2S} warning rule and triggered the evaluation of the rest of the rules. The 1_{3S} rule is not violated, but examination of the previous run determines that the control has violated the 2_{2S} rule. This is because for two runs in a row, the control results both exceeded 2 SD. In this example, the control results happened to demonstrate a low bias, but the 2_{2S} rule can also be violated if control results demonstrate a high bias by exceeding the $+2$ SD limit in a positive direction rather than a negative direction.

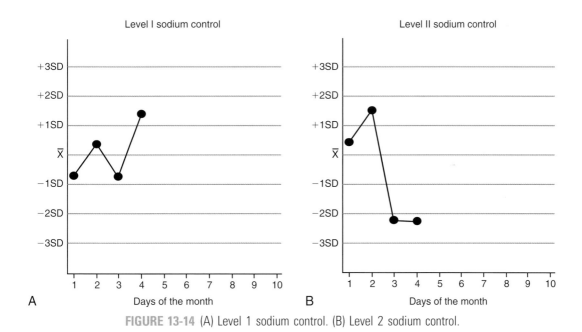

FIGURE 13-14 (A) Level 1 sodium control. (B) Level 2 sodium control.

Example 13-5d   The following are the results of 15 days of two levels of quality control for potassium. Are any Westgard rules violated during these 15 days?

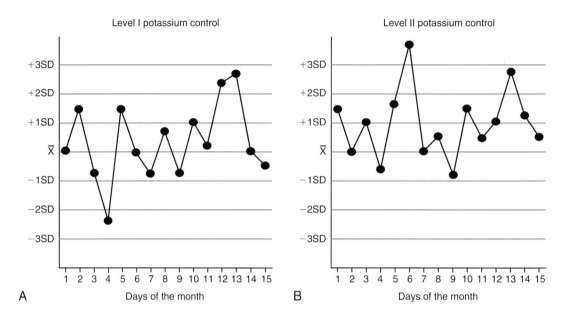

A

B

Westgard rules were violated on days 4, 6, 12, and 13. On day 4 of the Level 1 control, there was a 1_{2S} warning rule that was violated. On day 6, there was a 1_{3S} rule violation of the Level 2 control. On day 12, there was a 1_{2S} rule violation for Level 1, and on day 13, there was a 2_{2S} rule violation both between runs (Level 1) and within runs (both QC results exceeded the −2 SD cutoff).

Example 13-5e   A medical laboratory technician who worked in a physician office laboratory obtained the following glucose results for two levels of control over 20 days. Are any Westgard rules violated in those 20 days?

Level 1: mean = 80 mg/dL, 1 SD = 5 mg/dL
Level 2: mean = 220 mg/dL, 1 SD = 10 mg/dL

All results are in mg/dL.

	LEVEL 1		LEVEL 2
Day	Result	Day	Result
1	73	1	242
2	80	2	220
3	86	3	235
4	71	4	215
5	80	5	220
6	93	6	217
7	78	7	255
8	85	8	220
9	68	9	210
10	68	10	225
11	77	11	236
12	82	12	217

LEVEL 1		LEVEL 2	
Day	Result	Day	Result
13	77	13	232
14	82	14	240
15	98	15	245
16	72	16	225
17	80	17	235
18	81	18	187
19	76	19	219
20	75	20	231

For Level 1, there is a 1_{2S} warning on day 6, a 1_{2S} warning on day 9, and a 2_{2S} rule violation between runs on day 10. There is also a 1_{3S} rule violation on day 15, which is also a 2_{2S} rule violation since the Level 2 control exceeds 2 SD in the same positive direction.

For Level 2, there is a 1_{2S} warning on day 1, a 1_{3S} rule violation on day 7 and day 18, and a 2_{2S} rule violation within the run on day 15.

WHAT **The R_{4S} Rule**

The R_{4S} rule is violated when the difference, or range, between the two control values within a run is greater than 4 SD. For example, if one level of control was -2.2 SD from the mean, and the other level of control was $+2.0$ SD from the mean, the spread of the difference between the two levels is 4.2 SD. Therefore the R_{4S} rule would have been violated. The R_{4S} rule is violated when both control values violate the 1_{2S} rule but in opposite directions; that is, one control is elevated higher than the $+2$ SD limit and the other is less than the -2 SD limit. The R_{4S} rule is usually violated because of random error. The run is rejected and patient results are not reported until the method is in control.

HOW **Example 13-6**

Two levels of quality control for total serum amylase are charted on the Levey-Jennings charts shown in Figure 13-15. Notice the control results for day 12. Are any quality control rules violated on that day?

On day 12, the control result for Level 1 was $+2.1$ above the mean. This violated the 1_{2S} rule and triggered review of the other rules. The control result for Level 2 was -2.2 less than the mean. The spread, or range, between the two control results is 4.3, which violates the R_{4S} rule.

Example 13-6a   Given 4 days of QC results for two levels of QC for a uric acid assay, determine whether any Westgard rules are violated. If so, which one(s)?

Level 1: Mean $= 5.0$ mg/dL, 1 SD $= 0.9$ mg/dL
Level 2: Mean $= 9.1$ mg/dL, 1 SD $= 1.2$ mg/dL

QC LEVEL	DAY 1	DAY 2	DAY 3	DAY 4
1	5.1 mg/dL	5.5 mg/dL	4.7 mg/dL	3.1 mg/dL
2	8.7 mg/dL	9.5 mg/dL	9.0 mg/dL	11.7 mg/dL

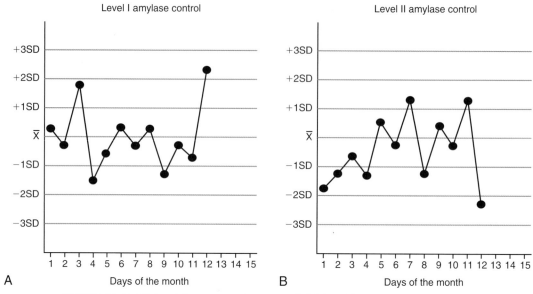

FIGURE 13-15 (A) Level 1 serum amylase control. (B) Level 2 serum amylase control.

For this example, you have to first determine the +/−1, 2, and 3 SD ranges for each level of control. Then you may plot them on a Levey-Jennings chart to better visualize them. On day 4 there is a R_{4S} rule violation as the QC1 was −2 SD and the QC2 was +2 SD, giving a range of over 4 SD. The R_{4S} rule typically is violated because of random error but is also one of the less common rule violations.

WHAT **The 4_{1S} Rule**

The 4_{1S} rule can be violated in two ways. The first is when with one level of control, four consecutive results fall on the same side of the mean and exceed +1 SD of the mean or −1 SD of the mean. This rule can also be used with two levels of control. The rule is violated when both levels of control for two runs in a row exceed +1 SD from the mean or −1 SD from the mean. This rule is somewhat like the rule for a shift; that is, the four results are on the same side of the mean (which is statistically unlikely) and exceed 1 SD (but not 2 SD). This rule demonstrates the importance of not only reviewing the immediate quality control results for rule violations but also reviewing the previous results to look for violations.

HOW *Example 13-7*

Two levels of control for total bilirubin are charted on the Levey-Jennings chart shown in Figure 13-16. Do any of the control results violate any Westgard rules? If so, which one(s)?

On day 4, the Level 1 control violated the 4_{1S} rule because the control result for that day was the fourth result to fall on the same side of the mean and exceed +1 SD of the mean. A systematic error is most likely the cause, and the run is rejected until the problem is corrected.

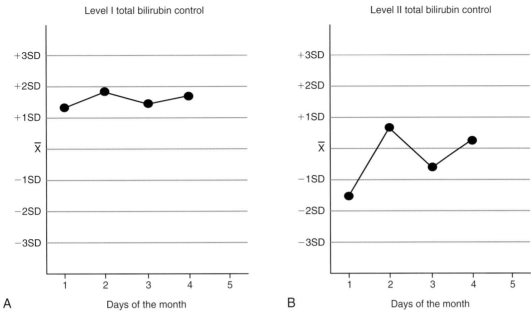

FIGURE 13-16 (A) Level 1 total bilirubin control. (B) Level 2 total bilirubin control.

HOW *Example 13-7a* Evaluate the Levey-Jennings charts of two levels of QC for a sodium assay over 10 days. Are any Westgard rules violated? If so, on which days and on which level of QC?

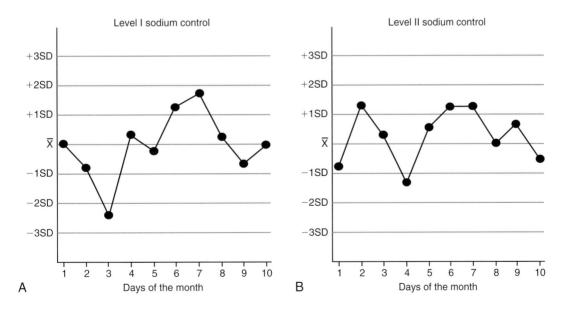

On day 3, there is a 1_{2S} warning rule violation for Level 1. On day 7, there is a 4_{1S} rule violation for the Level 1 and the Level 2 control.

HOW ***Example 13-7b*** Evaluate the following values for two levels of hemoglobin quality control over 10 days. Are any Westgard rules violated? If so, on which days and which level of QC?

Level 1: Mean = 8.0 mg/dL, 1 SD = 0.8 mg/dL
Level 2: Mean = 15 mg/dL, 1 SD = 1.2 mg/dL

All results are in mg/dL.

LEVEL 1		LEVEL 2	
Day	Result	Day	Result
1	7.9	1	15.5
2	10.7	2	14.2
3	7.6	3	16.1
4	6.1	4	12.0
5	8.4	5	15.0
6	9.3	6	16.2
7	9.0	7	13.0
8	9.2	8	16.8
9	9.3	9	15.7
10	7.5	10	15.0

The Westgard rules violated by these controls are as follows:

Level 1: Day 2 is a 1_{3S} rule violation, day 4 is a 1_{2S} warning rule, but that becomes a 2_{2S} rule violation when coupled with the 1_{2S} rule violation on the same day in the same direction for Level 2 control (a within run 2_{2S}). On day 9, there is a 4_{1S} rule violation for Level 1.

Level 2: The only Westgard rule violation is the 2_{2S} on day 4.

WHAT **The 10_X Rule**

The 10_X rule can also be violated in two ways. The first is when results of 10 consecutive runs for one level of quality control are all on the same side of the mean. The 10 results can fall in either a positive or negative direction. The second way this rule is violated is when the results are all on the same side of the mean for both levels of control for 5 days (or five runs) in a row. The 10_X rule detects shifts and is violated because of systematic error. As with all the other rule violations, patient results are not reported until the error is corrected. This rule is not normally used because it would mean that the QC was not accurately analyzed for at least 5 days to detect the shift that is occurring with the QC values. See Example 13-2 for a 10_X rule violation.

HOW ***Example 13-8***

The following are the Levey-Jennings charts (Figure 13-17) of two levels of control for serum total protein. Do the control results violate any Westgard rules? If so, which one(s)?
The Level 2 control results violate the 10_X rule on day 15. Level 1 control results do not violate any of the Westgard rules. A systematic error is occurring with the Level 2 control. The patient results should not be reported until the method is troubleshot.

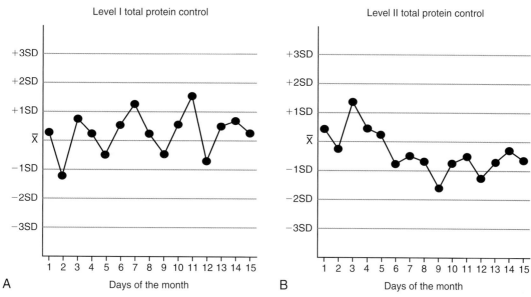

FIGURE 13-17 (A) Level 1 serum total protein control. (B) Level 2 serum total protein control.

Westgard Rules for Three Levels of Control

Three levels of controls are often used with automated cell counters in the hematology laboratory. As mentioned earlier, three levels of controls may also be used for certain chemistry analytes such as therapeutic drugs. The Westgard rules for using three levels of control are not much different from those for two levels. Instead of the 2_{2S} rule, the $(2 \text{ of } 3)_{2S}$ rule is used. This rule is violated when two of the three levels of control exceed 2 SD in the same direction. Instead of the 10_x rule, the 9_x rule is used. This rule is violated when nine results in a row for a single control all fall on the same side of the mean, or when the results for all three levels of control for three runs fall on the same side of the mean. The 4_{1S} rule is not used when using three levels of control. Figure 13-18 is a control schematic when using three levels of control.

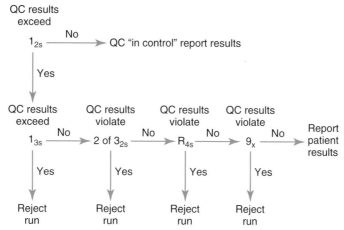

FIGURE 13-18 Quality control rule flow chart for three levels of control. (Redrawn from Westgard JO, Barry PL, Hunt MR, et al: A multi-rule Shewhart chart for quality control in clinical chemistry, *Clin Chem* 27:493–501, 1981.)

EXAMPLE PROBLEMS

This section is designed to be useful to both the student and the laboratory professional. Students can use the additional problems to master the material. The laboratory professional can use the examples as templates for solving laboratory calculations. By finding an example similar to the problem that you need to solve, substitute the numbers appropriate to your calculation into the equation.

1. **Q.** The mean for the Level 1 control for a glucose method is 98 mg/dL. One standard deviation is 5.0 mg/dL. The laboratory uses the +/−2 SD range for the criteria for quality control limits. (Assume that the laboratory operates only one shift.) For the first 10 days of the month, the following quality control results in units of mg/dL were obtained: 105, 106, 104, 107, 104, 105, 106, 106, 107, 108, 107. Is there anything wrong with the quality control results?

   A. The +/−2 SD range for this assay is from 88 mg/dL to 108 mg/dL. All of the quality control results fall within the +/−2 SD range. However, these results demonstrate a shift has occurred as all of the results are above the mean value of 98 mg/dL. The cause of the shift should be investigated and corrected.

2. **Q.** A small physician office laboratory uses the +/−2 SD cutoff for its quality control limits for its hematology analyzer. The mean for the white blood cell count Level 2 quality control is 8.0×10^9/L and the +/−2 SD range is from 7.0×10^9/L to 9.0×10^9/L. Ten Level 1 results were obtained on 10 consecutive days. Is there anything wrong with these results?

   Level 1 results (in units of 10^9/L): 7.5, 7.8, 7.9, 8.0, 8.1, 8.3, 8.5, 8.6, 8.7, 8.8.

   A. None of the results exceed the +/−2 SD quality control cutoff limits. However, the results demonstrate an upward trend is occurring as the results increase in value over time. Quality control results should demonstrate a random pattern of distribution, which these results do not demonstrate. The cause of the trend should be determined **and corrective action should be taken.**

3. **Q.** Using the Westgard multirules criteria and the following quality control results for the Level 1 and Level 2 sodium controls, are the results acceptable? The mean for the Level 1 sodium control is 135 mEq/L with a +/−2 SD range from 130 to 140 mEq/L. The mean for the Level 2 control is 150 mEq/L with a +/− 2 SD range from 145 to 155 mEq/L.

DAY	1	2	3	4	5	6	7
Level 1 control results:	135	136	131	135	136	138	133
Level 2 control results:	150	145	142	152	149	150	148

   A. On day 3, the Level 2 control exceeded the −2 SD cutoff of 145 mEq/L. However, the Level 1 control fell within acceptable limits. The Level 2 control violated the 1_{2S} rule. This rule is only a warning rule, which indicates that a potential problem may be developing. The results are acceptable, and any patient samples run that day could be reported.

4. **Q.** The following are Levey-Jennings charts for two levels of control for glucose. Notice the results for day 5. Are these results acceptable? What rule is violated?

A. On day 5, the result for the level 1 glucose control exceeded + 3 SD. This violates the 1_{3S} rule. The quality control results should not be accepted. Instead, the cause of the out of control result should be investigated.

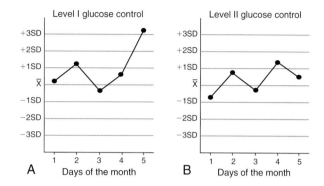

EXAMPLE 4 (A) Level 1 glucose control. (B) Level 2 glucose control.

5. **Q.** The following are the Levey-Jennings charts for the Level 1 and Level 2 potassium controls. Are any Westgard rules violated, and if so which one(s)?

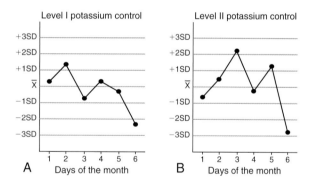

EXAMPLE 5 (A) Level 1 potassium control. (B) Level 2 potassium control.

A. On day 3, Level 2 violated the 1_{2S} warning rule. As no other rule was violated, the quality control results were acceptable that day. On day 6, results for both levels of control fall below the 2 SD cutoff but within 3 SD. This occurrence violates the 2_{2S} rule. This rule indicates that a systematic problem is affecting the method. The cause of the error should be investigated and corrective action should be taken.

6. **Q.** The following are the Levey-Jennings charts for Level 1 and Level 2 creatinine controls. Are any Westgard rules violated, and if so, which one(s)?

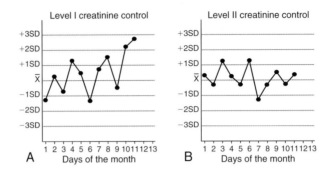

EXAMPLE 6 (A) Level 1 serum creatinine control. (B) Level II serum creatinine control.

A. On day 10, the Level 1 control exceeded +2 SD and therefore violated the 1_{2S} warning rule. However, the Level 2 control for that day did not violate any rules. Thus the quality control results for that day were acceptable. On day 11, the Level 1 creatinine control again violated the 1_{2S} rule as the control result again exceeded +2 SD. However, this violates the 2_{2S} rule, as two sequential quality control results exceeded 2 SD. Remember that the 2_{2S} rule applies not only to the quality control results for both levels of control measured during a run but also to one level of control between runs. Therefore it is always important to evaluate the control results with respect to previous control results when evaluating the results for possible rule violations.

7. Q. The following are the Levey-Jennings charts for the Level 1 and Level 2 amylase controls. Are any Westgard rules violated, and if so, which ones?

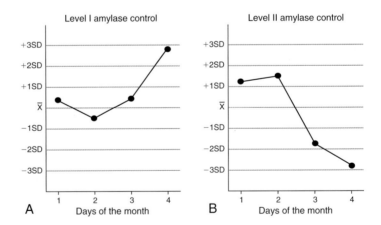

EXAMPLE 7 (A) Level 1 serum amylase control. (B) Level 2 serum amylase control.

A. The R_{4S} rule was violated on day 4 because there is a greater than 4 SD spread between the Level 1 and Level 2 control values. The R_{4S} rule is usually violated because of random error.

8. **Q.** The following are two Levey-Jennings charts for Level 1 and Level 2 cholesterol controls. Are any Westgard rules violated, and if so, which ones?

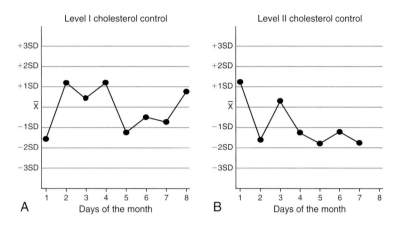

EXAMPLE 8 (A) Level 1 total cholesterol control. (B) Level 2 total cholesterol control.

   A. No rules are violated for the Level 1 control. However, the Level 2 cholesterol control violates the 4_{1S} rule on day 7.

9. **Q.** The following are the Levey-Jennings charts for the Level 1 and Level 2 uric acid controls. Are any Westgard rules violated, and if so, which ones?

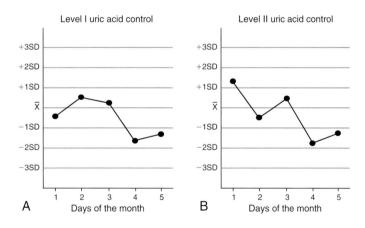

EXAMPLE 9 (A) Level 1 uric acid control. (B) Level 2 uric acid control.

   A. Notice the control results on day 5 for both levels of control. On day 5, the 4_{1S} rule was violated because both levels of control exceeded −1 SD for 2 days in a row. This is most likely not a random occurrence, but rather an indication that a shift may be occurring. The method should be investigated to determine the cause of the problem.

10. Q. The following are the Levey-Jennings charts for Level 1 and Level 2 total protein controls. Are any Westgard rules violated, and if so, which ones?

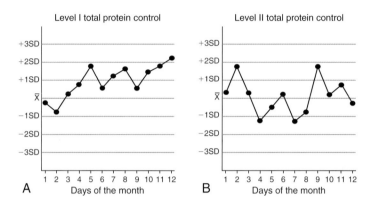

EXAMPLE 10 (A) Level 1 total protein control. (B) Level 2 total protein control.

A. On day 12 for Level 1 the 10_X rule was violated. This rule is violated when for 10 consecutive runs, the quality control results fall on the same side of the mean. This rule may be violated even if the results do not violate the 1_{2S} or 4_{1S} rules. Statistically, it is very unlikely that 10 values in a row will fall on the same side of the mean. Rather, there should be random variation, with some results higher than the mean and some results lower than the mean. The method should be evaluated to determine the systematic error that is causing the problem.

11. Q. The following are two Levey-Jennings charts for the Level 1 and Level 2 albumin controls. Are any Westgard rules violated, and if so, which ones?

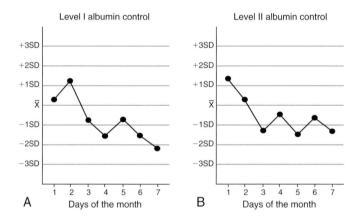

EXAMPLE 11 (A) Level 1 serum albumin control. (B) Level 2 serum albumin control.

A. On day 7, the 10_X rule was violated because on this day, for both control levels, the fifth consecutive control result fell on the same side of the mean. This is highly unlikely and strongly suggests that a shift is occurring. The cause of the problem should be investigated.

HOW   **PRACTICE PROBLEMS**

Solve the following practice problems to further master the material. Answers and explanations to some problems can be found in the Answer Key.

1. Describe what can cause a shift.

2. Describe what can cause a trend.

Use the Westgard multirules system to answer the following questions.

3. Descirbe how to read a Westgard rule to determine how many QC values are to be looked at and what SD the value(s) may have exceeded.

4. Describe the causes of a random error.

5. Describe the causes of a systematic error.

6. Can the R_{4S} rule be violated across runs for one level of control?

7. How can the 4_{1S} rule be violated by both QC levels?

8. How can the 10_X rule be violated?

9. Evaluate the following two levels of QC for a glucose method over 10 days to determine if there are any violations of Westgard rules. All values are in mg/dL.

Level 1: Mean = 83, 1 SD = 4
Level 2: Mean = 260, 1 SD = 8

Level 1:
Day 1: 77, Day 2: 79, Day 3: 84, Day 4: 87, Day 5: 76, Day 6: 74, Day 7: 80, Day 8: 66, Day 9: 74, Day 10: 73
Level 2:
Day 1: 280, Day 2: 265, Day 3: 277, Day 4: 258, Day 5: 280, Day 6: 263, Day 7: 264, Day 8: 273, Day 9: 275, Day 10: 271

10. Evaluate the following two levels of QC for a creatinine method over 10 days to determine if there are any violations of Westgard rules. All values are in mg/dL.

Level 1: Mean = 1.0, 1 SD = 0.2
Level 2: Mean = 5.4, 1 SD = 0.7

Level 1:
Day 1: 1.1, Day 2: 0.8, Day 3: 1.4, Day 4: 0.8, Day 5: 0.5, Day 6: 0.5, Day 7: 1.4, Day 8: 1.0, Day 9: 0.8, Day 10: 1.2
Level 2:
Day 1: 5.4, Day 2: 4.8, Day 3: 5.6, Day 4: 7.9, Day 5: 5.4, Day 6: 4.8, Day 7: 5.8, Day 8: 4.7, Day 9: 6.4, Day 10: 5.5

QUICK NOTES

- Quality control must be performed per good laboratory practice and CLIA'88 requirements.
- QC should be performed and accepted or rejected prior to testing patient specimens.

- Levy-Jennings charts are a visual method to determine if a QC value is in or out of control.
- Most modern laboratory analyzers have built-in Levey-Jennings charts so that many laboratory professionals no longer construct or hand plot QC on these charts. However, they should still be reviewed to ensure that there are no shifts or trends.
- A new Levey-Jennings chart must be made whenever there is a change in calibration that affects the mean and SD ranges of the QC or the QC lot number changes.
- Prior to changing lot numbers, 20 replicates of the new lot must be analyzed and a new mean and SD ranges determined.
- Westgard rules are a way to determine if the QC values obtained are acceptable. Westgard has a computerized version of the rules that many laboratories use.
- The 1_{2S} warning rule, the 1_{3S} rule, and the R_{4S} rule are usually caused because of random error.
- The 2_{2S}, 4_{1S}, and 10_x are usually caused because of systematic error.

BIBLIOGRAPHY

CFR49342: Revision to the Clinical Laboratory Improvement Amendments of 1988: Final Rule, Washington, DC, Oct 2004, US Government Printing Office.

Centers for Medicare & Medicaid Services: Individualized Quality Control Plan (IQCP). Available at http://www.cms.gov/Regulations-and-Guidance/Legislation/CLIA/Individualized_Quality_Control_Plan_IQCP.html.

Korpman RA, Bull BS: The implementation of a robust estimator of the mean for quality control on a programmable calculator or laboratory computer, *Am J Clin Pathol* 65:252, 1976.

Westgard JO, Barry PL: CLIA final rules. Available at https://www.westgard.com/clia-final-rule.htm.

Westgard JO, Barry PL, Hunt MR, et al: A multi-rule Shewhart chart for quality control in clinical chemistry, *Clin Chem* 27:493-501, 1981.

Westgard JO, Quam EF, Barry PL: Selection grids for planning quality control procedures, *Clin Lab Sci* 3:273-280, 1990.

Appendix 13-A   Regulatory Considerations

All CLIA regulations, other than those specifically designated as eligible for IQCP in Table 13-1, continue to be in force and must be followed.

Table 13-1 lists those specialties/subspecialties and general regulations for which the laboratory has the flexibility to develop control procedures using the IQCP procedure. Table 13-1 also lists those specialties/subspecialties and specialty/subspecialty regulations that are not eligible for IQCP.

- The first column lists the CLIA specialties/subspecialties: Bacteriology, Mycobacteriology, Mycology, Parasitology, Virology, Syphilis Serology, General Immunology, Routine Chemistry, Urinalysis, Endocrinology, Toxicology, Hematology, Immunohematology, Clinical Cytogenetics, Radiobioassay, Histocompatibility, Pathology, Histopathology, Oral Pathology, and Cytology.
- The second column indicates whether each specialty/subspecialty is eligible for IQCP. The specialties/subspecialties eligible for IQCP are Bacteriology, Mycobacteriology, Mycology, Parasitology, Virology, Syphilis Serology, General Immunology, Routine Chemistry, Urinalysis, Endocrinology, Toxicology, Hematology, Immunohematology, Clinical Cytogenetics, Radiobioassay, and Histocompatibility. The specialties/subspecialties not eligible for IQCP are Pathology, Histopathology, Oral Pathology, and Cytology.

- The third column lists the regulations that are eligible for IQCP and may be applied to the eligible specialty/subspecialties listed in column 1: §493.1256(d)(3)-(5) and §493.1256(e)(1)-(4).
- The fourth column lists the specialty/subspecialty regulations that are eligible for IQCP: §493.1261, §493.1262, §493.1263, §493.1264, §493.1265, §493.1267(b),(c), §493.1269, and §493.1278(b)(6), (c), (d)(6), (e)(3).
- The fifth column lists the specialty/subspecialty regulations that are not eligible for IQCP: §493.1267(a), (d), §493.1271, §493.1276, and §493.1278(a), (b)(1-5), (d)(1-5), (d)(7), (e)(1-2), (f),(g).

TABLE 13-1 Eligibility for IQCP

CLIA Specialty/ Subspecialty	Eligible for IQCP?	General Regulations Eligible for IQCP	Specialty/ Subspecialty Regulations Eligible for IQCP	Specialty/ Subspecialty Regulations NOT Eligible for IQCP
Bacteriology	Yes	§493.1256(d)(3)-(5) $493.1256(e)(I)-(4)	§493.1261	N/A
Mycobacteriology	Yes	§493.1256(d)(3)-(5) §493.1256(e)(1)-(4)	§493.1262	N/A
Mycology	Yes	§493.1256(d)(3)-(5) §493.1256(e)(1)-(4)	§493.1263	N/A
Parasitology	Yes	§493.1256(d)(3)-(5) §493.1256(e)(1)-(4)	§493.1264	N/A
Virology	Yes	§493.1256(d)(3)-(5) §493.1256(e)(1)-(4)	§493.1265	N/A
Syphilis Serology	Yes	§493.1256(d)(3)-(5) §493.1256(e)(1)-(4)	N/A	N/A
General Immunology	Yes	§493.1256(d)(3)-(5) §493.1256(e)(1)-(4)	N/A	N/A
Routine Chemistry	Yes	§493.1256(d)(3)-(5) §493.1256(e)(1)-(4)	§493.1267(b), (c)	§493.1267(a), (d)
Urinalysis	Yes	§493.1256(d)(3)-(5) §493.1256(e)(1)-(4)	N/A	N/A
Endocrinology	Yes	§493.1256(d)(3)-(5) §493.1256(e)(1)-(4)	N/A	N/A
Toxicology	Yes	§493.1256(d)(3)-(5) §493.1256(e)(1)-(4)	N/A	N/A
Hematology	Yes	§493.1256(d)(3)-(5) §493.1256(e)(1)-(4)	§493.1269	N/A
Immunohematology	Yes	§493.1256(d)(3)-(5) §493.1256(e)(1)-(4)	N/A	§493.1271
Clinical Cytogenetics	Yes	§493.1256(d)(3)-(5) §493.1256(e)(1)-(4)	N/A	§493.1276

Continued

TABLE 13-1 Eligibility for IQCP—cont'd

CLIA Specialty/ Subspecialty	Eligible for IQCP?	General Regulations Eligible for IQCP	Specialty/ Subspecialty Regulations Eligible for IQCP	Specialty/ Subspecialty Regulations NOT Eligible for IQCP
Radiobioassay	Yes	§493.1256(d)(3)-(5) §493.1256(e)(1)-(4)	N/A	N/A
Histocompatibility	Yes	§493.1256(d)(3)-(5) §493.1256(e)(1)-(4)	§493.1278(b)(6), (c), (d)(6), (e)(3)	§493.1278(a), (b)(1-5), (d) (1-5), (d)(7), (e)(1-2), (f), (g)
Pathology	No	None (Not eligible for IQCP)	N/A	N/A
Histopathology	No	None (Not eligible for IQCP)	N/A	N/A
Oral Pathology	No	None (Not eligible for IQCP)	N/A	N/A
Cytology	No	None (Not eligible for IQCP)	N/A	N/A

IQCP, Individualized Quality Control Plan.

CHAPTER 14

Comprehensive Laboratory Quality Assurance

OBJECTIVES

At the end of this chapter, the reader should be able to do the following:

1. Define the 10 CLIA standards that must be included in a laboratory's quality assurance protocol.
2. Define the true negatives, true positives, false negatives, and false positives for a method when determining the diagnostic value of that method.
3. Calculate the diagnostic sensitivity, specificity, efficiency, and positive and negative predictive value of a method.
4. Use Student's *t*-test to compare the difference between both paired and unpaired data sets.

5. Analyze the precision of methods by the use of the F test.
6. Define the terms used in linear regression analysis.
7. Calculate, using linear regression analysis, the slope, intercept, and degree of bias between two methods.
8. Calculate the standard error of the estimate associated with linear regression analysis.
9. Determine the coefficient of correlation associated with linear regression analysis.

WHAT ## CLIA REQUIREMENTS FOR COMPREHENSIVE LABORATORY QUALITY ASSURANCE FOR NONWAIVED METHODS

There are 10 standards listed in the Code of Federal Regulations (Subpart K, 42 CFR 493.1239) that define the components that must be included in a laboratory that performs nonwaived testing as part of its quality assurance program. Some of these standards have been discussed already in this book, and some of these standards are outside the scope of this book. They are:

1. Patient test management, which includes among its many components patient preparation, specimen collection, test requisition, and relevance and necessity for testing.

Determining which method to perform may fall under this section and will be discussed in this chapter.

2. Laboratory procedures, which must be signed by the laboratory director.
3. Quality control, which was covered in Chapter 13.
4. Proficiency testing, which will be discussed in this chapter.
5. Test method verification, which will be discussed in this chapter.
6. Calibration and calibration verification, which will be discussed in this chapter.
7. Personnel, which is outside the scope of this book.
8. Record and specimen retention, which is outside the scope of this book.
9. Communications, which is outside the scope of this book.
10. Complaints, which are outside the scope of this book.

WHAT DETERMINATION OF THE DIAGNOSTIC VALUE OF A METHOD

Diagnostic Sensitivity and Specificity

The goal of the clinical laboratory is to produce accurate and precise results that aid physicians in the diagnosis and treatment of disease states and processes. In addition, the laboratory tests should be able to distinguish between patients who have a disease and those who do not have the disease. Figure 14-1 is a graph of two sets of patients. The group on the left does not have the disease, whereas the group on the right has the disease. The best laboratory test will have no overlap between groups (i.e., a gray area in which the physician would not be able to diagnose if the patient had the disease). Figure 14-2 demonstrates a test that has an overlap between groups.

Diagnostic sensitivity is the probability that only patients with the disease will test positive for the disease. Diagnostic specificity is the probability that patients who do not have the disease will test negative for the disease. The best test will have 100% sensitivity and specificity.

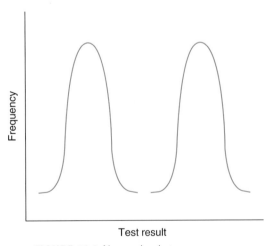

FIGURE 14-1 No overlap between groups.

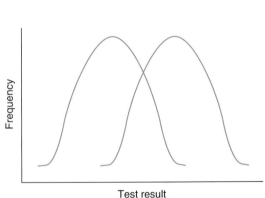

FIGURE 14-2 Overlap between groups.

The sensitivity and specificity of a method can be calculated by the following formulas:

$$\text{Sensitivity} = \frac{\text{True Positives}}{\text{True Positives} + \text{False Negatives}} \times 100$$

$$\text{Specificity} = \frac{\text{True Negatives}}{\text{True Negatives} + \text{False Positives}} \times 100$$

where:

True Positives (TP) = Number of individuals who actually have the disease and test positive
False Positives (FP) = Number of individuals who do not have the disease but test positive
True Negatives (TN) = Number of individuals who do not have the disease and test negative
False Negatives (FN) = Number of individuals who have the disease but test negative

HOW **Example 14-1**

A new kit was developed to detect the presence of group A *Streptococcus* in throat swabs. The manufacturer tested the kit on 600 pediatric patients with presumptive diagnoses of group A *Streptococcus*. Four hundred and seventy-five patients tested positive for group A *Streptococcus* with the kit. Of these 475 patients, 460 were verified by culture to be positive for group A *Streptococcus*. One hundred twenty-five children tested negative by the kit; of these, 20 were determined to be positive for group A *Streptococcus* by culture. What is the diagnostic sensitivity and specificity of this new kit?

To calculate the diagnostic sensitivity and specificity of this kit, first determine the number of true positives, true negatives, false positives, and false negatives.

- If 475 children tested positive by the kit, but only 460 of them were confirmed, then the number of true positives is 460 and the number of false positives is 15.

- Because 125 children tested negative by the kit but 20 were actually positive, then the number of true negatives is 105 and the number of false negatives is 20. Therefore, by using the formulas, the diagnostic sensitivity and specificity of this kit can be determined.

$$\text{Diagnostic sensitivity} = \frac{460}{460 + 20} \times 100$$

$$= \frac{460}{480} \times 100$$

$$= 95.8\%$$

$$\text{Diagnostic specificity} = \frac{105}{105 + 15} \times 100$$

$$= \frac{105}{120} \times 100$$

$$= 87.5\%$$

Therefore this method has a diagnostic sensitivity of 95.8% and a diagnostic specificity of 87.5%.

HOW   *Example 14-1a*   A new Ebola virus assay was quickly developed in response to an Ebola epidemic. Of the 800 individuals tested, 780 tested negative. Of these, two individuals were actually positive for the virus, so the FN = 2. Of the 20 individuals who initially tested positive, 17 were confirmed positive, therefore TP = 17. What is the diagnostic sensitivity and specificity of this new assay? Use Example 14-1 as a guide. The TN = 778 (780 − 2 FN) and the FP = 3 (20 − 17 TP).

$$\text{Diagnostic sensitivity} = \frac{17}{17+2} \times 100$$
$$= \frac{17}{19} \times 100$$
$$= 89.5\%$$
$$\text{Diagnostic specificity} = \frac{778}{778+3} \times 100$$
$$= \frac{778}{781} \times 100$$
$$= 99.6\%$$

The diagnostic sensitivity of this new kit is 89.5%, and its diagnostic specificity is 99.6%.

Example 14-1b   A tumor marker is being developed to detect early breast cancer. Of the 400 women who volunteered for the study, 350 tested negative for the marker. Of these women, three developed breast cancer. Therefore, there are 347 TN and 3 FN. The 50 women who tested positive for the marker underwent further tests; of these 50 women, 48 were diagnosed with early breast cancer (TP = 48), and the other two women were found to not have breast cancer (FP = 2). What is the diagnostic sensitivity and specificity of this new tumor marker?

$$\text{Diagnostic sensitivity} = \frac{48}{48+3} \times 100$$
$$= \frac{48}{51} \times 100$$
$$= 94.1\%$$
$$\text{Diagnostic specificity} = \frac{347}{347+2} \times 100$$
$$= \frac{347}{349} \times 100$$
$$= 99.4\%$$

The diagnostic sensitivity of this new tumor marker is 94.1%, and its specificity is 99.4%.

Efficiency

In addition to diagnostic sensitivity and specificity, the efficiency of the test can be calculated. The efficiency of a test is the number of patients correctly diagnosed for the disease or not having the disease—that is, true positives or true negatives. The following calculation can be used to determine the efficiency of a laboratory test:

$$\text{Efficiency} = \frac{\text{TP} + \text{TN}}{\text{TP} + \text{FP} + \text{FN} + \text{TN}} \times 100$$

Example 14-2

Using the data from Example 14-1, what is the efficiency of the new group A *Streptococcus* kit?
Analysis of the new kit revealed the following:

True positives = 460
False positives = 15
True negatives = 105
False negatives = 20

Using the formula to determine the efficiency of a test, the following equation is derived:

$$\text{Efficiency} = \frac{460 + 105}{460 + 15 + 20 + 105} \times 100$$

$$\text{Efficiency} = \frac{565}{600} \times 100$$

$$\text{Efficiency} = 94.2\%$$

Therefore the efficiency of the new *Streptococcus* kit is 94.2%.

Example 14-2a   Calculate the efficiency of a new method of troponin I that had the following information:

True positives = 590
False positives = 40
True negatives = 480
False negatives = 25
The efficiency is 94.3%.

Example 14-2b   Calculate the efficiency of a new method of detecting *Clostridium difficile* that had the following information:

True positives = 650
False positives = 35
True negatives = 440
False negatives = 50
The efficiency is 92.8%.

WHAT Predictive Value

The last calculation that is used to assess the diagnostic value of a test method is the predictive value of the test method. There are two types of predictive value. The first is the positive predictive value of a method. The positive predictive value is the ability of the method to correctly determine the presence of a disease in those patients who have the disease. That is, patients who are positive for the disease will test positive by the test method.

The negative predictive value is the ability of a method to correctly determine the absence of a disease in those patients who do not have the disease. These patients should test negative by the test method designed to detect the disease.

The positive predictive value is calculated with the following formula:

$$\text{Positive predictive value} = \frac{\text{True Positive}}{\text{True Positive} + \text{False Positive}} \times 100$$

The negative predictive value is calculated with the following formula:

$$\text{Negative predictive value} = \frac{\text{True Negative}}{\text{True Negative} + \text{False Negative}} \times 100$$

Example 14-3

A new assay was developed that promised to be able to detect prostate cancer in men before the development of any clinical symptoms. The manufacturer claimed that the new assay was more sensitive and specific than any existing tests for prostate cancer. In a large clinical trial, blood samples from 10,000 men who were asymptomatic for prostate cancer were tested using this new assay. Two thousand men tested positive for this assay and 8000 tested negative. Of the 2000 positives, 1900 (TP) later developed prostate cancer. Of the 8000 negatives, 30 (FN) later developed prostate cancer. What is the positive predictive value for this test?

To calculate positive predictive value, the following formula is used:

$$\text{Positive predictive value} = \frac{\text{True Positive}}{\text{True Positive} + \text{False Positive}} \times 100$$

The number of TPs for this test is 1900, while there were 100 FPs. Therefore the positive predictive value is as follows:

$$\text{Positive predictive value} = \frac{1900}{1900 + 100} \times 100$$

$$\text{Positive predictive value} = \frac{1900}{2000} \times 100$$

$$\text{Positive predictive value} = 95.0\%$$

The positive predictive value of 95.0% means that if a patient tested positive with this new method, there is a 95% chance that he actually has prostate cancer.

Example 14-3a   Using the data from Example 14-3, what would be the negative predictive value of this new prostate cancer test?

The negative predictive value is calculated by the following formula:

$$\text{Negative predictive value} = \frac{\text{True Negative}}{\text{True Negative} + \text{False Negative}} \times 100$$

Of the 10,000 men tested, 8000 tested negative. However, 30 of the men were false negatives, as they later developed prostate cancer. Therefore, there were 7970 true negatives. Using the formula, the negative predictive value is as follows:

$$\text{Negative predictive value} = \frac{7970}{7970 + 30} \times 100$$

$$\text{Negative predictive value} = \frac{7970}{8000} \times 100$$

$$\text{Negative predictive value} = 99.6\%$$

A negative predictive value of 99.6% means that if a patient tests negative, there is only a 0.4% chance that he actually has prostate cancer.

Example 14-3b   Calculate the negative and positive predictive value for the following colon cancer test: Out of 6600 adults with a family history of colon cancer, 6245 tested negative. Of these, 12 developed colon cancer. Of the 355 individuals who tested positive, 340 developed colon cancer.

There are 340 true positives, 15 false positives, 6233 true negatives, and 12 false negatives. Substituting the values into the formulas for negative and positive predictive values yields the following:

Positive predictive value = 340/(340 + 15) = 0.958 × 100 = 95.8%
Negative predictive value = 6233/(6233 + 12) = 0.998 × 100 = 99.8%

Example 14-3c   Calculate the positive and negative predictive value given the following data:

True positive = 855 False positive = 3
True negative = 340 False negative = 2
Positive predictive value = (855/855 + 3) = 0.9965 × 100 = 99.65%
Negative predictive value = (340/340 + 2) = 0.9942 × 100 = 99.42%

WHAT CLIA REQUIREMENTS FOR INSTRUMENT/METHOD QUALITY ASSURANCE

On January 23, 2003, the final rules for CLIA'88 were released that put the emphasis on quality back on the laboratory itself rather than on the manufacturer of the laboratory's instruments. The original CLIA rules that were passed in 1988 and released in 1992 allowed the laboratory to use the manufacturer's data for method validation, etc. The rule mandated method quality assurance studies be performed by the laboratory instead of relying on the manufacturer's data, such as method validation, accuracy, and precision studies. Except for personnel requirements, the 2003 final rules also changed the test categories of waived, moderate, and high complexity into waived and nonwaived categories. The final rules became effective after April 24, 2003.

The final rules stated that laboratories were not required to verify or establish performance specifications for any test system used by the laboratory before April 24, 2003. However, the laboratory was, and is, responsible to verify or establish performance specifications for any test system brought in after April 24, 2003. The rule further clarified what the laboratory must do to verify or establish performance specifications for unmodified test systems that were cleared or approved by the Food and Drug Administration (FDA) and those test systems that were developed in-house.

For unmodified FDA-approved or cleared systems the laboratory must:

A. Demonstrate that it can obtain performance specifications comparable to those established by the manufacturer for the following performance characteristics:
   1. Accuracy
   2. Precision
   3. Reportable range of test results for the test system
B. Verify that the manufacturer's reference intervals (normal values) are appropriate for the laboratory's patient population

For those tests that are developed in-house by the laboratory, or modified, or not cleared or approved by the FDA (including methods developed in-house and standardized methods such as textbook procedures, Gram stain, or potassium hydroxide preparations), or use a test system in which performance specifications are not provided by the manufacturer, the laboratory must, before reporting patient test results, establish for each test system the performance specifications for the following:

1. Accuracy
2. Precision
3. Analytical sensitivity
4. Analytical specificity to include interfering substances
5. Reportable range of test results for the test system
6. Reference intervals (normal values)
7. Any other performance characteristic required for test performance

In addition, Section 493.1281 of CLIA regulations states that, "if a laboratory performs the same test using different methodologies or instruments, or performs the same test at multiple testing sites, the laboratory must have a system that twice a year evaluates and defines the relationship between test results using the different methodologies, instruments, or testing sites." The same statistical tests that are used to determine accuracy can be used by the laboratory to meet this requirement. The Clinical Laboratory Standards Institute (CLSI) has a protocol to perform method comparisons, and James Westgard at https://www.westgard.com/lesson23.htm presents many factors to consider when performing a method comparison study.

WHAT **Determining Accuracy**

Accuracy is defined as the agreement between measurement and the true value. Accuracy studies are designed to detect systematic bias between two methods. A laboratory can determine the accuracy of a test method in a number of ways. The most common is to analyze 20 to 30 samples that span the reportable range of the method on both the new test method and a reference method. How can the laboratory determine if the results from an old analyzer and a new replacement analyzer are the same, or that the glucose result obtained in the emergency room satellite clinical laboratory would be the same result if analyzed on a different instrument in the main laboratory?

There are a number of inferential statistics that can be calculated to answer this question. Most laboratories today use computer programs specifically designed for the clinical laboratory to calculate these statistics. The information that follows is based on data that are normally distributed and has a sample number (n) value of at least 30. Information on using population statistics or nonparametric sample distributions can be found in many statistics textbooks.

WHAT ### Student's t-Test

The Student's *t*-test is useful to determine whether there is a statistical difference (or bias) between the two methods. The bias can be either positive (the new method's results are higher than the reference method) or negative (the new method's results are lower than the reference method).

WHAT   Student's *t*-test can be an indicator of the **accuracy** of a new method. Before describing the actual calculations involved, some basic information must first be given. In general, one method is considered the "reference" method and the other method is the "test" method. Two hypotheses can be formed: the null (H_o) and the alternate (H_a). The null hypothesis states that there is no statistically significant difference between methods (Method A is the same as Method B), and the alternate hypothesis states that there is a statistically significant difference between methods (Method A is not the same as Method B). Based on the statistical difference, the null hypothesis is either rejected or accepted. When the null hypothesis is accepted, in statistical terminology, it is a failure to reject the null hypothesis.

To correctly reject or fail to reject the null hypothesis, a probability level (or significance level) of rejection or acceptance has to be established. The probability level depends on the degree of certainty that is required. For example, if a 95% probability level is used for acceptance of the null hypothesis, the significance level of rejection is 5%. The significance level is often referred to as a fraction of 100; that is, 5% would be expressed as $P = 0.05$. There is a greater degree of certainty if a 99% probability level is used because then there is only a 1% significance level ($P = 0.01$). The probability level used will depend on the needs of each laboratory. The probability level determines the degree of certainty that is required. What is not yet established is the numerical limit or cutoff point at which the significance level is reached. The critical region establishes this limit. In a Gaussian distribution, the values are equally distributed around the mean. Statistically, if there is a 95% probability level, there is a 5% chance that a result will fall into the critical region.

Whether there are one or two critical regions depends on whether the test is one tailed or two tailed. A one-tailed test is demonstrated in Figure 14-3. In this type of test, Method A compared

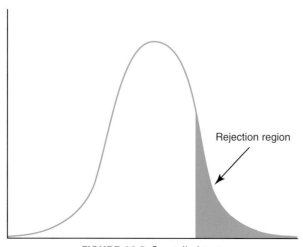

Rejection region

FIGURE 14-3 One-tailed test.

to Method B has results that are either statistically greater than or less than Method B. For example, the null hypothesis may state that Method A results are greater than Method B or Method A results are less than Method B. In a one-tailed test, the entire 5% rejection region is on one side of the distribution.

In comparison, a two-tailed test has two possible outcomes. Statistically, it may be proved that Method A is different from Method B. Method A may be greater or less than Method B as shown in Figure 14-4. In two-tailed tests, the 5% significance level is split between both tails of the distribution. Therefore, there is a 2.5% probability that a result will fall in each critical region.

WHAT   Statistically it has been determined that the actual numerical cutoff point for the 5% confidence limit for a two-tailed test with a sample size of at least 30 is the mean +/−1.96 SD, as shown in Figure 14-5. If a calculated t value is greater than 1.96 SD, it will fall into the critical region, and the null hypothesis will be rejected. If the calculated t value is less than 1.96 SD, statistically, there is a failure to reject the null hypothesis, and therefore the null hypothesis can be accepted.

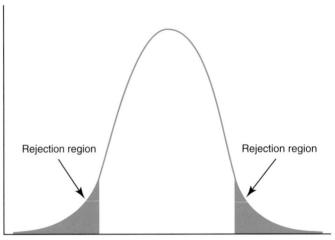

Rejection region   Rejection region

FIGURE 14-4 Two-tailed test.

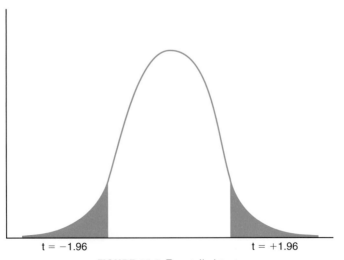

$t = -1.96$ $t = +1.96$

FIGURE 14-5 Two-tailed test.

The last piece of basic information to be discussed is the concept of degrees of freedom. The amount that any number can vary is dependent on the amount of restrictions placed on that number. In a group of 10 numbers (n = 10) with a mean of 50, nine of the numbers have no restrictions. The tenth number is restricted because, based on the values of the previous nine numbers, the value of the tenth number is fixed. Therefore the degrees of freedom in this example are 9, or n − 1.

There are two different calculations associated with Student's t-test depending on if the data are paired or unpaired. For most clinical laboratory applications, the formula for paired t-test is used. Student's t-test is the ratio of the difference of two means to the standard deviation of that difference.

WHAT **Paired t-Test**

The formula for the paired Student's t-test is as follows:

$$\text{Paired } t\text{-test} = \frac{\overline{d}}{\text{standard error of the mean (SE)}}$$

Where: $\overline{d}$ = difference between mean divided by n

$$\overline{d} = \frac{\sum \overline{X}_1 - \overline{X}_2}{n}$$

$$SE = \frac{\sqrt{\dfrac{\sum d^2 - \left[\sum (\overline{X}_1 - \overline{X}_2)\right]^2 \div n}{n-1}}}{\sqrt{n}}$$

$$d^2 = \sum (\overline{X}_1 - \overline{X}_2)^2$$

Combined, the formula for the paired Student's t-test becomes:

$$\text{Paired } t\text{-test} = \frac{\dfrac{\sum (\overline{X}_1 - \overline{X}_2)}{n}}{\sqrt{\dfrac{\sum d^2 - \left[\sum (\overline{X}_1 - \overline{X}_2)\right]^2 \div n]}{n-1}}} \div \sqrt{n}$$

HOW **Example 14-4**

A laboratory wants to purchase a new chemistry analyzer that has a higher throughput than the current analyzer. The laboratory was able to temporarily obtain the instrument to conduct method comparison studies. As part of this study, 30 patient samples were split into two aliquots. Each aliquot was analyzed for glucose on both analyzers. Is there a statistically significant difference ($P = 0.05$) between analyzers?

Aliquot	Glucose Results (mg/dL)	
	Analyzer A (Current Analyzer)	**Analyzer B (New Analyzer)**
1.	85	86
2.	198	195
3.	110	113
4.	140	142
5.	245	210
6.	103	99
7.	87	78
8.	96	99
9.	375	364
10.	68	64
11.	210	215
12.	105	103
13.	117	112
14.	184	193
15.	180	168
16.	157	153
17.	293	287
18.	83	81
19.	72	79
20.	102	112
21.	76	65
22.	89	93
23.	371	401
24.	125	120
25.	310	290
26.	138	153
27.	68	71
28.	90	96
29.	546	472
30.	193	184

To answer this question, it is helpful to phrase it as the null and alternate hypothesis.

H_o = there is no statistically significant difference between glucose results from both analyzers
H_a = there is a statistically significant difference between glucose results from both analyzers

To calculate the paired t-test value, first obtain the difference between samples (d) and the difference between means (d^2).

Aliquot	Glucose Results (mg/dL)			
	Analyzer A	Analyzer B	d	d^2
1.	85	86	−1	1
2.	198	195	3	9
3.	110	113	−3	9
4.	140	142	−2	4
5.	245	210	35	1225
6.	103	99	4	16
7.	87	78	9	81
8.	96	99	−3	9
9.	375	364	11	121
10.	68	64	4	16
11.	210	215	−5	25
12.	105	103	2	4
13.	117	112	5	25
14.	184	193	−9	81
15.	180	168	12	144
16.	157	153	4	16
17.	293	287	6	36
18.	83	81	2	4
19.	72	79	−7	49
20.	102	112	−10	100
21.	76	65	11	121
22.	89	93	−4	16
23.	371	401	−30	900
24.	125	120	5	25
25.	310	290	20	400
26.	138	153	−15	225
27.	68	71	−3	9
28.	90	96	−6	36
29.	546	472	74	5476
30.	193	184	9	81

$$\sum = 118 = d \quad \sum = 9264 = d^2$$

$$\overline{d} = \frac{118}{30}$$

$$\overline{d} = 3.9$$

Next, substitute into the Student's t-test formula the data from the problem.

$$\text{Paired } t\text{-test value} = \frac{\dfrac{\sum(\bar{X}_1 - \bar{X}2)}{n}}{\sqrt{\dfrac{\sum d^2 - \left[\sum(\bar{X}_1 - \bar{X}_2)\right]^2 \div n}{n-1}}} \div \sqrt{n}$$

$$\text{Paired } t\text{-test value} = \frac{\dfrac{118}{30}}{\sqrt{\dfrac{9264 - \left[118^2 \div 30\right]}{29}}} \div \sqrt{30}$$

$$\text{Paired } t\text{-test value} = \frac{3.9}{\sqrt{\dfrac{9264 - 464.1}{29}}} \div \sqrt{30}$$

$$\text{Paired } t\text{-test value} = \frac{3.9}{\dfrac{\sqrt{303.4}}{\sqrt{30}}}$$

$$\text{Paired } t\text{-test value} = \frac{3.9}{\dfrac{17.4}{5.5}}$$

$$\text{Paired } t\text{-test value} = \frac{3.9}{3.2}$$

$$\text{Paired } t\text{-test value} = 1.219$$

The last step is to determine if the calculated t value exceeds the value obtained from the Student's t table in Appendix 14-A. This is a two-tailed test because we are testing to determine if the two methods are different. We are not testing to determine if one method is greater than or less than the other. Using the Student's t table, find the column under "Area" in two tails at the $P = 0.05$ significance level. As we have 30 samples, the degrees of freedom are 29. Next, find the number 29 under the column "df." Look across the row until it intersects the 0.05 significance column. The number 2.045 is our tabulated t value. Our calculated t value is 1.219. Any calculated t value greater than 2.045 would fall into the rejection portion of the t distribution. As 1.219 is less than 2.045, we fail to reject the null hypothesis; that is, we accept the null hypothesis. Therefore, there is no statistical difference between the glucose results obtained on the new and the old analyzer.

Example 14-4a A laboratory performs a comparison of the serum potassium values obtained by a point of care analyzer used in the emergency room to the chemistry analyzer used in the core laboratory. Perform a t-test to determine if there is a statistical difference between the two methods. All values are in milliequivalents per liter.

Aliquot	Reference (Core Lab Analyzer)	Emergency Room Analyzer
1.	4.5	4.6
2.	4.3	4.3
3.	4.8	4.7
4.	5.6	5.4

Aliquot	Reference (Core Lab Analyzer)	Emergency Room Analyzer
5.	5.7	5.7
6.	4.1	4.2
7.	5.5	5.5
8.	6.1	5.9
9.	5.8	5.6
10.	6.2	6.3
11.	5.9	5.7
12.	3.4	3.3
13.	3.9	4.1
14.	4.2	4.5
15.	4.7	4.9
16.	6.0	6.2
17.	5.8	5.2
18.	3.9	4.1
19.	4.8	4.6
20.	4.2	4.2

The Student's t-test value is 0.677, which is within the 95% confidence limit. Therefore we "fail to reject the null hypothesis that there is a statistical difference between the two methods." What this means is that there is no statistical difference between the result obtained by the point of care instrument and the result obtained by the core laboratory instrument.

HOW   *Example 14-4b*   A new hematology analyzer was being evaluated to replace an older instrument. Is there a statistical difference between the hemoglobin results ($P = 0.05$)? For example purposes only, 10 comparisons are given.

Aliquot	Current Analyzer	New Analyzer
1.	15.2	16.0
2.	16.5	17.0
3.	14.1	14.0
4.	17.3	17.4
5.	10.2	8.9
6.	11.3	11.6
7.	9.7	9.4
8.	10.0	10.3
9.	13.4	13.2
10.	12.5	12.7

The Student's t-test value is 0.87, which means there is no statistically significant difference between methods.

WHAT   *Unpaired t-Test*

The paired *t*-test is useful when duplicate aliquots of the same samples are analyzed on two different analyzers to determine if there is a difference between analyzers. The paired *t*-test has some limitations in its application. Generally the same technologist analyzes the samples on both instruments to minimize any variations in testing. The sample size is identical for both analyzers as well. Sometimes a different situation occurs in which two different groups are compared to determine if there is a difference between them. For example, if 15 men and 20 women who suffered from hay fever received a new drug that promised to reduce the number of eosinophils in peripheral blood, the researchers would want to be able to combine the results obtained to determine if the new drug did in fact reduce the number of eosinophils. The unpaired Student's *t*-test may allow them to combine the data. The null hypothesis would be that there is no statistically significant difference between the effect of the new drug on the eosinophil counts on men and women. The alternate hypothesis would be that there is a difference between the effect of the new drug on men and women. As most clinical laboratories, if using Student's *t*-test, will use the paired *t*-test, the calculation of the unpaired Student's *t*-test will not be discussed. For those laboratory professionals who use the unpaired Student's *t*-test, information on performing the test is found in many biostatistics books.

WHAT   *Linear Regression Analysis by the Method of Least Squares*

Student's *t*-test is a useful but limited statistical tool when comparing methods. It may indicate that there is indeed a statistical difference between methods, but it cannot give information on the cause of the difference. One statistical tool that is used often in the clinical laboratory for method comparison is linear regression analysis. As with Student's *t*-test, one method is considered the reference method; the other, newer method is considered the test method. In linear regression, analysis samples are tested by both methods. Then the results obtained from each method are plotted on linear graph paper. The results for the reference method are plotted on the *x* axis, and the results of the test method are plotted on the *y* axis. If, for each sample tested, the results for both test and reference method were identical, there would be perfect correlation between methods and a perfectly linear line as demonstrated in Figure 14-6.

Linear regression analysis uses the following equation to determine the placement of the regression line:

$$y_c = mx + b$$

where:

m = the slope of the line
x = result of reference method
b = the expected y intercept if x is 0
y_c = predicted y intercept derived from equation

The slope of the line (m) is calculated by the following formula:

$$m = \frac{n(\sum xy) - (\sum x)(\sum y)}{n(\sum x^2) - (\sum x)^2}$$

The y intercept (b) is calculated by the following formula:

$$b = \bar{y} - (m\bar{x})$$

There are some assumptions made when performing linear regression analysis. It is assumed that the reference method is accurate and precise, that random error is held to a minimum, that each method is performing to its best, and that there are no other factors that may interfere in the analysis of either method that might lead to erroneous conclusions. Most regression

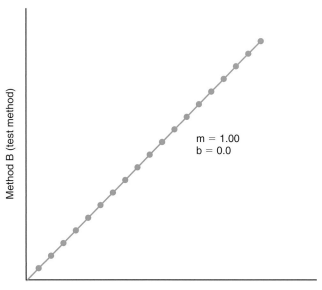

$m = 1.00$
$b = 0.0$

Method B (test method)

Method A (reference method)

FIGURE 14-6 Linear regression demonstrating perfect correlation between methods.

analysis is performed using computer software such as Excel. The manually performed examples that follow are provided to help explain how the regression formula is calculated.

HOW   ***Example 14-5***

A new method for total calcium was developed, and linear regression analysis was performed between the new method and the reference calcium method. Using the CLSI guidelines, 40 patient samples were analyzed by both methods. The concentration of the patient samples used in this study encompassed the full analytical range of both methods. Using the regression analysis formula, what is the slope and calculated y intercept? Note: Not all data points are shown, but all necessary information is given.

Total Calcium Results (mg/dL)

No.	A(x)	B(y)	x^2	y^2	xy
			Methods		
1.	8.4	8.5	70.56	72.25	71.40
2.	9.2	9.4	84.64	88.36	86.48
3.	8.3	8.1	68.89	65.61	67.23
.	.	.	.	.	.
.	.	.	.	.	.
38.	8.2	8.5	67.24	72.25	69.70
39.	8.8	8.8	77.44	77.44	77.44
40.	9.0	9.0	81.00	81.00	81.00
	$\Sigma = 352.7$	$\Sigma = 351.8$	$\Sigma = 3126.87$	$\Sigma = 3111.34$	$\Sigma = 3117.68$
	$\bar{x} = 8.82$	$\bar{y} = 8.80$			

Using the formula for the slope of the line and substituting into it the values from the problem yields the following equation:

$$m = \frac{40(3117.68) - (352.7)(351.8)}{40(3126.87) - (352.7)^2}$$

$$m = \frac{124707.20 - 124079.86}{125074.8 - 124397.29}$$

$$m = \frac{627.34}{677.51}$$

$$m = +0.926$$

Using the formula to determine the y intercept, the following equation is derived:

$$b = 8.80 - (+0.926)(8.82)$$

$$b = 8.80 - 8.17$$

$$b = +0.630$$

If there were perfect correlation between the two methods, then y would equal x. If this were true, then by the equation of the line $y = mx + b$, the slope (m) would be 1.00 and the y intercept (b) would be zero. The value of the slope indicates the presence of **proportional error**, whereas the y intercept value indicates the constant error or bias of the test method compared with the reference method. The positive sign of the slope indicates that the line follows an upward direction. The equation of the line can be used to calculate the y value. As $y = mx + b$, then $y = (+0.926)(x) + (+0.630)$. If, for example, $x = 10$, then the calculated value of y would be $y = (+0.926)(10) + (+0.630)$ or 9.89. The proportional error of +0.926 means that for every 1.00 increase of x, y increases by only +0.926. Using the same example, if $x = 11$, then $y = (+0.926)(11) + (+0.630)$ or 10.816. The proportional error of +0.926 is verified by subtracting 9.89 from 10.816. This means that x increased by 1, from 10 to 11, whereas y increased only +0.926, from 9.89 to 10.816. Graphically, this can be demonstrated by Figures 14-7 and 14-8. Figure 14-7 is a graph of an ideal regression line where slope is 1.00 and the y intercept is at 0,0. In the previous example, the slope does not equal 1.00, and the y intercept is not at 0,0. Figure 14-8 illustrates the regression line of the example.

The degree of variability around the regression line is calculated by the standard error of the estimate (SEE). The SEE is also referred to as the standard deviation of the test method compared to the reference method. The SEE is an indication of the random error associated with the method and theoretically should be zero. The SEE is calculated with the following formula:

$$SEE = \sqrt{\frac{\sum (y_m - y_c)^2}{n - 2}}$$

where:

y_m = the measured value of y
y_c = the calculated value of y obtained from the regression formula

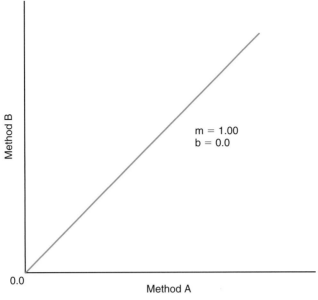

FIGURE 14-7 Perfect correlation.

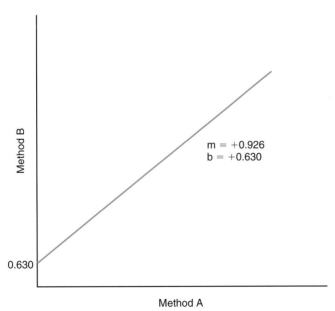

FIGURE 14-8 Linear regression analysis of Example 14-5.

HOW   **_Example 14-5a_**   Using the data from Example 14-5, the SEE can be calculated. The first step is to calculate the y value for each calcium value. This is accomplished by using the following formula:

$$y_c = mx + b$$

The total calcium results are as follows:

Total Calcium Results (mg/dL)

No.	Method A (x)	Method B (y)
1.	8.4	8.5
2.	9.2	9.4
3.	8.3	8.1
.	.	.
.	.	.
37.	9.2	8.6
38.	8.2	8.5
39.	8.8	8.8
40.	9.0	9.0

$m = +0.926$ and $b = +0.630$; therefore, $y_c = (+0.926)x + (+0.630)$.

Substituting the measured value of x for each calcium result yields the following calculated y values:

No.	A(x)	Method $y_c = (+0.926)x + (+0.630)$	y_c
1.	8.4	$y_c = (+0.926)(8.4) + (+0.630) =$	8.4
2.	9.2	$y_c = (+0.926)(9.2) + (+0.630) =$	9.2
3.	8.3	$y_c = (+0.926)(8.3) + (+0.630) =$	8.3
.	.	. . . .	.
.	.	. . . .	.
38.	8.2	$y_c = (+0.926)(8.2) + (+0.630) =$	8.2
39.	8.8	$y_c = (+0.926)(8.8) + (+0.630) =$	8.8
40.	9.0	$y_c = (+0.926)(9.0) + (+0.630) =$	9.0

Next, the values of $y_m - y_c$ and $(y_m - y_c)^2$ for each sample must be calculated:

No.	Method B(y)	y_c	$y_m - y_c$	$(y_m - y_c)^2$
1.	8.5	8.4	0.1	0.01
2.	9.4	9.2	0.2	0.04
3.	8.1	8.3	−0.2	0.04
.	.	.	.	.
.	.	.	.	.
38.	8.5	8.2	0.3	0.09
39.	8.8	8.8	0.0	0.00
40.	9.0	9.0	0.0	0.00
				$\Sigma = 2.74$

The last step is to substitute into the SEE formula the sum of the squared differences between measured and calculated y values:

$$SEE = \sqrt{\frac{\sum (y_m - y_c)^2}{n - 2}}$$

$$SEE = \sqrt{\frac{2.74}{38}}$$

$$SEE = 0.2684$$

What this means is that any predicted y value will deviate 0.2684 from its calculated value 68% of the time and 0.5368 (2 × 0.2684) from its calculated y value 95% of the time.

WHAT   The last calculation used with linear regression analysis is the Pearson coefficient of correlation (r). This statistic is useful to determine the relationship between the test methods: Are they related at all, and do they deviate in the same or a different direction? If the results from the test method correspond exactly to the results of the reference method, the linear regression analysis would show a perfectly straight line with a slope of 1.00 and a y intercept of zero. Consequently, there would be perfect correlation as well. The correlation coefficient ranges from −1 to +1. A positive 1 correlation means that both methods increase in the same direction, whereas a negative 1 correlation means that as one method increases, the other decreases. A correlation of zero means that there is no relationship at all between methods. In this case, the data points would be scattered in all directions around the regression line. In the clinical laboratory, two methods usually are considered to have perfect correlation with an r value of +1.

The formula to calculate the correlation coefficient is as follows:

$$r = \frac{\sum (x - \bar{x})(y - \bar{y})}{\sqrt{\left[\left(\sum x - \bar{x}\right)^2\right]\left[\left(\sum y - \bar{y}\right)^2\right]}}$$

Permutations of this calculation can be performed to simplify the calculation and use values that have already been obtained from other linear regression calculations.

The following equations may be substituted into the correlation formula:

$$\sum (x - \bar{x})(y - \bar{y}) = \sum xy - \frac{\left(\sum x\right)\left(\sum y\right)}{n}$$

$$\left(\sum x - \bar{x}\right)^2 = \sum x^2 - \frac{\left(\sum x\right)^2}{n}$$

$$\left(\sum y - \bar{y}\right)^2 = \sum y^2 - \frac{\left(\sum y\right)^2}{n}$$

Combined, the correlation coefficient formula becomes:

$$r = \frac{\sum xy - \frac{(\sum x)(\sum y)}{n}}{\sqrt{\left[\sum x^2 - \frac{(\sum x)^2}{n}\right]\left[\sum y^2 - \frac{(\sum y)^2}{n}\right]}}$$

HOW   **Example 14-6**

Using the same data from Example 14-5a, what is the correlation coefficient value?

Total Calcium Results (mg/dL)

No.	A (x)	B (y)	x²	y²	xy
			Methods		
1.	8.4	8.5	70.56	72.25	71.40
2.	9.2	9.4	84.64	88.36	86.48
3.	8.3	8.1	68.89	65.61	67.23
.	.	.	.	.	.
.	.	.	.	.	.
38.	8.2	8.5	67.24	72.25	69.70
39.	8.8	8.8	77.44	77.44	77.44
40.	9.0	9.0	81.00	81.00	81.00
	Σ = 352.7	Σ = 351.8	Σ = 3126.87	Σ = 3111.34	Σ = 3117.68
	x̄ = 8.82	ȳ = 8.80			

The formula for the correlation coefficient is as follows:

$$r = \frac{\sum xy - \frac{(\sum x)(\sum y)}{n}}{\sqrt{\left[\sum x^2 - \frac{(\sum x)^2}{n}\right]\left[\sum y^2 - \frac{(\sum y)^2}{n}\right]}}$$

Substituting into the formula the values obtained by the previous calculations, the following equation is derived:

$$r = \frac{3117.68 - \frac{(352.7)(351.8)}{40}}{\sqrt{\left[3126.87 - \frac{(352.7)^2}{40}\right]\left[3111.34 - \frac{(351.8)^2}{40}\right]}}$$

$$r = \frac{3117.68 - 3102.00}{\sqrt{(3126.87 - 3109.93) \times (3111.34 - 3094.08)}}$$

$$r = \frac{15.68}{\sqrt{(16.94)(17.26)}}$$

$$r = \frac{15.68}{17.10}$$

$$r = 0.917$$

Therefore the two calcium test methods have a correlation of +0.917, which indicates a good correlation.

Example 14-6a   Using a computer software program, calculate the slope, correlation coefficient, and standard error of the estimate for the following set of glucose values measured on (A) a reference method and (B) the new analyzer the laboratory would like to adopt.

	Values for A (all values are in mg/dL)	Values for B (all values are in mg/dL)
1.	100	101
2.	112	113
3.	155	153
4.	125	121
5.	141	138
6.	220	230
7.	250	242
8.	148	136
9.	111	109
10.	77	81
11.	65	64
12.	89	85
13.	146	137
14.	155	161
15.	122	121
16.	107	105
17.	128	128
18.	147	150
19.	122	119
20.	88	87

The correlation coefficient is 0.99361, the slope is 0.991073, the y intercept is 2.501995, and the SEE is 5.079739. The y intercept shows that there is a constant systematic error of -0.85 mg/dL for the new analyzer compared to the current analyzer.

WHAT   *Accuracy Study to Determine Proportional Systematic Error: Recovery Experiment*
A recovery experiment is designed to determine if there is a proportional systematic error in a method. In a recovery experiment, 20 to 30 samples with known values are split into two aliquots. One aliquot is called the reference aliquot and the other is spiked with a known amount (no more than 10% of the known value). The reference aliquot is spiked with the same volume used in the test aliquot but with diluents so that the total volumes of each aliquot are the same.

The test and reference aliquots are tested in triplicate, and the average result for each aliquot is used for statistical purposes. The recovery experiment calculation for each pair of aliquots is:

Spiked value − control value = recovered concentration

Percent recovery = (Concentration recovered divided by the concentration added) × 100

The acceptable recovery = 95%

HOW   *Example 14-7*

A recovery experiment was performed on a sodium assay. Twenty paired samples had 5 mEq/L sodium added to the 100 mcL test volume; 100 mcL of diluent was added to the paired reference samples. The paired samples were analyzed, and the following results were obtained. Calculate the percent recovery. All values are in milliequivalents per liter and are the average of the triple replicates.

	Reference Aliquot	Test Aliquot
1.	145	150
2.	148	152
3.	141	146
4.	144	149
5.	145	149
6.	138	143
7.	135	139
8.	140	145
9.	155	159
10.	153	158
11.	145	150
12.	144	149
13.	150	155
14.	144	149
15.	139	143
16.	152	156
17.	150	155
18.	145	150
19.	144	149
20.	147	152

Using the percent recovery calculation, the following results can be obtained:

	Reference Aliquot	Test Aliquot	Recovered Conc	% Recovery
1.	145	150	5	100
2.	148	152	4	80
3.	141	146	5	100
4.	144	149	5	100
5.	145	149	5	100
6.	138	143	5	100
7.	135	139	4	80
8.	140	145	5	100
9.	155	159	4	80
10.	153	158	5	100
11.	145	150	5	100
12.	144	149	5	100
13.	150	155	5	100
14.	144	149	5	100
15.	139	143	4	80
16.	152	156	4	80
17.	150	155	5	100
18.	145	150	5	100
19.	144	149	5	100
20.	147	152	5	100

Although there are values less than 100%, the average percent recovery was 95%.

WHAT *Accuracy Study to Determine Constant Systematic Error: Interference Study*

An interference study is performed to determine if the addition of a known interferent will result in an inaccurate result. Common interferents are bilirubin, hemoglobin (hemolysis), and lipids. Other interferents can be common cancer drugs, contrast media, or anticoagulants. Samples are paired as in the percent recovery experiment with one aliquot being the test aliquot and receiving the interferent and the other aliquot receiving an equal volume of diluents (reference aliquot). Samples should be tested over the analytical range of the instrument that is being evaluated. The calculation to be performed for each pair is as follows:

Average of test aliquot result − Average of reference aliquot = bias

The average bias is then compared with the amount of error that is allowable for the test. Some laboratories use the CLIA allowable ranges for proficiency testing that is found in Appendix 14-B.

WHAT **Determining Precision**

Precision is defined as the ability of a method to produce the same value for replicate measurements of a test sample. The precision of a method can be determined by its standard deviation and coefficient of variation. The F test can also be an indicator of precision.

CLIA mandates that precision studies be performed as part of the method validation process. Usually before a new method is adopted, both a between-run and a within-run precision study is performed. The within-run precision can be performed by analyzing the same aliquot of material 20 times during one analytical run and then calculating the standard deviation and coefficient of variation (see Chapter 12). The between-run precision studies can be short term (a few days) to much longer (a few weeks). The within-run precision study will help to determine if there is random error present in the method. The between-run precision study will help determine if there is systematic error in the method. The laboratory must determine what is the allowable standard deviation and coefficient of variation for the method being evaluated. Frequently, laboratories will use the CLIA criteria for acceptance used for proficiency testing evaluation for this determination.

WHAT **F Test**

A very simple statistic to calculate is the F test. This test can provide an idea of the precision of a new method. As with Student's t-test, the F test has an associated probability table for assessment of the F value. Unlike Student's t-test, there are separate F probability tables for each separate probability. Appendix 14-C contains an F probability table for $P = 0.05$. The formula for the F value is as follows:

$$\text{Calculated F value} = \frac{\text{Larger Variance}}{\text{Smaller Variance}}$$

Once the F value has been calculated, it must be compared to the appropriate F score from the F table. The tabulated F score is dependent on the degrees of freedom for each of the two measurements. Each degree of freedom for each method is calculated by $n - 1$.

HOW **Example 14-8**

A method comparison of hemoglobin values between two hematology analyzers was performed. The Level I control was analyzed 30 times on each analyzer. The mean, standard deviation, and coefficient of variation for each analyzer were calculated. The standard deviation of Analyzer A was 2.1, and the standard deviation of Analyzer B was 1.8. Using the F test, determine if there is a statistical difference in the precision of Analyzer B compared to Analyzer A.

The formula for the F test is as follows:

$$\text{Calculated F value} = \frac{\text{Larger Variance}}{\text{Smaller Variance}}$$

The SD is the square root of the variance. By squaring each SD value, the variance for each method can be determined.

$$\text{Analyzer A: SD of } 2.1 \ (2.1)^2 = \text{variance of } 4.41$$

$$\text{Analyzer B: SD of } 1.8 \ (1.8)^2 = \text{variance of } 3.24$$

$$\text{Calculated F value} = \frac{4.41}{3.24}$$

$$\text{Calculated F value} = 1.36$$

Next, the calculated F value is compared to the tabulated F value obtained from Appendix 14-C. Each method has an n of 30; therefore each method's degree of freedom is 29. To use the F table, because there are 29 degrees of freedom for Analyzer A, use the column with the heading "24." Find number 29 in the column marked "Denominator degrees of freedom." The number at the intersection of both columns is 1.90. This is the F cutoff value. The calculated F value is 1.36, which is lower than the cutoff value. Therefore we fail to reject H_0 and there is no statistical difference in precision between analyzers.

WHAT DETERMINATION OF REPORTABLE RANGE OR LINEARITY OF A METHOD

CLIA mandates that the linearity or reportable range of each moderate-complexity and high-complexity test system used in the laboratory must be determined by the laboratory.

According to the CLIA Interpretive Guidelines 493.1253(b)(1)(i)(C) Appendix C, Subpart K, Part 1, the reportable range can be determined by analyzing low and high calibration materials or control materials or evaluating known samples of abnormally high or abnormally low values. A minimum of three replicates of at least five concentrations across the reportable range should be analyzed. A best-fit line can be drawn with the x axis being the known value and the y axis being the average of the replicate values. Patient results higher than the highest reportable range value must be diluted and reanalyzed or reported out as higher than whatever the value of the highest reportable value. Patient values that fall below the lowest reportable limit value can be reported out as "less than...."

WHAT VERIFICATION OF REFERENCE INTERVALS

When physicians order tests from the laboratory, the identity of the actual instrument or method that will be used to analyze the specimen is unknown to them. To allow the physician to compare the patient result with a reference point, the laboratory report must include the normal or reference range or interval concentration for each compound analyzed in the laboratory. When a laboratory changes methods or instruments, either because of increased speed and convenience or decreased cost, the result obtained on the new analyzer or method should not significantly differ from the result that would have been obtained from the old analyzer. If the results differ, the laboratory must establish new normal or reference interval concentrations for each compound analyzed on the new instrument or method. Samples must be included in the study of all ages and genders that are analyzed in the laboratory. The CLSI currently recommends a minimum of 120 samples from each group that is analyzed by the method. The laboratory must ensure that the samples to be tested are representative of their patient population. For example, a laboratory should not use samples from individuals older than 50 for their reference intervals if the laboratory only analyzes samples obtained from pediatric patients.

The samples are analyzed, and a mean and standard deviation are established. The new reference interval typically includes 95% of the results.

WHAT PROFICIENCY TESTING

Proficiency testing is a quality assurance tool to assess the accuracy and precision of the laboratory's methods and instrumentation. CLIA'88 has mandated the use of proficiency testing three times a year for all laboratories performing moderate-complexity or high-complexity testing. There are many organizations and companies that supply laboratories with proficiency test samples. Each proficiency test consists of a number of samples that must be analyzed in the same manner as patient samples. The laboratory analyzes the samples, records the results on the supplied form, and sends the results to the agency.

The criteria for acceptable results depends on the analyte. Some analytes have a target value with a small variable interval. Appendix 14-B lists the acceptable ranges established by the Health Care Financing Administration for many analytes. Each sample is scored as acceptable or unacceptable depending on if it falls inside or outside of the acceptable intervals or values.

Other analytes may use the criteria of comparing each result with the peer group's results. In this method, a peer group standard deviation is established, which is termed the standard deviation index (SDI). The SDI is calculated by the following formula:

$$SDI = \frac{\text{Result from Lab} - \text{Peer Group Result}}{\text{Standard Deviation of Peer Group}}$$

HOW   **EXAMPLE PROBLEMS**

This section is designed to be useful to both the student and the laboratory professional. Students can use the additional problems to master the material. The laboratory professional can use the examples as templates for solving laboratory calculations. By finding an example similar to the problem that you need to solve, substitute the numbers appropriate to your calculation into the equation.

Use the following situation to answer Example Problems 1 to 5.

Situation: A new urine pregnancy test kit was developed and tested on 400 women attending an ob/gyn clinic. Two hundred twenty women tested positive. Of these, 216 pregnancies were confirmed by other means. Of the remaining 180 women who tested negative, 5 women were confirmed pregnant by other means.

1. **Q.** What is the diagnostic sensitivity of this new assay?
   A. Diagnostic sensitivity is calculated by the following formula:

$$\text{Sensitivity} = \frac{\text{True Positives (TP)}}{\text{True Positives (TP)} + \text{False Negatives (FN)}} \times 100$$

   The number of true positives is 216, whereas the number of false negatives is 5. Therefore the diagnostic sensitivity of this kit is as follows:

$$\text{Sensitivity} = \frac{216}{216 + 5} \times 100$$

$$\text{Sensitivity} = \frac{216}{221} \times 100$$

$$\text{Sensitivity} = 0.977 \times 100$$

$$\text{Sensitivity} = 97.7\%$$

2. **Q.** What is the diagnostic specificity of the new pregnancy kit?
   A. The formula for diagnostic specificity is as follows:

$$\text{Specificity} = \frac{\text{True Negatives (TN)}}{\text{True Negatives (TN)} + \text{False Positives (FP)}} \times 100$$

The number of true negatives is 175, whereas the number of false positives is 4. Therefore the diagnostic specificity of this kit is as follows:

$$\text{Specificity} = \frac{175}{175 + 4} \times 100$$

$$\text{Specificity} = \frac{175}{179} \times 100$$

$$\text{Specificity} = 0.978 \times 100$$

$$\text{Specificity} = 97.8\%$$

3. **Q.** What is the efficiency of this new kit?
   A. The efficiency of a test is the number of patients correctly diagnosed as having or not having the disease or condition. The formula for efficiency is as follows:

$$\text{Efficiency} = \frac{TP + TN}{TP + FP + FN + TN} \times 100$$

$$TP = 216, FP = 4$$

$$TN = 175, FN = 5$$

Substituting into the formula the obtained values yields:

$$\text{Efficiency} = \frac{216 + 175}{216 + 4 + 5 + 175} \times 100$$

$$\text{Efficiency} = \frac{391}{400} \times 100$$

$$\text{Efficiency} = 0.978 \times 100$$

$$\text{Efficiency} = 97.8\%$$

4. **Q.** What is the positive predictive value of this kit?
   A. The positive predictive value is the ability of the test to correctly determine the presence of a disease or condition in those patients who have the disease or condition. It is calculated by the following formula:

$$\text{Positive predictive value} = \frac{TP}{TP + FP} \times 100$$

Therefore the positive predictive value of this new kit is as follows:

$$\text{Positive predictive value} = \frac{216}{216 + 4} \times 100$$

$$\text{Positive predictive value} = \frac{216}{220} \times 100$$

$$\text{Positive predictive value} = 0.982 \times 100$$

$$\text{Positive predictive value} = 98.2\%$$

5. **Q.** What is the negative predictive value of this new pregnancy kit?

   A. The negative predictive value is the ability of the test to correctly determine the absence of the disease or condition in patients whose tests proved negative for the disease or condition. The negative predictive value is calculated by the following formula:

$$\text{Negative predictive value} = \frac{TN}{TN + FN} \times 100$$

As there were 175 true negatives and five false negatives, the negative predictive value of this kit is as follows:

$$\text{Negative predictive value} = \frac{175}{175 + 5} \times 100$$

$$\text{Negative predictive value} = \frac{175}{180} \times 100$$

$$\text{Negative predictive value} = 0.972 \times 100$$

$$\text{Negative predictive value} = 97.2\%$$

6. **Q.** What is the null and alternate hypothesis in inferential statistics?

   A. Inferential statistics are statistical analyses in which groups of data are compared to determine if there are significant differences between them. The null hypothesis (H_o) states that there is no statistically significant difference between the groups of data. The alternate hypothesis (H_a) states that there is a statistically significant difference between the two data groups.

7. **Q.** What is Student's t-test?

   A. Student's t-test is used in the clinical laboratory to compare the means of two methods. Student's t-test can detect bias between the methods—that is, if one method yields higher or lower values than the other.

8. **Q.** What is the difference between a one-tailed and a two-tailed Student's t-test?

   A. A one-tailed Student's t-test is used when one method is tested to determine if it yields data that are greater than or less than the other method. For example, the laboratory may only be interested in determining if the test method yields higher values than the reference method. In contrast, a two-tailed test determines if there is a difference between the methods, either higher or lower.

9. **Q.** What are degrees of freedom?

   A. The degrees of freedom used in statistical analyses are the amount that any number can vary within the group of numbers. The amount that any individual number can vary is dependent on the number of restrictions placed on that number. In general, the degree of freedom is calculated by n − 1 (i.e., the total number of data points minus 1).

10. **Q.** A laboratory received a new hematology analyzer. Before putting this analyzer into service, the supervisor analyzed for the total white blood count (WBC) using a normal control 30 times on each analyzer. If the sum of the difference between samples (d) is 115, and the difference between means (d^2) is 1980, calculate the paired t value and determine if there is a statistically significant difference at $P < 0.05$.

A. The paired Student's t-test is calculated by the following formula:
where

$$\sum(\overline{X}_1 - \overline{X}_2) = d$$

$$\text{Paired } t\text{-test value} = \cfrac{\cfrac{\sum(\overline{X}_1 - \overline{X}_2)}{n}}{\sqrt{\cfrac{\sum d^2 - \left[\sum(\overline{X}_1 - \overline{X}_2)\right]^2 \div n}{n-1}}} \div \sqrt{n}$$

Substituting into the formula the values from the problem yields the following:

$$\text{Paired } t\text{-test value} = \cfrac{\cfrac{115}{30}}{\sqrt{\cfrac{1980 - \cfrac{(115)^2}{30}}{29}}} \div \sqrt{30}$$

$$\text{Paired } t\text{-test value} = \cfrac{3.83}{\sqrt{\cfrac{1980 - 440.8}{29}}} \div \sqrt{30}$$

$$\text{Paired } t\text{-test value} = \cfrac{3.83}{\sqrt{53.1} \div \sqrt{30}}$$

$$\text{Paired } t\text{-test value} = \cfrac{3.83}{\cfrac{7.28}{5.5}}$$

$$\text{Paired } t\text{-test value} = \cfrac{3.83}{1.32}$$

$$\text{Paired } t\text{-test value} = 2.902$$

The two-tailed Student's t table in Appendix 14-A can be used to determine if the calculated t value is statistically significant. The significance level is 0.05, and as there were 30 values, the number of degrees of freedom is 29 ($n-1$). The tabulated value is 2.045. As our calculated value is larger than the tabulated value, the null hypothesis cannot be accepted. Therefore, there is a statistically significant (at $P < 0.05$) difference between the two hematology analyzers for total WBC counts.

11. Q. Two coagulation analyzers were compared for precision analysis. The same control was used to analyze 30 replicate prothrombin times on both analyzers. The mean standard deviation and coefficient of variation was performed on the data generated from each analyzer. The standard deviation of Analyzer A was 2.1, and the standard deviation of Analyzer B was 1.9. Using the F test, determine if there is a statistically significant difference (at $P < 0.05$) in the precision of Analyzer A compared with Analyzer B.

A. The F test is the ratio of the larger variance divided by the smaller variance of two methods. The variance is the square of the standard deviation value. Therefore the variance of each analyzer is as follows:

Analyzer A SD = 2.1, variance = $(2.1)^2 = 4.41$
Analyzer B SD = 1.9, variance = $(1.9)^2 = 3.61$

$$F\ value = \frac{large\ variance}{smaller\ variance} = \frac{4.41}{3.61}$$

F value = 1.22

Next, use the F table in Appendix 14-C. Each method has an n of 30; therefore each analyzer has a degree of freedom value of 29. From the F table, the critical value is 1.90. Because the calculated value is less than the tabulated value, the conclusion is that there is no significant difference in the precision of the analyzers.

For Example Problems 12 to 14, use the following information:

Situation: A new method (Method B) for serum creatinine was evaluated to determine if the results correlated with the current method (Method A). A method comparison study using CLSI guidelines was performed. Forty patient samples with values that were distributed across the detectable range of each analyzer were measured on each analyzer. Statistical analysis of the data yielded the following:

Σ Method A = 72 mg/mL
Σ Method B = 74 mg/mL
Mean of Method A (x) = 1.8 mg/mL
Mean of Method B (y) =1.9 mg/mL
$\Sigma x^2 = 134$ mg/dL
$\Sigma y^2 = 141$ mg/dL
$\Sigma xy = 137$ mg/dL

12. **Q.** What is the slope of the regression line?
    A. The linear regression line is calculated by the formula y = mx + b, where m is the slope of the line. The slope is calculated by the following formula:

$$m = \frac{n(\sum xy) - (\sum x)(\sum y)}{n(\sum x^2) - (\sum x)^2}$$

Substituting the data into the formula yields the following:

$$m = \frac{40(137) - (72)(74)}{40(134) - (72)^2}$$

$$m = \frac{5480 - 5328}{5360 - 5184}$$

$$m = \frac{152}{176}$$

$$m = +0.864$$

13. **Q.** What is the y intercept?

    A. The y intercept (b) is calculated by the following formula:

    $$b = \bar{y} - (mx)$$

    Substituting the data obtained into the formula yields the following:

    $$b = 1.9 - [(+0.864)(1.8)]$$
    $$b = 0.35$$

14. **Q.** What is the coefficient of correlation?

    A. The coefficient of correlation (r) can mathematically determine if there is a relationship between two methods. Another name for r is the correlation coefficient. The calculation for r is as follows:

    $$r = \frac{\sum xy - \dfrac{(\sum x)(\sum y)}{n}}{\sqrt{\left[\sum x^2 - \dfrac{(\sum x)^2}{n}\right]\left[\sum y^2 - \dfrac{(\sum y)^2}{n}\right]}}$$

    Substituting the data provided into the formula yields the following:

    $$r = \frac{137 - \dfrac{(72)(74)}{40}}{\sqrt{\left[134 - \dfrac{(72)^2}{40}\right]\left[141 - \dfrac{(74)^2}{40}\right]}}$$

    $$r = \frac{137 - 133.2}{\sqrt{[4.4][4.1]}}$$

    $$r = \frac{3.8}{4.2}$$

    $$r = 0.905$$

_{HOW} **PRACTICE PROBLEMS**

Solve the following practice problems to further master the material. Answers and explanations to some problems can be found in the Answer Key.

Given the following information for a new diagnostic test, answer questions 1 to 5. From an evaluative study of 1000 persons, the following statistics were generated.

TP = 950
TN = 45
FP = 1
FN = 4

1. What is the diagnostic sensitivity of the new test?

2. What is the diagnostic specificity of the new test?

3. What is the efficiency of the new test?

4. What is the positive predictive value of the new test?

5. What is the negative predictive value of the new test?

6. Given the variance of Method A = 2.7 (n = 50) and the variance of Method B = 4.2 (n = 50), is there a statistically significant ($P < 0.05$) difference in precision between Method A and Method B?

Use the following information to answer questions 7 to 10.

   Two methods were compared using 50 duplicate samples for linear regression analysis. The data are as follows:

Sum of Method A (reference) = 60
Sum of Method B (test) = 80
Mean of Method A = 4.5
Mean of Method B = 5.1
Sum of (Method A)^2 = 3600
Sum of (Method B)^2 = 6400
Sum of xy = 4800

7. What is the slope of the regression line?

8. What is the y intercept of the regression line?

9. How is the standard error of the estimate calculated?

10. What information does the correlation coefficient of the regression line infer?

QUICK NOTES

- Diagnostic sensitivity is the probability that only patients with a disease will test positive for that disease.
- Diagnostic specificity is the probability that patients who do not have the disease will test negative for that disease.
- The positive predictive value of a test method is its ability to correctly determine the presence of disease only in those patients who have the disease.
- The negative predictive value of a test method is its ability to determine the absence of disease in those patients who test negative for the disease.
- A Student's t-test compares the means of two methods to determine if there is a statistically significant difference between them.
- Most method comparisons use some type of software such as Excel to perform method comparison calculations, but it is always helpful to understand the math behind the calculations.
- The F test can determine the precision of a new method by dividing the larger variance by the smaller variance and obtaining an F value. That value then must be compared to the appropriate F score from an F table or by using Excel.

BIBLIOGRAPHY

Burtis CA, Bruns DE, editors: *Tietz fundamentals of clinical chemistry and molecular diagnostics*, ed 7, St Louis, 2015, Elsevier.

Clinical Laboratory Improvement Amendment of 1988: *Final rule*, Washington, DC, 1988, US Government Printing Office.

Clinical Laboratory Standards Institute: *C28-Ac3 (Electronic Document) Defining, establishing, and verifying reference intervals in the clinical laboratory*, ed 3, Villanova, PA, 2012.

Clinical Laboratory Standards Institute: *EP09-A3 (Electronic Document) Method comparison and bias estimation using patient samples*, ed 3, Villanova, PA, 2013.

Laboratory Requirements, Clinical Laboratory Improvement Amendment of 1988: *Code of Federal Regulations 42CFR493*, Washington, DC, 1988, US Government Printing Office.

Westgard J: *Basic method validation*. Available at https://www.westgard.com/lesson23.htm.

Westgard J: *Final CLIA rule*. Available at https://www.westgard.com/clia-final-rule.htm.

Appendix 14-A

Percentage points of the *t* distribution. (This table gives the values of *t* for differing *df* that cut off specified proportions of the area in one and in two tails of the *t* distribution.)

	Area in Two Tails				
	.10	.05	.02	.01	.001
	Area in One Tail				
df	.05	.025	.01	.005	.0005
1	6.314	12.706	31.821	63.657	636.619
2	2.920	4.303	6.965	9.925	31.598
3	2.353	3.182	4.541	5.841	12.941
4	2.132	2.776	3.747	4.604	8.610
5	2.015	2.571	3.365	4.032	6.859
6	1.943	2.447	3.143	3.707	5.959
7	1.895	2.365	2.998	3.499	5.405
8	1.860	2.306	2.896	3.355	5.041
9	1.833	2.262	2.821	3.250	4.781
10	1.812	2.228	2.764	3.169	4.587
11	1.796	2.201	2.718	3.106	4.437
12	1.782	2.179	2.681	3.055	4.318
13	1.771	2.160	2.650	3.012	4.221
14	1.761	2.145	2.624	2.977	4.140
15	1.753	2.131	2.602	2.947	4.073
16	1.746	2.120	2.583	2.921	4.015
17	1.740	2.110	2.567	2.898	3.965
18	1.734	2.101	2.552	2.878	3.922
19	1.729	2.093	2.539	2.861	3.883
20	1.725	2.086	2.528	2.845	3.850
21	1.721	2.080	2.518	2.831	3.819
22	1.717	2.074	2.508	2.819	3.792
23	1.714	2.069	2.500	2.807	3.767
24	1.711	2.064	2.492	2.797	3.745
25	1.708	2.060	2.485	2.787	3.725
26	1.706	2.056	2.479	2.779	3.707
27	1.703	2.052	2.473	2.771	3.690
28	1.701	2.048	2.467	2.763	3.674

Area in Two Tails					
29	1.699	2.045	2.462	2.756	3.659
30	1.697	2.042	2.457	2.750	3.646
40	1.684	2.021	2.423	2.704	3.551
60	1.671	2.000	2.390	2.660	3.460
120	1.658	1.980	2.358	2.617	3.373
∞	1.645	1.960	2.326	2.576	3.291

Adapted from Pearson ES, Hartley HO: Table 12: Percentage points of the t-distribution, p. 146. In: *Biometrika tables for statisticians*, vol 1, ed 3, 1966, with permission of the Biometrika Trustees.

Appendix 14-B CLIA '88 Criteria for Acceptable Performance

Analyte or Test	Criteria for Acceptable Performance
Immunology Laboratory	
α_1-Antitrypsin	Target value +/− 3 SD
α-Fetoprotein (tumor marker)	Target value +/− 3 SD
Antinuclear antibodies	Target value +/− 2 dilutions or positive or negative
Antistreptolysin O	Target value +/− 2 dilutions or positive or negative
Antihuman immunodeficiency virus	Reactive or nonreactive
Complement C3	Target value +/− 3 SD
Complement C4	Target value +/− 3 SD
Hepatitis (HBsAg, HBc, HBeAg)	Reactive or nonreactive
IgA	Target value +/− 3 SD
IgE	Target value +/− 3 SD
IgG	Target value +/− 25%
IgM	Target value +/− 3 SD
Infectious mononucleosis	Target value +/− 2 dilutions or positive or negative
Rheumatoid fever	Target value +/− 2 dilutions or positive or negative
Rubella	Target value +/− 2 dilutions or immune or nonimmune or positive or negative
Chemistry Laboratory	
ALT	Target value +/− 20%
Albumin	Target value +/− 10%
Alkaline phosphatase	Target value +/− 30%
Amylase	Target value +/− 30%
AST	Target value +/− 20%
Bilirubin (total)	Target value +/− 0.4 mg/dL or +/− 20% (greater)
Blood gas Po_2	Target value +/− 3 SD
Pco_2	Target value +/− 5 mm Hg or +/− 8% (greater)
pH	Target value +/− 0.04
Calcium, total	Target value +/− 1.0 mg/dL
Chloride	Target value +/− 5%
Cholesterol, total	Target value +/− 10%
Cholesterol, HDL	Target value +/−30%

Analyte or Test	Criteria for Acceptable Performance
Creatine kinase	Target value +/−30%
Creatine kinase isoenzymes	MB elevated (presence or absence) or target value +/−3 SD
Creatine	Target value +/−0.3 mg/dL or +/−15% (greater)
Glucose (excluding waived glucose methods)	Target value +/−6 mg/dL or 10% (greater)
Iron, total	Target value +/−20%
LDH	Target value +/−20%
LDH isoenzymes	LDH1/LDH2 (+ or −) or target value +/−30%
Magnesium	Target value +/−25%
Potassium	Target value +/−0.5 mmol/L
Sodium	Target value +/−4 mmol/L
Total protein	Target value +/−10%
Triglycerides	Target value +/−5%
Urea nitrogen	Target value +/−2 mg/dL or +/− 9% (greater)
Uric acid	Target value +/−17%

Endocrinology

Cortisol	Target value +/− 25%
Free thyroxine	Target value +/− 3 SD
HCG	Target value +/− 3 SD, positive or negative
T3 uptake	Target value +/− 3 SD
Triiodothyronine	Target value +/− 3 SD
Thyroid stimulating hormone	Target value +/− 3 SD
Thyroxine	Target value +/− 20% or 1.0 mg/dL (greater)

Toxicology

Alcohol, blood	Target value +/− 25%
Blood lead	Target value +/− 10% or 4 mcg/dL (greater)
Carbamazepine	Target value +/− 25%
Digoxin	Target value +/− 20% or +/− 2 ng/mL (greater)
Ethosuximide	Target value +/− 20%
Gentamicin	Target value +/− 25%
Lithium	Target value +/− 0.3 mmol/L or +/− 20% (greater)
Phenobarbital	Target value +/− 20%
Phenytoin	Target value +/− 25%
Primidone	Target value +/− 25%
Procainamide (and metabolite)	Target value +/− 25%

Analyte or Test	Criteria for Acceptable Performance
Quinidine	Target value +/− 25%
Tobramycin	Target value +/− 25%
Theophylline	Target value +/− 25%
Valproic acid	Target value +/− 25%
Hematology	
Cell identification	90% or greater consensus on ID
WBC differential	Target +/− 3 SD based on the percentage of different types of WBCs in the sample
Erythrocyte count	Target value +/− 6%
Hematocrit (excluding spun Hcts)	Target value +/− 6%
Hemoglobin	Target value +/− 7%
Leukocyte count	Target value +/− 15%
Platelet count	Target value +/− 25%
Fibrinogen	Target value +/− 20%
Partial thromboplastin time	Target value +/− 15%
Prothrombin time	Target value +/− 15%
Immunohematology	
ABO grouping	100% accuracy
D (Rho) typing	100% accuracy
Unexpected antibody detection	80% accuracy
Compatibility testing	100% accuracy
Antibody identification	80% accuracy

From 57 CFR: Clinical Laboratory Improvement Amendment of 1988: Final Rule. US Government Printing Office, Washington, DC, 1988.

Appendix 14-C

Denominator Degrees of Freedom	F.95 Numerator Degrees of Freedom								
	1	2	3	4	5	6	7	8	9
1	161.4	199.5	215.7	224.6	230.2	234.0	236.8	238.9	240.5
2	18.51	19.00	19.16	19.25	19.30	19.33	19.35	19.37	19.38
3	10.13	9.55	9.28	9.12	9.01	8.94	8.89	8.85	8.81
4	7.71	6.94	6.59	6.39	6.26	6.16	6.09	6.04	6.00
5	6.61	5.79	5.41	5.19	5.05	4.95	4.88	4.82	4.77
6	5.99	5.14	4.76	4.53	4.39	4.28	4.21	4.15	4.10
7	5.59	4.74	4.35	4.12	3.97	3.87	3.79	3.73	3.68
8	5.32	4.46	4.07	3.84	3.69	3.58	3.50	3.44	3.39
9	5.12	4.26	3.86	3.63	3.48	3.37	3.29	3.23	3.18
10	4.96	4.10	3.71	3.48	3.33	3.22	3.14	3.07	3.02
11	4.84	3.98	3.59	3.36	3.20	3.09	3.01	2.95	2.90
12	4.75	3.89	3.49	3.26	3.11	3.00	2.91	2.85	2.80
13	4.67	3.81	3.41	3.18	3.03	2.92	2.83	2.77	2.71
14	4.60	3.74	3.34	3.11	2.96	2.85	2.76	2.70	2.65
15	4.54	3.68	3.29	3.06	2.90	2.79	2.71	2.64	2.59
16	4.49	3.63	3.24	3.01	2.85	2.74	2.66	2.59	2.54
17	4.45	3.59	3.20	2.96	2.81	2.70	2.61	2.55	2.49
18	4.41	3.55	3.16	2.93	2.77	2.66	2.58	2.51	2.46
19	4.38	3.52	3.13	2.90	2.74	2.63	2.54	2.48	2.42
20	4.35	3.49	3.10	2.87	2.71	2.60	2.51	2.45	2.39
21	4.32	3.47	3.07	2.84	2.68	2.57	2.49	2.42	2.37
22	4.30	3.44	3.05	2.82	2.66	2.55	2.46	2.40	2.34
23	4.28	3.42	3.03	2.80	2.64	2.53	2.44	2.37	2.32
24	4.26	3.40	3.01	2.78	2.62	2.51	2.42	2.36	2.30
25	4.24	3.39	2.99	2.76	2.60	2.49	2.40	2.34	2.28
26	4.23	3.37	2.98	2.74	2.59	2.47	2.39	2.32	2.27
27	4.21	3.35	2.96	2.73	2.57	2.46	2.37	2.31	2.25
28	4.20	3.34	2.95	2.71	2.56	2.45	2.36	2.29	2.24
29	4.18	3.33	2.93	2.70	2.55	2.43	2.35	2.28	2.22
30	4.17	3.32	2.92	2.69	2.53	2.42	2.33	2.27	2.21
40	4.08	3.23	2.84	2.61	2.45	2.34	2.25	2.18	2.12

Denominator Degrees of Freedom	F.95								
	Numerator Degrees of Freedom								
	1	2	3	4	5	6	7	8	9
60	4.00	3.15	2.76	2.53	2.37	2.25	2.17	2.10	2.04
120	3.92	3.07	2.68	2.45	2.29	2.17	2.09	2.02	1.96
∞	3.84	3.00	2.60	2.37	2.21	2.10	2.01	1.94	1.88

Source: Corty EW: *Using and interpreting statistics: A practical text for the health, behavioral, and social sciences*, St Louis, 2007, Mosby.

Denominator Degrees of Freedom	F.95									
	Numerator Degrees of Freedom									
	10	12	15	20	24	30	40	60	120	∞
1	241.9	243.9	245.9	248.0	249.1	250.1	251.1	252.2	253.3	254.3
2	19.40	19.41	19.43	19.45	19.45	19.46	19.47	19.48	19.49	19.50
3	8.79	8.74	8.70	8.66	8.64	8.62	8.59	8.57	8.55	8.53
4	5.96	5.91	5.86	5.80	5.77	5.75	5.72	5.69	5.66	5.63
5	4.74	4.68	4.62	4.56	4.53	4.50	4.46	4.43	4.40	4.36
6	4.06	4.00	3.94	3.87	3.84	3.81	3.77	3.74	3.70	3.67
7	3.64	3.57	3.51	3.44	3.41	3.38	3.34	3.30	3.27	3.23
8	3.35	3.28	3.22	3.15	3.12	3.08	3.04	3.01	2.97	2.93
9	3.14	3.07	3.01	2.94	2.90	2.86	2.83	2.79	2.75	2.71
10	2.98	2.91	2.85	2.77	2.74	2.70	2.66	2.62	2.58	2.54
11	2.85	2.79	2.72	2.65	2.61	2.57	2.53	2.49	2.45	2.40
12	2.75	2.69	2.62	2.54	2.51	2.47	2.43	2.38	2.34	2.30
13	2.67	2.60	2.53	2.46	2.42	2.38	2.34	2.30	2.25	2.21
14	2.60	2.53	2.46	2.39	2.35	2.31	2.27	2.22	2.18	2.13
15	2.54	2.48	2.40	2.33	2.29	2.25	2.20	2.16	2.11	2.07
16	2.49	2.42	2.35	2.28	2.24	2.19	2.15	2.11	2.06	2.01
17	2.45	2.38	2.31	2.23	2.19	2.15	2.10	2.06	2.01	1.96
18	2.41	2.34	2.27	2.19	2.15	2.11	2.06	2.02	1.97	1.92
19	2.38	2.31	2.23	2.16	2.11	2.07	2.03	1.98	1.93	1.88
20	2.35	2.28	2.20	2.12	2.08	2.04	1.99	1.95	1.90	1.84
21	2.32	2.25	2.18	2.10	2.05	2.01	1.96	1.92	1.87	1.81
22	2.30	2.23	2.15	2.07	2.03	1.98	1.94	1.89	1.84	1.78
23	2.27	2.20	2.13	2.05	2.01	1.96	1.91	1.86	1.81	1.76
24	2.25	2.18	2.11	2.03	1.98	1.94	1.89	1.84	1.79	1.73
25	2.24	2.16	2.09	2.01	1.96	1.92	1.87	1.82	1.77	1.71
26	2.22	2.15	2.07	1.99	1.95	1.90	1.85	1.80	1.75	1.69
27	2.20	2.13	2.06	1.97	1.93	1.88	1.84	1.79	1.73	1.67
28	2.19	2.12	2.04	1.96	1.91	1.87	1.82	1.77	1.71	1.65
29	2.18	2.10	2.03	1.94	1.90	1.85	1.81	1.75	1.70	1.64
30	2.16	2.09	2.01	1.93	1.89	1.84	1.79	1.74	1.68	1.62
40	2.08	2.00	1.92	1.84	1.79	1.74	1.69	1.64	1.58	1.51
60	1.99	1.92	1.84	1.75	1.70	1.65	1.59	1.53	1.47	1.39
120	1.91	1.83	1.75	1.66	1.61	1.55	1.50	1.43	1.35	1.25
∞	1.83	1.75	1.67	1.57	1.52	1.46	1.39	1.32	1.22	1.00

Infrequently Performed Calculations

OBJECTIVES

At the end of this chapter, the reader should be able to do the following:

1. Calculate the concentrations of anhydrous solutions given the hydrated form and vice versa.
2. Determine the density of solutions based on the specific gravity (SG) of the solution.
3. Calculate the concentrations of unknown samples by single-standard and factor method.
4. Calculate how to make working standards from a stock standard.
5. Calculate the analyte concentration per volume of collection of urine analytes.
6. Calculate the quantity of analyte collected in urine per unit of time of collection.
7. Calculate the quantity of analyte measured in milligrams per deciliter into grams per day.

ANHYDROUS VERSUS HYDROUS SOLUTIONS

Another type of solution may consist of hydrated chemical salts dissolved in a solvent. As the difference between the hydrous and the anhydrous form of a chemical is the amount of water molecules present in the hydrated form, it may be necessary to be able to interchange between the two. Sometimes, in the laboratory, only one of the forms of a chemical is available. You must be able to interchange the two forms to arrive at the form that you need. The basic formula for interchanging between hydrous and anhydrous chemicals is as follows:

$$\frac{\text{anhydrous chemical molecular weight}}{\text{hydrated chemical molecular weight}} = \frac{\text{gram of anhydrous chemical}}{\text{gram of hydrous chemical}}$$

Notice that it is a ratio and proportion calculation. Ratio and proportion are used whenever the same concentration of a solution but different quantities of the solution are necessary. In anhydrous as opposed to hydrous forms of a chemical, the ratio and proportion are used to ensure that the same concentration of the chemical is used regardless of its water content.

HOW   **Example 15-1**

Suppose you needed to make a $12.0\%^{w/v}$ solution of $CuSO_4$, but only $CuSO_4 \cdot H_2O$ was available. How much of the $CuSO_4 \cdot H_2O$ should you use? The gram molecular weight of $CuSO_4$ is 159.61, whereas the gram molecular weight of $CuSO_4 \cdot H_2O$ is 177.63.

The first step is to determine the amount of grams in a $12.0\%^{w/v}$ solution. A $12\%^{w/v}$ solution contains 12.0 g in 100 mL of solvent. Using the formula for interchanging hydrous and anhydrous chemicals, the following equation is derived:

$$\frac{159.61 \text{ gmw } (CuSO_4)}{177.63 \text{ gmw } (CuSO_4 \cdot H_2O)} = \frac{12.0(CuSO_4)}{X \text{ g hydrated}}$$

By crossmultiplying, the following equation is derived:

$$(159.61)(X) = (177.63)(12.0)$$
$$(159.61)(X) = 2131.56$$
$$X = 13.4 \text{ g}$$

Therefore 13.4 g of $CuSO_4 \cdot H_2O$ qs to 100 mL of solvent will result in a $12.0 \%^{w/v}$ solution of $CuSO_4$.

Example 15-1a   You need to make a $5\%^{w/v}$ solution of $CaCl_2$, but only $CaCl_2 \cdot 2H_2O$ is available. How do you make the $5\%^{w/v}$ solution?

To make this solution, use the formula for interchanging between anhydrous and hydrous chemicals:

$$\frac{110.98 \text{ gmw } (CaCl_2)}{147.02 \text{ gmw } (CaCl_2 \cdot 2H_2O)} = \frac{5.0 \text{ g}(CaCl_2)}{X \text{ g hydrated}}$$
$$X = 6.62 \text{ g of } CaCl_2 \cdot 2H_2O \text{ qs to } 100 \text{ mL}$$

Example 15-1b   You need to make a $25\%^{w/v}$ solution of $CaSO_4$, but only $CaSO_4 \cdot 2H_2O$ is available. How do you make this solution?

To make this solution, use the formula for interchanging between anhydrous and hydrous chemicals:

$$\frac{136.15 \text{ gmw } (CaSO_4)}{172.17 \text{ gmw } (CaSO_4 \cdot 2H_2O)} = \frac{25.0 \text{ g } (CaSO_4)}{X \text{ g hydrated}}$$
$$X = 31.6 \text{ g of } CaSO_4 \cdot 2H_2O \text{ qs to } 100 \text{ mL}$$

Example 15-1c   You need to make a 25%$^{w/v}$ solution of Na_2CO_3, but only $NaCO_3 \cdot H_2O$ is available. How do you make this solution?

To make this solution, use the formula for interchanging between anhydrous and hydrous chemicals:

$$\frac{105.99 \text{ gmw } (Na_2CO_3)}{124.00 \text{ gmw } (Na_2CO_3 \cdot H_2O)} = \frac{25.0 \text{ g } (Na_2CO_3)}{X \text{ g hydrated}}$$

$$X = 29.2 \text{ g of } Na_2CO_3 \cdot H_2O \text{ qs to } 100 \text{ mL}$$

Example 15-1d   A buffer solution needs to be prepared. The directions call for 2.50 g of anhydrous Na_2HPO_4 to be dissolved into 100 mL of deionized water. Only $Na_2HPO_4 \cdot 7H_2O$ is available in the chemical storeroom. How much of the $Na_2HPO_4 \cdot 7H_2O$ should be used to prepare the solution?

The molecular weight of Na_2HPO_4 is 141.96, whereas the molecular weight of the hydrous form is 268.10 because there are 7.00 water molecules attached to the salt. By substituting into the ratio formula the data from the problem, the following equation is derived:

$$\frac{141.96 \text{ gmw } (Na_2HPO_4)}{268.10 \text{ gmw } (Na_2HPO_4 \cdot 7H_2O)} = \frac{2.50 \text{ g } (Na_2HPO_4)}{X \text{ g } (Na_2HPO_4 \cdot 7H_2O)}$$

Crossmultiplying the equation yields the following:

$$(141.96)(X) = (2.50)(268.10)$$

$$(141.96)(X) = 670.25$$

$$X = \frac{670.25}{141.96}$$

$$X = 4.72 \text{ g } Na_2HPO_4 \cdot 7H_2O$$

Therefore 4.72 g of $Na_2HPO_4 \cdot 7H_2O$ can be dissolved into solvent and qs to 100 mL.

WHAT **DENSITY CALCULATIONS**

Some acids and bases may have the specific gravity (SG) of the chemical on the chemical label. This is important when the mass concentration per milliliter of the acid or base must be known. The SG is the ratio of the density of the chemical in terms of grams per milliliter compared with pure water at 4°C. Pure water has a density of 1.000 at 4°C or 1.000 g/1.00 mL of pure water. Thus, using pure water, there is a direct relationship between mass and volume.

NOTE: The SG of a solution is equal to the density of the solution (grams per milliliter of solution).

HOW   *Example 15-2*

A bottle of HCl has the following values listed on its label: SG = 1.19 and assay 37.0% ($^{w/w}$).
How many grams of HCl are there per milliliter?

To solve this problem, first determine the concentration of HCl per milliliter. Because the hydrochloric acid has a concentration of 37.0%$^{w/w}$, we can conclude the following:

$$37.0\%^{w/w} = \frac{37.0 \text{ g}}{100.0 \text{ g solution}}$$

Using ratio and proportion, next determine the quantity of HCl per 1 g of solution.

$$\frac{37.0 \text{ g}}{100.0 \text{ g solution}} = \frac{X \text{ g}}{1.00 \text{ g solution}}$$

Crossmultiplying the equation yields the following:

$$(37.0)(1.00) = (100.0)(X)$$
$$37.0 = (100.0)(X)$$
$$X = 0.370$$

There are 0.370 g of HCl in 1.00 g of solution. Remember that a solution is composed of a solute and a solvent. In this case, HCl is the solute, and water is the solvent. We want to know the actual weight of HCl per milliliter of solution, not just the purity of the solution (0.370 g per 1.00 mL of solution or 37.0%). As the SG is known, and SG by definition is the weight of a substance per 1.00 mL, we can determine the amount of grams per milliliter of HCl.

Given: SG = 1.19

Remember: This means that there are 1.19 g of HCl per 1.00 mL of solution and that 37.0% of the mass of 1.19 g is HCl.

$$\left(\frac{1.19 \text{ g HCl solution}}{1.00 \text{ mL solution}}\right)\left(\frac{0.370 \text{ g HCl}}{1.00 \text{ g HCl solution}}\right) = \frac{0.440 \text{ g HCl}}{1.00 \text{ mL solution}}$$

Using significant figures, there are 0.440 g of HCl in 1.00 mL of solution.

Example 15-2a   A 1.00 L bottle of sulfuric acid (H_2SO_4) is labeled 92.0%$^{w/w}$, with a specific gravity of 1.84. How many grams of sulfuric acid are found per milliliter?

As in Example 15-2, first determine the concentration of H_2SO_4/mL. We know that if a solution is 92.0%$^{w/w}$, then there are 92.0 g in 100.0 g of solution. Therefore, using ratio and proportion, we can determine the amount of g of H_2SO_4 in 1 g of solution.

$$\frac{92.0 \text{ g}}{100.0 \text{ g solution}} = \frac{X \text{ g}}{1.00 \text{ g solution}}$$

Crossmultiplying the equation yields the following:

$$(92.0)(1.00) = (100.0)(X)$$
$$92.0 = (100.0)(X)$$
$$X = 0.920$$

Therefore, there are 0.920 g of H_2SO_4 in 1 g of solution. But we want to know the amount of g of H_2SO_4/mL of solution. The specific gravity of this H_2SO_4

solution is 1.84, which means that there are 1.84 g of H_2SO_4/1.0 mL of solution. But, only 92.0% of that 1.84 g actually is H_2SO_4. Use the following formula to determine the amount of g of H_2SO_4 in 1.00 mL of solution:

$$\left(\frac{1.84 \text{ g } H_2SO_4 \text{ solution}}{1.00 \text{ mL solution}}\right)\left(\frac{0.920 \text{ g } H_2SO_4}{1.00 \text{ g } H_2SO_4 \text{ solution}}\right) = \frac{1.69 \text{ g } H_2SO_4}{1.00 \text{ mL solution}}$$

Therefore, there actually are 1.69 g of H_2SO_4/mL of solution.

Example 15-2b   A solution of nitric acid (HNO_3) has a purity of 70.0%$^{w/w}$ and a specific gravity of 1.42. How many grams of nitric acid are there per milliliter?

This is solved in the same way as the two previous examples. The amount of grams of HNO_3 per 1.0 g of solution is 0.700 because the purity of the solution is 70.0%$^{w/w}$. The specific gravity tells us that there are 1.42 g of nitric acid in 1.0 mL solution. Combining both of these facts (multiplying the density by the purity) can tell us how many grams of nitric acid are in 1.00 mL:

$$\left(\frac{1.42 \text{ g } HNO_3 \text{ solution}}{1.00 \text{ mL solution}}\right)\left(\frac{0.700 \text{ g } HNO_3}{1.00 \text{ g } HNO_3 \text{ solution}}\right) = \frac{0.994 \text{ g } HNO_3}{1.00 \text{ mL solution}}$$

Therefore, there are 0.994 g of nitric acid in 1.00 mL of solution.

Example 15-2c   A 1.00 L bottle of acetic acid (CH_3COOH) is labeled 99.7%$^{w/w}$, SG 1.06. How many grams of acetic acid are found in 100.0 mL of the acetic acid solution?

Remember:

$$99.7\%^{w/w} = \frac{99.7 \text{ g } CH_3COOH}{100.0 \text{ g solution}} \quad \text{OR} \quad \frac{0.997 \text{ g acetic acid}}{1.00 \text{ g solution}}$$

The SG tells us that for every 1.00 mL of solution there is 1.06 g of acetic acid.

By multiplying the density of the solution by the percent purity of the solution, the actual quantity of grams per 1.00 mL can be determined.

$$\left(\frac{1.06 \text{ g solution}}{1.00 \text{ mL solution}}\right)\left(\frac{0.997 \text{ g } CH_3COOH}{1.00 \text{ g solution}}\right) = 1.06 \text{ g per } 1.00 \text{ mL of solution.}$$

As we want to know the amount present in 100 mL, using ratio and proportion yields:

$$\frac{1.06 \text{ g solution}}{1.00 \text{ mL solution}} = \frac{X \text{ g}}{100.0 \text{ mL solution}} =$$

$$X = 106.0 \text{ g acetic acid per } 100.0 \text{ mL solution}$$

Therefore, there are 106.0 g of acetic acid in 100.0 mL of solution.

WHAT   In the laboratory, the SG of a particular acid or base becomes important when mass concentrations of the acid or base are required. To make a particular molar concentration of an acid or base solution, the amount of grams of the acid or base need to be known. Alternatively, a solution may be labeled for its SG and percent purity, but the molarity of the solution may not be labeled and might need to be known.

Example 15-3

What is the molarity of a 1.00 L 97.0%$^{w/w}$, SG 1.84 solution of H_2SO_4?
   Okay, take a deep breath; it is not as hard to figure out as it looks!
   The first step to solve this problem is to determine the amount of grams of H_2SO_4/1.00 g of solution.

$$97.0\%^{w/w} = \frac{97.0 \text{ g } H_2SO_4}{100.0 \text{ g solution}} = \frac{0.97 \text{ g } H_2SO_4}{1.00 \text{ g solution}}$$

Next, determine the *actual* amount of g/1.00 mL based on the SG (or density) of the solution.

$$SG = 1.84 = \frac{1.84 \text{ g}}{1.00 \text{ mL}}$$

As there are 0.97 g of H_2SO_4 in 1.00 g of solution, and there are 1.84 g of solution (H_2SO_4 and solvent) per 1.00 mL of solution, then:

$$(1.84)(0.97) = \frac{1.78 \text{ g } H_2SO_4}{1.00 \text{ mL of solution}}$$

As we want to find molarity, next convert the grams per milliliter into grams per liter:

$$\frac{1.78 \text{ g } H_2SO_4}{1.00 \text{ mL}} = \frac{X \text{ g } H_2SO_4}{1000.0 \text{ mL}}$$

$$X = \frac{1780.0 \text{ g } H_2SO_4}{1.00 \text{ L}}$$

Next, use the molarity formula to solve for molarity:

$$M = \frac{\left(\dfrac{1780 \text{ g } H_2SO_4}{98.08 \text{ g}}\right)}{1.00 \text{ L of solution}}$$

$$M = 18.1$$

Therefore the molarity of this solution is 18.1 mol/L.

Example 15-3a   In Example 15-2, it was determined that there were 0.440 g of HCL in 1.00 mL of solution. What is the molarity of this solution?

To solve, first convert the amount of grams per milliliter into grams per liter:

$$\frac{0.440 \text{ g HCl}}{1.00 \text{ mL}} = \frac{X \text{ g HCl}}{1000.0 \text{ mL}}$$

$$X = \frac{440.0 \text{ g HCl}}{1.00 \text{ L}}$$

There are 440.0 g HCl in 1.00 L. Next, solve for the molarity:

$$M = \frac{\left(\dfrac{440.0 \text{ g HCl}}{36.46 \text{ g}}\right)}{1.00 \text{ L of solution}}$$

$$M = 12.07 \text{ or } 12.1$$

Therefore a 37%$^{w/w}$ solution of HCl with a density of 1.19 has a molarity of 12.1.

Example 15-3b   Using the data from the nitric acid example, there were 0.994 g of nitric acid in 1.00 mL. What is the molarity of this solution?

A 0.994 g/mL solution is equal to a 994 g/L solution. The gram molecular weight of nitric acid is 63.02. Therefore:

$$M = \frac{\left(\dfrac{994 \text{ g HNO}_3}{63.02 \text{ g}}\right)}{1.00 \text{ L of solution}}$$

$$M = 15.77$$

Therefore this solution has a molarity of 15.77.

Example 15-3c   How many grams of a stock solution of HNO$_3$ are needed to make 1.00 L of a 1.50 M solution? The stock solution has an SG of 1.42 and a purity of 70.0%$^{w/w}$.

Solve this problem by first using the molarity formula to calculate grams per liter:

$$1.50 \text{ M} = \frac{\left(\dfrac{X \text{ g HNO}_3}{63.02 \text{ g molecular weight}}\right)}{1.00 \text{ L of solution}}$$

$$X = 94.52 \text{ pure g of HNO}_3 \text{ needed}$$

However, the stock nitric acid solution is only 70.0% pure, meaning that for every 100 mL of stock solution, 70.0 mL is nitric acid, and 30.0 mL is water. As the stock nitric acid solution is not pure, divide 94.5 by 0.70 (70%) to arrive at the amount of stock solution necessary to be comparable to a pure solution.

$$94.5 \div 0.70 = 135.0 \text{ g stock solution}$$

Therefore you would need 135.0 g of this stock nitric acid to make 1.0 L of a 1.5 M solution.

Another way to make the same solution is to determine the volume of stock nitric acid necessary to make this solution. The volume can be calculated because we know the SG.

Because this is not a pure solution, we have calculated that we need 135.0 g nitric acid.

Next, as the SG is 1.42, meaning 1.42 g per 1.0 mL of solution, the g of nitric acid are divided by the SG:

$$\frac{135\ g}{1.42\ g/mL} = 95.07\ mL\ \text{stock nitric acid}$$

Therefore 95.07 mL of stock solution are diluted or qs to 1.00 L with water.

NOTE: The example demonstrates two different ways in which a solution with the same volume and concentration can be prepared. The first method used 135.0 g of the stock solution, whereas the second method used 95.1 mL of the stock solution. The conditions inherent to the experiment determine which method is used.

SPECTROPHOTOMETRY

WHAT **Single-Standard Method for Determining the Concentration of Unknowns**

Beer's law states that A = abc, and as b and c are constants, in practice, A α c. If an assay is performed using a single standard and patient and quality control specimens, the absorbances of the patient and quality control samples can be compared to the standard. A ratio and proportion calculation can determine the concentrations of our patient and quality control samples.

HOW *Example 15-4*

A manual glucose assay is performed using a single 150 mg/dL standard. Upon analysis, the absorbance of the standard is 0.465. The absorbance of a patient's sample is 0.338. What is the concentration of the patient's sample?

To solve this problem, use ratio and proportion:

$$\frac{\text{standard absorbance}}{\text{standard concentration}} = \frac{\text{unknown absorbance}}{\text{unknown concentration}}$$

$$\frac{0.465}{150\ mg/dL} = \frac{0.338}{X}$$

Using algebra and crossmultiplying:

$$(0.465)(X) = (0.338)(150\ mg/dL)$$

$$(0.465)(X) = 50.7\ mg/dL$$

$$X = \frac{50.7}{0.465}$$

$$X = 109\ mg/dL$$

Therefore the patient specimen has a glucose concentration of 109 mg/dL. By convention, glucose values tend to be reported to the nearest whole number.

Example 15-4a   A manual serum creatinine is performed in an MLT student laboratory experiment. A 5.0 mg/dL standard is used, and the following results were obtained: absorbance of the standard = 1.142, absorbance of the unknown = 0.778. What is the concentration of the unknown?

$$\text{Remember:} \frac{\text{standard absorbance}}{\text{standard concentration}} = \frac{\text{unknown absorbance}}{\text{unknown concentration}}$$

Using ratio and proportion, the following formula is derived:

$$\frac{1.142}{5.0 \text{ mg/dL}} = \frac{0.778}{X}$$

$$(1.142)X = (0.778)(5.0)$$

$$X = 3.4 \text{ mg/dL}$$

Therefore the concentration of the unknown is 3.4 mg/dL. By convention, creatinine values tend to be reported to the nearest one-tenth.

Example 15-4b   Given a standard concentration of 300 mg/dL with an absorbance equal to 1.262 and an unknown concentration's absorbance of 0.715, what is the concentration of the unknown?

Using ratio and proportion, the concentration of the unknown is 170 mg/dL.

WHAT By manipulating the ratio and proportion calculation, the following formula can be derived to determine the concentration of unknowns using a single-point standard:

$$\text{Conc. of unknown} = \frac{(\text{concentration of standard})(\text{absorbance of unknown})}{\text{absorbance of standard}}$$

NOTE: This formula should not be used if the absorbance of the unknown is higher than the absorbance of the standard.

Dilute the unknown and reanalyze or use a standard with a higher concentration. It is assumed that with a single-point standard assay, the reaction is linear up to the standard concentration. However, absorbances beyond the absorbance of the standard cannot be assumed to be linear.

HOW   **Example 15-5**

The absorbance of a 40.0 mg/dL blood urea nitrogen (BUN) standard is 0.758. The absorbance of the patient's serum specimen is 0.220. What is the patient's serum BUN concentration?
   Use the formula to determine the concentration of BUN in the patient's serum:

$$\text{Conc.of unk.} = \frac{(\text{Conc.std.})(\text{Abs.unk.})}{\text{Abs.std.}}$$

$$X = \frac{(40.0 \text{ mg/dL})(0.220)}{0.758}$$

$$X = 11.6 \text{ mg/dL BUN}$$

Therefore the patient's serum BUN concentration is 11.6 mg/dL.

Example 15-5a   Given the absorbance of a 150 mg/dL standard is 0.425, and the absorbance of QC Level 1 is 0.205, calculate the concentration of QC Level 1.

Using the formula from Example 15-5, and substituting into it the values from this problem, the following formula is derived:

$$\text{Conc.of unk.} = \frac{(\text{Conc.std.})(\text{Abs.unk.})}{\text{Abs.std.}}$$

$$X = \frac{(150 \text{ mg/dL})(0.205)}{0.425}$$

$$X = 72 \text{ mg/dL}$$

The concentration of QC Level 1 is 72 mg/dL.

Example 15-5b   Given the absorbance of a 250 mg/dL standard is 0.750, and the absorbance of QC Level 2 is 0.680, what is the concentration of QC Level 2?

Using the same formula and substituting into it the values of this new problem, the concentration of QC Level 2 is 227 mg/dL. It would be correct to round up to 230 mg/dL but QC values are an exception to the significant figures rule.

WHAT **Factor Method to Determine the Concentrations of Unknowns**

If a single-point standard is used in a manually performed assay and a number of unknowns need concentrations calculated, the mathematics involved can become quite tedious. Notice that within the formula, once the assay is performed, there are two constants: the concentration of the standard and the absorbance of the standard. By mathematically manipulating the formula, a factor can be derived. The concentration of an unknown can be determined by multiplying the absorbance of the unknown by the factor. Using the factor simplifies the mathematics involved when calculating the concentrations of multiple unknowns.

$$\text{Conc. of unknown} = \frac{(\text{concentration of standard})(\text{absorbance of unknown})}{\text{absorbance of standard}}$$

By dividing the concentration of the standard by the absorbance of the standard, a factor is derived. The remaining unknown concentrations in the run can be calculated quickly by multiplying this factor by each individual absorbance.

$$\text{Concentration of unknown} = (\text{Factor})(\text{absorbance of unknown})$$

HOW **Example 15-6**

Glucose was analyzed in three patient samples and two control samples using a manual method. The single standard used had a concentration of 200 mg/dL and an assayed absorbance of 0.448. Calculate the concentration of the five unknowns given the following absorbance readings for each:

Sample 1: Absorbance = 0.295
Sample 2: Absorbance = 0.210
Sample 3: Absorbance = 0.300
Sample 4: Absorbance = 0.350
Sample 5: Absorbance = 0.270

Each of these unknowns could be calculated as in Example 15-4. However, calculating six unknowns by this method is time consuming. Using a factor speeds up the calculations involved in multiple samples. To calculate the factor for this assay, divide the concentration of the standard by the obtained absorbance of the standard:

$$\text{Factor} = \frac{200}{0.448} = 446$$

Next, use the factor 446 and multiply each sample absorbance to obtain the sample concentration:

Sample 1: 446 × 0.295 = 132 mg/dL
Sample 2: 446 × 0.210 = 94 mg/dL
Sample 3: 446 × 0.300 = 134 mg/dL
Sample 4: 446 × 0.350 = 156 mg/dL
Sample 5: 446 × 0.270 = 120 mg/dL

Example 15-6a Using the factor method and the information given in the table, complete the table by calculating the concentrations of three unknowns that were analyzed using the single-point standard method. The factors were rounded to match the significant figures of the standards.

Sample No.	Standard Concentration	Absorbance of Standard	Factor	Absorbance of Unknown	Concentration of Unknowns
Standard	12.0 mg/dL	1.455	8.2		
Unknown No. 1			8.2	1.215	
Unknown No. 2			8.2	0.637	
Unknown No. 3			8.2	0.283	

Sample No.	Standard Concentration	Absorbance of Standard	Factor	Absorbance of Unknown	Concentration of Unknowns
Standard	12.0 mg/dL	1.455	8.2		
Unknown No. 1			8.2	1.215	10.0 mg/dL
Unknown No. 2			8.2	0.637	5.2 mg/dL
Unknown No. 3			8.2	0.283	2.3 mg/dL

Example 15-6b Using the factor method and the information given in the table, complete the table by calculating the concentrations of three unknowns that were analyzed using the single-point standard method.

Sample No.	Standard Concentration	Absorbance of Standard	Factor	Absorbance of Unknown	Concentration of Unknowns
Standard	80 mg/dL	0.850	94		
Unknown No. 1			94	0.515	
Unknown No. 2			94	0.780	
Unknown No. 3			94	0.625	
Sample No.	Standard Concentration	Absorbance of Standard	Factor	Absorbance of Unknown	Concentration of Unknowns
Standard	80 mg/dL	0.850	94		
Unknown No. 1			94	0.515	48 mg/dL
Unknown No. 2			94	0.780	73 mg/dL
Unknown No. 3			94	0.625	59 mg/dL

Example 15-6c Using the factor method and the information given in the table, complete the table by calculating the concentrations of three unknowns that were analyzed using the single-point standard method.

Sample No.	Standard Concentration	Absorbance of Standard	Factor	Absorbance of Unknown	Concentration of Unknowns
Standard	500 mg/dL	1.280	391		
Unknown No. 1			391	1.145	
Unknown No. 2			391	1.080	
Unknown No. 3			391	0.849	
Sample No.	Standard Concentration	Absorbance of Standard	Factor	Absorbance of Unknown	Concentration of Unknowns
Standard	500 mg/dL	1.280	391		
Unknown No. 1			391	1.145	448 mg/dL
Unknown No. 2			391	1.080	422 mg/dL
Unknown No. 3			391	0.849	332 mg/dL

WHAT Preparing Working Standards for Standard Curves Used for Manual Methods

The standards used for standard curves are obtained usually either by buying them directly from a vendor or obtaining one concentration of standard and, by performing dilutions, preparing a series of working standards. When performing dilutions of the standard, it is important to remember that there is a limited supply of the standard. Therefore the limiting factor for the dilutional series is the total quantity of standard available to dilute. When the standard that must be used or that is available contains only 3 mL, it serves no useful purpose to devise a dilutional scheme that requires 5 mL of standard. To prepare a series of working standards, the calculation of C1V1 = C2V2 is used. (Refer to Chapter 5 for additional information.)

HOW   *Example 15-7*

A medical laboratory scientist needs to prepare a standard curve for a total protein assay. The stock standard has a concentration of 10.0 g/dL. Five working standards are necessary with concentrations of 8.0 g/dL, 6.0 g/dL, 4.0 g/dL, and 2.0 g/dL and a total volume of 2 mL each. Deionized water is used as the diluent. What is the medical laboratory scientist's next step?

The formula C1V1 = C2V2 is used to solve this problem.

Where: C1 = original concentration (stock concentration of 10.0 g/dL)

$$V1 = \text{unknown volume needed}$$

$$C2 = \text{working standard concentration}$$

$$V2 = \text{volume of working standard}$$

To determine how to prepare the 8.0 g/dL working standard, substitute the data that are known into the equation:

$$(10 \text{ g/dL})(X \text{ volume}) = (8 \text{ g/dL})(2 \text{ mL})$$

$$(10)(X) = 16$$

$$X = \frac{16}{10}$$

$$X = 1.6 \text{ mL}$$

Therefore, to prepare the 8.0 g/dL working standard, add 1.6 mL of the 10.0 g/dL stock standard to 0.4 mL of deionized water to make a total volume of 2.0 mL.

How is the 6.0 g/dL working standard prepared?

Use the same formula and substitute into it the 6.0 g/dL instead of the 8.0 g/dL:

$$(10)(X) = (6)(2)$$

$$(10)(X) = 12$$

$$X = \frac{12}{10}$$

$$X = 1.2 \text{ mL}$$

Therefore add 1.2 mL of the 10.0 g/dL stock standard and 0.8 mL of deionized water together to prepare the 6.0 g/dL working standard.

How is the 4.0 g/dL standard prepared?

Use the same formula as earlier:

$$(10)(X) = (4)(2)$$

$$(10)(X) = 8$$

$$X = \frac{8}{10}$$

$$X = 0.8 \text{ mL}$$

Therefore 0.8 mL of the 10.0 g/dL stock standard is added to 1.2 mL of deionized water to prepare the 4.0 g/dL working standard.

How is the 2.0 g/dL working standard prepared?

Again, use the same formula:

$$(10)(X) = (2)(2)$$

$$(10)(X) = 4$$

$$X = \frac{4}{10}$$

$$X = 0.4 \text{ mL}$$

To prepare the 2.0 g/dL standard, add 0.4 mL of the 10.0 g/dL stock standard to 1.6 mL of deionized water.

Notice that the total volume of the 10.0 g/dL standard that is used to prepare the working standards is only 4 mL.

Example 15-7a An MLT student had to make four working standards with a total volume of 3.0 mL from a 300 mg/dL standard. The concentrations of the working standards were 200, 150, 75, and 50 mg/dL. How would this student prepare these standards?

By using the C1V1 = C2V2 formula, the standard volumes and diluent volumes for each working standard are listed in the following table.

Standard Concentration	Amount of Standard Needed	Amount of Diluent Needed
300 mg/dL		
200 mg/dL	2 mL of 300 mg/dL standard	1 mL diluent
150 mg/dL	1.5 mL of 300 mg/dL standard	1.5 mL diluent
75 mg/dL	0.75 mL of 300 mg/dL standard	2.25 mL diluent
50 mg/dL	0.5 mL of 300 mg/dL standard	2.5 mL diluent

Example 15-7b A series of four working standards with a 2.0 mL volume had to be prepared from a 40.0 mg/dL standard. The concentrations of the working standards are 30, 20, 10, and 5 mg/dL. How are these working standards prepared?

By using the C1V1 = C2V2 formula, the standard volumes and diluent volumes for each working standard are listed in the following table.

Standard Concentration	Amount of Standard Needed	Amount of Diluent Needed
40 mg/dL (2 mL total volume)		
30 mg/dL	1.5 mL of 40 mg/dL standard	0.5 mL diluent
20 mg/dL	1.0 mL of 40 mg/dL standard	1.0 mL diluent
10 mg/dL	0.5 mL of 40 mg/dL standard	1.50 mL diluent
5 mg/dL	0.25 mL of 40 mg/dL standard	1.75 mL diluent

Example 15-7c A series of four working standards with a 3.0 mL volume had to be prepared from a 15.0 mg/dL standard. The concentrations of the working standards are 12.0, 9.0, 7.0, and 5.0 mg/dL. How are these working standards prepared?

By using the C1V1 = C2V2 formula, the standard volumes and diluent volumes for each working standard are listed in the following table.

Standard Concentration	Amount of Standard Needed	Amount of Diluent Needed
15.0 mg/dL		
12.0 mg/dL	2.4 mL of 15 mg/dL standard	0.6 mL diluent
9.0 mg/dL	1.8 mL of 15 mg/dL standard	1.2 mL diluent
7.0 mg/dL	1.4 mL of 15 mg/dL standard	1.6 mL diluent
5.0 mg/dL	1.0 mL of 15 mg/dL standard	2.0 mL diluent

WHAT % OXYGEN SATURATION

A blood gas analysis usually contains the following values: pH, pO_2, pCO_2, HCO_3^-, base excess, and % oxygen saturation. The first three are measured by the blood gas analyzer and the last three are calculations. The % oxygen saturation, or % SO_2, can also be determined by pulse oximetry or estimated from a nomogram. The % SO_2 calculation is dependent on the hemoglobin concentration and its ability to bind oxygen. Each molecule of hemoglobin can bind four molecules of oxygen, and if a person is healthy, his or her % SO_2 ranges from 96% to 98%. A % SO_2 above 100% is almost impossible for someone who is breathing room air and most likely would be found in patients on respirators. The % SO_2 is rarely calculated by the laboratory professional.

$$\%SO_2 = \frac{cO_2\ Hb}{cO_2\ Hb + cHHb}$$

where:
$cO_2\ Hb$ = the concentration of oxyhemoglobin
$cHHB$ = the concentration of deoxyhemoglobin

WHAT QUANTITATIVE CHEMICAL ANALYSES IN URINE SPECIMENS

The chemistry tests performed during a urinalysis are qualitative in nature but may indicate a problem if they are abnormal. To follow up on an abnormal result, a physician may request a 24-hour quantitative analysis of a constituent found in urine. For example, a 24-hour sample collected for total protein analysis or for urea may be ordered. The urine sample is analyzed for the particular constituent, but additional mathematical calculations must be performed before the result is recorded. Because the volume and duration of collection of the urine sample is variable, the urine result must be standardized to allow for comparison of results. Most urine results are recorded as quantity of analyte per unit of time (usually 24 hours). Occasionally a urine sample will be collected for a shorter period. In that case, the quantitative urine result can be reported as "quantity per volume of collection" or as "quantity per unit of time."

Calculating the Analyte Concentration per Volume of Collection of Urine Analytes

In general, if a nonelectrolyte is measured in urine, it is reported in units of milligrams per day or in the international units of millimoles per day. Urine electrolytes are generally reported in units of milliequivalents per day or millimoles per day. If urine is not collected for a full 24 hours, or a 1-day period, the results may be extrapolated for a 24-hour collection for compounds that are uniformly excreted during a 24-hour period and reported in terms of per-volume quantity collected or quantity per total time collected. To calculate the quantity per volume of collection, a ratio and proportion calculation can be performed.

HOW **Example 15-8**

A urine specimen collected over 12 hours with a volume of 800.0 mL is analyzed for creatinine. The creatinine result is 90.0 mg/dL. What is the creatinine result reported as milligrams per volume of collection?

To solve this problem, a ratio and proportion calculation is performed. Remember: Units must be the same; therefore convert deciliter into milliliter terms (1 dL = 100 mL).

$$\frac{90 \text{ mg}}{100 \text{ mL}} = \frac{X \text{ mg}}{800 \text{ mL}}$$

Crossmultiplying, the equation yields:

$$(90)(800) = (100)(X)$$
$$72{,}000 = 100 \text{ X}$$
$$720 = \text{X}$$

Therefore, there is 720 mg creatinine per 800 mL of urine.

Example 15-8a Calculate the amount of creatinine reported as milligrams per volume of collection in a 24-hour urine specimen with a total volume of 1250.0 mL and a urine creatinine of 110 mg/dL.

Remember that the units of mg/dL have to be converted to mg/mL and substitute into the previous equation the values given in this problem to solve:

$$\frac{110 \text{ mg}}{100 \text{ mL}} = \frac{X \text{ mg}}{1250 \text{ mL}}$$

Solving for X yields a result of 1375 mg creatinine per 1250 mL of urine in a 24-hour period.

Example 15-8b Calculate the amount of urea in terms of milligrams per volume of collection in a 24-hour urine specimen, with a total volume of 1100 mL and a urine urea concentration of 150 mg/dL.

$150 \text{ mg/dL} \times 1 \text{dL}/100 \text{ mL} = 1.5 \text{ mg/mL} \times 1100 \text{ mL} = 1650 \text{ mg (total)}$ of urea

$1100 \text{ mg} \times 1 \text{L}/1000 \text{ mL} = 1.1 \text{L}$

$1650 \text{ mg urea} \times 1 \text{g}/1000 \text{ mg} = 1.65 \text{ g urea per } 1.1 \text{ L urine in a 24-hr period}$

The concentration is 1650 mg of urea per 1100 mL of urine or 1.65 g of urea per 1.1 L of urine.

WHAT **Calculating the Quantity of Analyte Collected in Urine per Unit of Time of Collection**

This calculation is nearly identical to the previous calculation, with the exception of reporting as milligrams per collection period. Unless a time other than 24 hours is specified, the unit of time of 24 hours will be used in the following examples.

HOW **Example 15-9**

Using the same data from Example 15-8, calculate the quantity of creatinine collected in terms of milligrams per collection period.

The amount of creatinine in 800 mL within a 12-hour period was calculated to be 720 mg/800 mL. As the 800 mL was collected over 12 hours, the result can also be equally recorded as 720 mg/12 hr or 60 mg/hr creatinine.

Example 15-9a   Convert the result obtained from Example 15-8a into terms of mg of creatinine/unit of 24 hours.

The result is 1375 mg/24 hr.

Example 15-9b   Convert the result of Example 15-8b 1.65 g per 1.1 L into g/L of urea per 24 hours.

The result is 1.65 g/24 hr.

WHAT **Converting the Quantity of Analyte Measured in Milligrams per Deciliter into Grams per 24 hours**

The quantity of an analyte measured in milligrams per deciliter can be converted to the concentration of analyte in gram units per 24 hours by using the following conversion formula. Note that if it is a 24-hour collection, the last fraction within the problem becomes 24/24, or 1, and can be dropped from the equation:

$$\left(\frac{X \text{ analyte mg}}{dL}\right)\left(\frac{mL}{\text{collected}}\right)\left(\frac{1 \text{ dL}}{100 \text{ mL}}\right)\left(\frac{1 \text{ g}}{1000 \text{ mg}}\right)\left(\frac{24 \text{ hr}}{\text{collection time (hrs)}}\right) = g/24 \text{ hr}$$

HOW **Example 15-10**

A urine urea value of 60 mg/dL is obtained from urine collected for 24 hours with a volume of 1500 mL. What is the urine urea value reported as grams per 24 hours?

Substituting into the conversion formula, the following formula is derived:

$$\left(\frac{60 \text{ mg}}{dL}\right)\left(\frac{1500 \text{ mL}}{24 \text{ hr}}\right)\left(\frac{1 \text{ dL}}{100 \text{ mL}}\right)\left(\frac{1 \text{ g}}{1000 \text{ mg}}\right) = \frac{(60 \text{ g})(1500)(1)}{100,000} = 0.9g/24 \text{ hr}$$

Therefore the urine urea concentration is 0.9 g/24 hours of collection.

Example 15-10a   Calculate the urine urea value reported as grams per 24 hours given a urine urea value of 75 mg/dL from a urine sample collected for 24 hours with a volume of 2100 mL.

Using the formula shown in Example 15-10 and substituting into it the values from this problem:

$$\left(\frac{75 \text{ mg}}{\text{dL}}\right)\left(\frac{2100 \text{ mL}}{24 \text{ hr}}\right)\left(\frac{1 \text{ dL}}{100 \text{ mL}}\right)\left(\frac{1 \text{ g}}{1000 \text{ mg}}\right) = \frac{(75 \text{ g})(2100)(1)}{100,000} = 1.6\text{g/24hr}$$

The result is 1.6 g/24 hours.

Example 15-10b   Calculate the urine protein value reported as grams per day given a urine protein value of 400 mg/dL from a 24-hour urine sample with a volume of 550 mL. Use the formula shown in Example 15-10a and substitute into it the values for this problem.

The answer is 2.2 g/24 hours.

WHAT **OSMOTIC FRAGILITY**

Hereditary spherocytosis is a genetically inherited condition in which the RBCs have an abnormal spherical shape. This abnormal shape leads to increased RBC destruction by the spleen, resulting in chronic anemia. In addition, the abnormal shape causes the RBCs to be particularly sensitive to changes in low plasma osmolality. The osmotic fragility test places RBCs in increasingly hypotonic saline solutions. The amount of hemolysis is quantitated for each of the hypotonic saline solutions. Spherocytes will exhibit increased fragility compared with normal RBCs.

The osmotic fragility test is no longer performed in many hospital hematology laboratories. Instead the samples are sent to reference laboratories for the test to be performed. However, a brief description of how to perform the test may help the clinical laboratory student better understand the test itself.

To perform an osmotic fragility test, heparinized blood is added to commercially prepared hypotonic saline solutions. The blood is mixed with the solutions and incubated at room temperature for 20 minutes. The individual solutions are transferred to centrifuge tubes and centrifuged at 2000 rpm for 5 minutes. The supernatant is decanted to appropriately labeled tubes for each hypotonic solution. A spectrophotometer is set at a wavelength of 540 nm and zeroed using deionized water. The absorbance of each hypotonic solution is recorded. The percent hemolysis for each tube is calculated using the following formula:

$$\text{Percent (\%) hemolysis} = \frac{\text{Absorbance}_{(\text{test})} - \text{Absorbance}_{(0.85\% \text{ tube})}}{\text{Absorbance}_{(0.00\% \text{ tube})} - \text{Absorbance}_{(0.85\% \text{ tube})}} \times 100$$

The percent hemolysis is calculated for each of the hypotonic solutions. Spherocytes will hemolyze faster than normal cells with an initial hemolysis at 0.65% NaCl (compared with 0.45% NaCl for normal RBCs) with complete hemolysis at 0.45% NaCl (normal RBCs have complete hemolysis at 0.35% NaCl).

EXAMPLE PROBLEMS

This section is designed to be useful to both the student and the laboratory professional. Students can use the additional problems to master the material. The laboratory professional can use the examples as templates for solving laboratory calculations. By finding an example similar to the problem that you need to solve, substitute the numbers appropriate to your calculation into the equation.

1. **Q.** A $27.0\%^{w/v}$ solution of $CaCl_2$ is needed. However, only $CaCl_2 \cdot 3H_2O$ is available. How many grams of $CaCl_2 \cdot 3H_2O$ are necessary to prepare the solution?

   A. This problem can be solved using ratio and proportion. The gram molecular weight of $CaCl_2$ is 110.98, and the gram molecular weight of $CaCl_2 \cdot 3H_2O$ is 165.04. The following formula is used:

   $$\frac{\text{anhydrous chemical gmw}}{\text{hydrous chemical gmw}} = \frac{\text{gram of anhydrous chemical}}{\text{gram of hydrous chemical}}$$

   By substituting into the equation the data from the problem, the equation is as follows:

   $$\frac{110.98 \text{ gmw}}{165.04 \text{ gmw}} = \frac{27.0 \text{ g}}{X \text{ g}}$$

   Crossmultiplying yields the following:

   $$(110.98)(X) = (165.04)(27.0)$$
   $$(110.98)(X) = 4456.08$$
   $$X = 40.15 \text{ g}$$

   Therefore 40.15 g of $CaCl_2 \cdot 3H_2O$ dissolved (or qs) in 100 mL of water will yield a $27.0\%^{w/v}$ solution of $CaCl_2$.

2. **Q.** How many grams of H_2SO_4 are present in 1.00 mL of a concentrated acid solution with a SG of 1.84 and an assay purity of $96.0\%^{w/w}$?

   A. The SG of a solution is the density of the solution and is calculated as the number of grams of the solution in 1.00 mL of solution. Therefore, within 1.00 mL of solution, there are 1.84 g of the solution. The purity of the solution is 96.0%, meaning that within the 100 g total weight of the solution, 96.0 g of the solution consist of H_2SO_4.

   The purity of the solution must be taken into account when determining the amount of grams of H_2SO_4 per 1.00 mL. This can be done by ratio and proportion. Therefore, there are 1.77 g H_2SO_4 present in 1.00 mL of a $96.0\%^{w/w}$ solution of H_2SO_4.

3. **Q.** What is the molarity of a concentrated acetic acid (CH_3CO_2H) solution with a specific gravity of 1.06 and an assay purity of $99.7\%^{w/w}$?

   A. First, determine the amount of grams per milliliters of solution as demonstrated in the previous example. Next, determine the quantity of acetic acid in 1.00 L:

   $$\frac{1.06 \text{ g } CH_3CO_2H}{1.00 \text{ mL of solution}} = \frac{X \text{ g } CH_3CO_2H}{1000 \text{ mL of solution}}$$

Crossmultiplying the equation yields:

$$(1.06)(1000) = (1.00)(X)$$
$$1060 = X$$

Therefore, there are 1060 g of acetic acid per 1.00 L of solution. Last, use the molarity formula to determine the molarity of the solution:

$$X\,M = \frac{\left(\dfrac{1060\ \text{g acetic acid}}{60.06\ \text{gmw}}\right)}{1.00\ \text{L of solution}}$$

$$X\,M = 17.65$$

Therefore a concentrated acetic acid solution with a purity of $99.7\%^{w/w}$ and a density of 1.06 has a molarity of 17.65.

4. **Q.** A creatinine assay was performed that yielded an absorbance of 0.483 for the single 5.0 mg/dL creatinine standard. The absorbance of a patient's sample was 0.375. What is the concentration of creatinine in the patient's sample?

   A. The following formula is used when determining the concentration of unknowns when a single standard is used:

$$\text{Conc. of unknown} = \frac{(\text{conc. of standard})(\text{Abs. of unknown})}{\text{absorbance of standard}}$$

Substituting the data into the equation from the problem yields the following:

$$\text{Conc. of unknown} = \frac{(5.0\ \text{mg/dL})(0.375)}{0.483}$$

$$\text{Concentration of unknown} = 3.9\ \text{mg/dL}$$

5. **Q.** A glucose assay was performed that yielded an absorbance of 1.150 for the single 200 mg/dL standard. The absorbance of a patient's sample was 0.632. What is the patient's glucose concentration?

   A. To solve this problem, use the same formula as in Example Problem 4:

$$\text{Conc. of unknown} = \frac{(\text{conc. of standard})(\text{Abs. of unknown})}{\text{absorbance of standard}}$$

$$\text{Conc. of unknown} = \frac{(200\ \text{mg/dL})(0.632)}{1.150}$$

$$\text{Conc. of unknown} = 110\ \text{mg/dL}$$

6. **Q.** A total cholesterol assay using a single standard was performed on four patient samples and two controls. The cholesterol concentration of the standard was 300 mg/dL, with a measured absorbance of 0.963. The absorbance values for each control and patient are listed in the following table. Using the factor method of calculating concentrations, what is the concentration of each control and patient sample?

Sample Identification	Absorbance
Control I	0.532
Control II	0.765
Patient 1	0.624
Patient 2	0.815
Patient 3	0.480
Patient 4	0.550

   A. To solve this problem, the concentration of each of the samples can be calculated using the formula used in Example Problems 4 and 5. However, performing the same calculation multiple times can be quite tedious. Notice that the absorbance and concentration of the standard are fixed within the calculation and do not change. A factor can be calculated by dividing the concentration of the standard by its absorbance. This factor can then be multiplied by the individual absorbances of each unknown sample, thereby simplifying the calculations that must be performed.

$$\text{Factor} = 300 \text{ mg/dL} \div 0.963 = 312$$
$$\text{Control I} = 0.532 \times 312 = 166 \text{ mg/dL}$$
$$\text{Control II} = 0.765 \times 312 = 239 \text{ mg/dL}$$
$$\text{Patient 1} = 0.624 \times 312 = 195 \text{ mg/dL}$$
$$\text{Patient 2} = 0.815 \times 312 = 254 \text{ mg/dL}$$
$$\text{Patient 3} = 0.480 \times 312 = 150 \text{ mg/dL}$$
$$\text{Patient 4} = 0.550 \times 312 = 172 \text{ mg/dL}$$

7. **Q.** How should a standard curve of a glucose assay in which five standards are used be constructed? The concentration and absorbance of each standard is as follows: 50 mg/dL Abs. 0.150; 100 mg/dL Abs. 0.300; 150 mg/dL Abs. 0.450; 300 mg/dL Abs. 0.900; 500 mg/dL Abs. 1.500.
   A. A standard curve is constructed by placing absorbance values on the y axis and the concentration of the standards on the x axis. Linear graph paper is used for the standard curve when plotting absorbance versus concentration. A well-constructed standard curve consists of at least four to six different concentrations of standards whose values are spread throughout the linear range of the assay. A dot or circle is placed at the intersection on the graph of the absorbance and concentration values for each of the standards. A best-fit line is then drawn through the dots. A best-fit line is one in which, rather than "connect the dots," the line is drawn in such a manner that an equal amount of standards fall above and below the line. The standard curve line is never drawn past the dot or circle that represents the highest standard. The standard curve line should also be drawn from the lowest concentration to the x and y axis zero intersect. Figure 15-1 shows the standard curve.

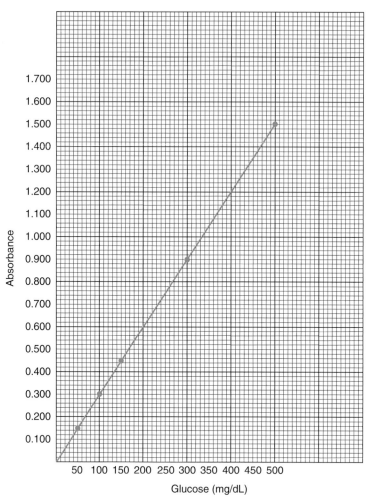

FIGURE 15-1 Standard curve of glucose assay.

8. **Q.** A procedure calls for a standard curve to be developed from a stock standard containing a total volume of 3.0 mL and a concentration of 20 mg/dL. How would 2.0 mL of a working standard with a concentration of 5.0 mg/dL be prepared?

A. Standard curves may be prepared by diluting a single stock standard into a series of working standards. To determine the volume needed to perform the dilutions, the formula C1V1 = C2V2 is used. To solve this problem, C1 is the known stock standard concentration of 20 mg/dL; V1 is the unknown quantity of the stock standard that is needed; C2 is the concentration of the working standard, which in this example is 5.0 mg/dL; and V2 is the volume of the working standard needed, which in this example is 2.0. Combining this data into the formula yields the following:

$$(20 \text{ mg/dL})(X \text{ mL}) = (5.0 \text{ mg/dL})(2.0 \text{ mL})$$

$$20 X = 10$$

$$X = \frac{10}{20}$$

$$X = 0.5 \text{ mL}$$

Therefore 0.5 mL of the 20 mg/dL stock standard is diluted with diluent to a total volume of 2.0 mL to prepare 2.0 mL of a working standard with a concentration of 5.0 mg/dL.

9. **Q.** A urine specimen collected over 6 hours has a volume of 475 mL and a potassium value of 35 mEq/L. What is the potassium result in terms of volume of collection?

   A. This problem is solved using ratio and proportion. Note: The collection volume in milliliters must be expressed in liter terms to keep comparable units.

$$\frac{35 \text{ mEq}}{1 \text{ L}} = \frac{X \text{mEq}}{0.475 \text{ L}}$$

Crossmultiplying the equation:

$$(35 \text{ mEq})(0.475 \text{L}) = (1 \text{L})(X \text{ mEq/L})$$
$$16.6 \text{ mEq} = X$$

Therefore this patient's urine contains 17 mEq of potassium total in 475 mL of urine.

10. **Q.** What is the urine potassium value for the patient in Example Problem 9 in terms of milliequivalents of potassium per 6 hours?

   A. Whenever a urine specimen is collected in a time period of less than 24 hours, the results can be recorded as concentration per volume collected, concentration per time collected, and concentration extrapolated to a 24-hour collection period. The results for concentration per volume collected and concentration per time collected are similar, only the units are different. In the previous example, 17 mEq of potassium in 475 mL of urine was collected in 6 hours. The result can be recorded as 17 mEq/475 mL or as 17 mEq/6 hours. Both are equivalent results.

11. **Q.** A 12-hour urine specimen with a volume of 1750 mL was collected for sodium analysis. The sodium result is 80 mEq/L. What is the patient's sodium result in terms of quantity per total volume?

   A. The patient's urine volume is 1750 mL, and the quantity of sodium is 80 mEq/L. Using ratio and proportion, the amount of sodium found within the 1750 mL of specimen can be calculated:

$$\frac{80 \text{ mEq}}{1000 \text{ mL}} = \frac{X \text{ mEq}}{1750 \text{ mL}}$$

Crossmultiplying the equation:

$$(X)(1000) = (80)(1750)$$
$$(X)(1000) = 140,000$$
$$X = 140 \text{ mEq/1750 mL}$$

12. **Q.** Refer to Example Problem 11. What is the patient's sodium value in terms of mEq/12 hr?

   A. As the urine was collected over 12 hours, and the volume collected within that time period is 1750 mL, the terms 140 mEq/1750 mL and 140 mEq/12 hours are equivalent. Therefore the sodium value in terms of mEq/12 hours is 140 mEq/12 hours.

PRACTICE PROBLEMS

Solve the following practice problems to further master the material. Answers and explanations to some problems can be found in the Answer Key.

1. If anhydrous NaH_2PO_4 was unavailable, how many grams of $NaH_2PO_4 \cdot 3H_2O$ would be needed to prepare 100 mL of a 15.0%$^{w/v}$ solution of NaH_2PO_4?

2. If anhydrous $CuSO_4$ was unavailable, how many grams of $CuSO_4 \cdot 5H_2O$ would be needed to make 75.0 mL of a 20.0%$^{w/v}$ solution of $CuSO_4$?

3. Determine how many grams are present in 1.00 mL of a concentrated NH_4OH solution with a density of 0.91 and a purity of 28.0%$^{w/w}$.

4. Determine the molarity of a solution of concentrated nitric acid (HNO_3) with a density of 1.42 and a purity of 70.0%$^{w/w}$.

A glucose assay was performed with a single glucose standard of 300 mg/dL. If the standard had an absorbance value of 1.250, calculate the concentration of the following samples given their absorbances:

5. Absorbance = 0.681, glucose concentration = ?

6. Absorbance = 1.120, glucose concentration = ?

Given the urine collection times, volumes, and analyte concentration, express the following in terms of concentration per volume of collection.

7. Sodium concentration of 35 mEq/L, collected over 12 hours, 900 mL volume

8. Glucose concentration of 50 mg/dL, collected over 24 hours, 1500 mL volume

9. Creatinine concentration of 525 mg/dL, collected over 24 hours, 1825 mL volume
Express the following in terms of concentration per time.

10. Creatinine value of 1000 mg/1750 mL collected over 24 hours

11. Potassium result of 40 mEq/500 mL collected over 12 hours

12. To determine urine concentration per volume of collection, use ratio and proportion. For example: if in 24 hours the sodium concentration was 35 mEq/L in a 900 mL specimen, using ratio and proportion, the following equation is derived:

$$\frac{35 \text{ mEq}}{1000 \text{ mL}} = \frac{X \text{ mEq}}{900 \text{ mL}}$$

Crossmultiplying the equation yields the following:

$$(35)(900) = (1000)(X)$$
$$31,500 = 1000X$$
$$32 = X$$

The sodium concentration can be expressed as 32 mEq/900 mL.

Appendix

Greek Alphabet Appendix

Greek Letter Uppercase/Lowercase	Name	Pronunciation
A / α	Alpha	al'-fah
B / β	Beta	bay'-tah
Γ / γ	Gamma	gam'-ah
Δ / δ	Delta	del'-ta
E / ε	Epsilon	ep'-si-lon
Z / ζ	Zeta	zay'-tah
H / η	Eta	ay'-tah
Θ / θ	Theta	thay'-tah
I / ι	Iota	eye'-o-tah
K / κ	Kappa	cap'-ah
Λ / λ	Lambda	lamb'-dah
M / μ	Mu	mew
N / ν	Nu	new
Ξ / ξ	Xi	sai
O / o	Omicron	om'-ah-cron
Π / π	Pi	pie
P / ρ	Rho	row
Σ / σ	Sigma	sig'-ma
T / τ	Tau	tawh
Y / υ	Upsilon	up'-si-lon
Φ / φ	Phi	figh
X / χ	Chi	kigh
Ψ / ψ	Psi	sigh
Ω / ω	Omega	o'-may-gah

Math Terms Glossary

Accuracy study to determine constant systematic error: Interference study. A known concentration of an analyte is added to an aliquot of sample. A paired aliquot does not have the interferent placed in it. Both aliquots are measured. At least three paired sample analytes are measured and the results averaged:

Average of test aliquot result − Average of reference aliquot = bias

Acid: A substance that will donate a hydrogen ion (or proton).

Anhydrous solutions: Solutions made with dry chemicals that do not contain any water molecules.

Anion Gap:

$$([Na^+] + [K^+]) - ([Cl^-] + [HCO_3^-])$$

Note: Some calculations remove the potassium from the equation.

Antilog: The inverse logarithm of a number.

Average molecular weight, base pair:

Substance	Average Molecular Weight of a Base Pair
Molecular Weight of dsDNA	660 pg/pmol
Molecular Weight of ssDNA, RNA, and Nucleotides	330 pg/pmol

Base: A substance that will accept the hydrogen ion or donate a hydroxyl ion.

Beer's law: $A = abc$, where A equals absorbance, **a** equals absorptivity coefficient, **b** equals pathlength, and **c** equals concentration.

Buffer: A solution of weak acids or bases and their salts that resist changes in pH.

Calculated LDL cholesterol: The formula used to calculate LDL cholesterol is only accurate if the triglyceride concentration is greater than 400 mg/dL. The LDL formula is:

LDL cholesterol = Total cholesterol
$$- (HDL + Triglyceride/5)$$

Celsius: Developed in 1742 by Anders Celsius, this scale sets freezing at $0°$ and boiling at $100°$ Celsius. Also referred to as centigrade, although there are slight differences between the two.

Coefficient of variation: A measurement of precision. The formula is:

$$\frac{\text{Standard Deviation}}{\text{Mean}} \times 100$$

Concentration calculations C1V1 = C2V2: Used when making a concentrated stock solution less concentrated. C1 is the concentration of the stock, V1 is the volume that is to be calculated, C2 is the concentration of the new solution, and V2 is the volume of the new solution.

Conjugate acid and conjugate base: A substance that has donated a hydrogen ion is called a conjugate acid, and the newly formed base is called the conjugate base. A common conjugate acid/conjugate base pair is the carbonic acid/bicarbonate buffer system.

Corrected clearance test: Used to correct for body size. The patient's height and weight are used to calculate body surface area in m². The corrected clearance formula is:

$$UV/P \times 1.73 \text{ m}^2/\text{Patient's m}^2$$

Correction of the WBC count for nucleated RBCs:

$$\frac{\text{Automated WBC count} \times 100}{(\text{NRBC per 100 WBCs}) + 100}$$

Correlation coefficient: This is measured by r and perfect correlation between methods has a value of 1.000:

$$r = \frac{\sum(x - \bar{x})(y - \bar{y})}{\left[(\sum x - \bar{x})^2\right]\left[(\sum y - \bar{y})^2\right]}$$

Denominator: The bottom value in a fraction.

Determining concentration of CFUs in a urine culture: Urine that is cultured in the microbiology laboratory to rule out a urinary tract infection can be inoculated onto an agar plate using two different types of calibrated loops. One can hold 0.01 mL of urine, and the other can hold 0.001 mL of urine. When the colonies grow, they are counted. If the 0.01 loop is used, then the number of colonies, or CFUs, per milliliter on the plate is multiplied by 100. If the 0.001 loop is used, then the number of CFUs on the plate is multiplied by 1000.

Determining contamination, possible infection, and probable infection in a urine specimen: Urine that contains less than 10^3 CFUs/mL is indicative of contamination. Urine that contains between 10^3 and 10^5 CFUs/mL is indicative of a possible infection. Urine that contains more than 10^5 CFUs/mL is indicative of a probable infection.

Determining fresh frozen plasma increments: For every two units of fresh frozen plasma a patient receives, clotting factors should be elevated by 15% to 20%.

Determining hematocrit increments: For a patient who is not actively bleeding, for every unit of packed RBCs the patient receives, hematocrit should rise two to three percentage points.

Determining hemoglobin increments: For a patient who is not actively bleeding, each unit of packed RBCs should increase the hemoglobin by 1 g/dL.

Determining platelet increments: For each unit of platelets a patient receives, platelet count should rise by 10,000 mcL.

Diagnostic sensitivity: The probability that only patients with the disease have the disease.

Diagnostic specificity: The probability that patients who do not have the disease test negative for the disease.

$$\text{Sensitivity} = \frac{\text{True Positives}}{\text{True Positives} + \text{False Negatives}} \times 100$$

$$\text{Specificity} = \frac{\text{True Negatives}}{\text{True Negatives} + \text{False Positives}} \times 100$$

Difference: The answer to a subtraction problem.

Diluent: The liquid that a sample is placed into in order to make a dilution.

Dilution factor: The reciprocal of the dilution that was performed.

Dissociation constant Ka: This constant determines the relative strength of an acid or base. The formula is:

$$Ka = ([H+][A^-])/[HA]$$

where [H+] is the hydrogen ion concentration in mol/L, [A⁻] is the salt of the acid in mol/L, and [HA] is the undissociated acid in mol/L.

dsDNA: Double-stranded DNA, the DNA that is in our cells.

Efficiency: The number of patients correctly diagnosed for the disease or not having the disease:

$$\text{Efficiency} = \frac{\text{TP} + \text{TN}}{\text{TP} + \text{FP} + \text{FN} + \text{TN}} \times 100$$

Predictive Value:

Positive predictive value: the ability of a test method to correctly determine the presence of a disease in those patients who have the disease.

$$\text{Positive Predictive Value} = \frac{\text{True Positive}}{\text{True Positive} + \text{False Positive}} \times 100$$

Negative predictive value: The ability of a test method to correctly determine the absence of a disease in patients who do not have the disease.

Negative Predictive Value

$$= \frac{\text{True Negative}}{\text{True Negative} + \text{False Negative}} \times 100$$

End-point chemical reactions: The absorbance of the reactions are measured at the completion of the reaction.

Equivalent weight: The amount of replaceable hydrogen ions, hydroxyl ions, or charge, for the element or compound. It is calculated by dividing the gram molecular weight of an element or compound by its valence.

Estimated glomerular filtration rate (GFR): Modified Modification of Diet in Renal Disease (MDRD) equation:

$$\text{GFR}\left(\text{mL/min/1.73 m}^2\right) = 175 \times (\text{Serum}$$
$$\text{creatinine})^{-1.154} \times (\text{Age})^{-0.203} \times (0.742 \text{ if}$$
$$\text{female}) \times (1.210 \text{ if African American})$$
$$(\text{conventional units})$$

Crockoft-Gault equation:

$$\text{Creatinine clearance (mL/min)} = (140 - \text{age})$$
$$\times \text{weight in kg} \times (0.85 \text{ if female})$$
$$\text{serum creatinine (mg/dL)} \times 72$$

Exponent: A way to simplify complex mathematical problems. They are written as x^a where x is called the **base** and a is called the **exponent**. The base is the number that is to be multiplied by itself, and the exponent determines how many times it will be multiplied.

F test: An indicator of precision. The variances of two methods are compared:

$$\text{F} - \text{Test} = \frac{\text{Larger Variance}}{\text{Smaller Variance}}$$

Fahrenheit: A temperature scale developed by Daniel Gabriel Fahrenheit in 1724, where freezing is $32°$ and boiling is at $212°$ Fahrenheit.

First-order reactions: The enzyme reagent is in excess and the substrate concentration (the analyte to be measured) is the limiting factor.

Hemacytometer:

$$\text{No. cells/mm}^3 = \frac{\text{No. cells counted} \times \text{depth}}{\text{factor} \times \text{dilution factor}}$$
$$\frac{}{\text{Total area covered}}$$

Henderson-Hasselbalch equation:

$$\text{pH} = \text{pKa} + \log\left[A^-\right]/[HA]$$

Hydrated solutions: Solutions made with dry chemicals that contain water molecules in their chemical structure.

International Normalized Ratio (INR): The INR allows comparisons of prothrombin results from different laboratories:

$$\text{INR} = \frac{\text{Patient's PT value}^{\text{ISI}}}{\text{Laboratory's mean PT value}}$$

Kelvin: William Thomson, also known as Lord Kelvin, developed the thermodynamic scale of temperature in 1852.

Kinetic chemical reactions: Chemical reactions where the change in the absorbance rate is measured.

Kleihauer-Betke acid elution test: A measurement of the quantity of fetal cells in the maternal circulation using a blood smear made from the mother that is placed in an acid buffer to elute out the hemoglobin A inside the mother's RBCs. RBCs with hemoglobin F (fetal cells) will stain pink when the slide is stained with Wright stain:

$$\% \text{ fetal cells} = \frac{\text{No. fetal cells counted}}{1000 \text{ adult cells counted}} \times 100$$

Linear regression: Used to compare one set of data with another. The formula to determine the regression line is:

$$y_c = mx + b$$

where:

m = the slope of the line
x = result of reference method
b = the expected y intercept if x is 0
y_c = predicted y intercept derived from equation

The slope of the line (m) is calculated by the following formula:

$$m = \frac{n(\sum xy) - (\sum x)(\sum y)}{n(\sum x^2) - (\sum x)^2}$$

The y intercept (b) is calculated by the following formula:

$$b = y - (mx)$$

Logarithm: The inverse of the exponential function $y = a^x$. Logarithms consist of two parts: the **characteristic**, which is a whole number; and the **mantissa**, which is the decimal part.

Metric system: A measurement system developed in the late 18th century based on fixed standards and a uniform scale of 10. The standard unit of length is the meter; volume is the liter, and mass is the gram.

Mol: One mole is the gram weight of the solute divided by its gram molecular weight.

Molality: Similar to molarity but based on weight, not volume. It contains 1 mol of solute in 1 kg of solution.

Molarity: A 1 Molar solution contains 1 mol of solute in 1 L of solution.

Negative number: A number with a value less than zero.

Normality: A 1 Normal solution contains 1 equivalent weight in 1 L of solution.

Nucleotide: The basic building block of DNA and RNA. It contains a sugar molecule, a phosphate group, and a nitrogen-containing base. In DNA the bases are adenine (A), guanine (G), cytosine (C), and thymine (T). In RNA thymine is replaced by uracil (U).

Number of units or vials of RhIG:

$$\text{Vials of RhIG} = \frac{\% \text{ fetal cells} \times 50}{30}$$

Numerator: The top value in a fraction.

Oligonucleotide: A short ssDNA strand used in PCR procedures.

Osmolal gap: The osmolal gap is the mathematical difference between the measured osmolality and the calculated osmolality.

Osmolality: The osmolality of a solution is based on the number of dissolved particles in the solution. Serum osmolality is calculated as follows:

$$(\text{mOsmol/kg } H_2O) = 1.86(Na+) + (\text{glucose})/18 + (\text{BUN})/2.8$$

Osmotic fragility:

$$\% \text{ Hemolysis} = \frac{\text{Absorbance}_{(test)} - \text{Absorbance}_{(0.85\% \text{ tube})}}{\text{Absorbance}_{(0.00\% \text{ tube})} - \text{Absorbance}_{(0.085\% \text{ tube})}} \times 100$$

Percent volume/volume: The percent volume/volume of a solution is calculated by dividing the number of milliliters of a solute by 100 mL of solution.

Percent weight/volume: The percent weight/volume of a solution is calculated by dividing the grams of solute by 100 mL of solution.

Percent weight/weight: The percent weight/weight of a solution is calculated by dividing the grams of solute by 100 g of solution.

Polymerase chain reaction (PCR): A method to increase (or amplify) an amount of DNA so that it can be measured or studied.

Positive number: A number with a value greater than zero.

Product: The answer to a multiplication problem.

Proficiency testing SDI: When a proficiency testing result is sent to the proficiency testing vendor, the result is compared to the results obtained by all other subscribers with the same method and instrumentation. The standard deviation index (SDI) is calculated for each analyte and method. A laboratory must fall within an acceptable range of the SDI for each analyte, to get a score of satisfactory for the proficiency testing for that analyte. The formula for the SDI is:

$$SDI = \frac{\text{Result from Lab} - \text{Peer Group Result}}{\text{Standard Deviation of Peer Group}}$$

qs: *Quantum satis* or quantity sufficient. This term refers to the addition of a solvent to the calibration mark of a volumetric pipette or flask.

Quotient: The answer to a division problem.

Ratio: The relationship of one number to another number.

Recovery experiment calculations: Used to determine if there is a proportional systematic error in a method:

$$\text{Spiked Value} - \text{control value} = \text{recovered concentration}$$

$$\text{Percent recovery} = (\text{Concentration recovered divided by the concentration added}) \times 100$$

The acceptable recovery $= 95\%$

Red blood cell indices: Mean corpuscular volume; a calculation of the size of the RBCs:

MCV (fL)
$$= (\text{Hematocrit } (\%) \times 10)/\text{RBC count} (10^{12}/L)$$

Mean corpuscular hemoglobin: a calculation of the hemoglobin concentration in the RBCs:

$$\text{MCH (picograms)} = \frac{\text{Hemoglobin } (g/dL) \times 10}{\text{RBC count } (10^{12}/L)}$$

Mean corpuscular hemoglobin concentration: a ratio of the hemoglobin to the hematocrit:

$$\text{MCHC} = \frac{\text{Hemoglobin } (g/dL) \times 100}{\text{Hematocrit } (\%)}$$

Red cell distribution width: A measurement of the degree of anisocytosis present in a blood specimen:

$$\text{RDW } (\%) = \frac{\text{Standard deviation of MCV}}{\text{Mean MCV}} \times 100$$

Refractometer correction for 1.0 g/dL or higher of glucose in urine: For each 1.0 g/dL of glucose add 0.004 to the specific gravity reading.

Refractometer correction for 1.0 g/dL or higher of protein in urine: For each 1.0 g/dL of protein add 0.003 to the specific gravity measurement.

Renal clearance test: The formula for renal clearance tests is UV/P, where U is the urine concentration of the analyte being measured in mg/dL, V is the volume of urine in milliliters per minute, and P is the plasma concentration of the analyte. The most common analyte used for clearance tests is creatinine.

Reticulocyte correction for increased reticulocyte production:

Reticulocyte production index (RPI)
$$= \frac{\text{Reticulocyte count} \times \text{reticulocyte index}}{\text{Maturation factor (from Table 8-5)}}$$

Reticulocyte count: Slide method:

$$\% \text{ reticulocytes} = \frac{\text{No. of reticulocytes counted per 1000 RBCs}}{1000} \times 100$$

Miller disk method:

$$\% \text{ reticulocytes} = \frac{\text{No. of reticulocytes in squares Nos.1 and 2}}{(\text{No. RBCs in square No. 2}) \times 9} \times 100$$

Rule of three: The hemoglobin times 3 should equal the hematocrit, and the hemoglobin divided by 3 should equal the red blood cell count.

Scientific notation: A way to simplify the calculation. A number is written in such a way that it is larger than 1 but less than 10 and in integral power of 10 (e.g., 3400 can be written as 3.4×10^3). The number 3.4 is called the **mantissa number**.

Shift: A term that describes when quality control results are all distributed on one side of the mean or the other for 5 to 7 consecutive days.

Significant figure: A method to determine the exactness of a value.

Solution: A mixture of a **solute** and a **solvent**. A solute may be a dry solid or a liquid and it is placed into the solvent to form the solution.

Specific gravity of a chemical: The ratio of the density of the chemical in terms of gram per milliliter compared with pure water at $4°C$.

ssDNA: Single-stranded DNA, used for DNA replication procedures.

Standard deviation: The square root of the variance.

Probabilities associated with standard deviations (SD) and quality control material:

+/− 1 SD = 68.2%, which means that statistically 68.2% of the time a quality control value will fall within +/− 1 SD from the mean control value.

+/− 2 SD = 95.5%, which means that statistically 99.5% of the time a quality control value will fall within +/− 2 SD from the mean control value.

+/− 3 SD = 99.7%, which means that statistically 99.7% of the time a quality control value will fall within +/− 3 SD from the mean control value.

Standard error of the estimate (SEE):

$$SEE = \frac{\sqrt{\sum (y_m - y_c)^2}}{n - 2}$$

where:

y_m = the measured value of y
y_c = the calculated value of y obtained from the regression formula

STET buffer: A common buffer in the molecular biology lab; it contains 100 mM sodium chloride, 10 mM tris-HCl, 1 mM EDTA, and 5% triton X-100, and has a pH of 8.0.

Strong acids: Acids that will completely dissociate when in solution.

Strong bases: Bases that will completely dissociate when in solution.

Student's _t_-test: Used to determine if there is a statistically significant difference between two sets of data:

$$\text{Paired } t\text{-test} = \frac{\dfrac{\sum (\bar{X}_1 - \bar{X}_2)}{n}}{\sqrt{\dfrac{\sum d^2 - \left[\sum (\bar{X}_1 - \bar{X}_2)\right]^2 \div n}{n - 1}}} \div \sqrt{n}$$

Sum: The answer to the addition of a group of numbers.

Système Internationale: Also known as the International System of Units, this measurement system, developed in 1960 and then revised in 1971, further standardized measurements. The standard unit of length is meter, concentration is mole, and mass is kilogram.

TE buffer: A common buffer in the molecular biology lab; it contains a combination of tris buffer and EDTA.

Terms that describe central tendency: Mean: The average of a set of numbers. Median: The middle number in a ranked set of numbers. Mode: The number that occurs the most frequency.

Titer: The inverse of a dilution used in which a reaction occurred when testing antigen-antibody interactions.

To convert from mg/dL to picomoles/mcL:

where: n = number of nucleotides
X = micrograms per mL of substance (dsDNA, ssDNA, RNA, or nucleotides)

$$\frac{X \text{ mcg Substance}}{mL} \times \frac{pmol}{\text{base pair weight of substance in pg}} \times \frac{1mL}{1000 \text{ mcL}} \times \frac{10^6 \text{ pg}}{1 \text{ mcg}} \times \frac{1}{n} = X \text{ pmol/mcL Substance}$$

To convert from picomoles/mcL to mcg/mL:

where: N = number of nucleotides
X = number of picomoles/mcL of substance (dsDNA, ssDNA, RNA, or nucleotide)

$$\frac{X \text{ pmol Substance}}{mcL} \times \frac{\text{base pair weight of substance in pg}}{pmol} \times \frac{1000 \text{ mcL}}{1 \text{ mL}} \times \frac{1 \text{ mcg}}{10^6 \text{ pg}} \times n = X \text{ mcg/mL Substance}$$

Trend: A term that describes when quality control results either increase or decrease consistently over a period of 5 to 7 days.

Tris buffer: A common buffer in the molecular biology lab. Its chemical formula is tris(hydroxymethyl)aminomethane.

US Customary System of Measurement: Based on Old English methods of measurements. This system uses a variety of terms to describe measurements, such as *inches* and *yards* for length; *teaspoons, tablespoon, cups,* and *pecks* for liquid or dry measurements; and *ounces* and *pounds* for measurements of mass.

Variance: An indication of the precision of a set of numbers. The variance formula is:

$$s^2 = \frac{\sum (X_d - \overline{X})^2}{n - 1}$$

where:

s^2 = variance
Σ = the sum of the numbers within the parentheses
X_d = an individual data point within the group
$\overline{X}$ = the mean of the group of numbers
n = the total amount of numbers within the group

Westgard multirules: A set of quality control (QC) rules that help the laboratory personnel decide when a QC value is "in control" or "out of control."

1_{2S}: A warning rule where one of two QC values fall outside of the plus 2 or minus 2 SD value. It is indicative of random error.

1_{3S}: A rule that results in rejection of the QC results if one or more of the two QC values fall outside of plus or minus 3 SD values. It is indicative of random error.

2_{2S}: A rule that can be violated in two ways. The first is if two different levels of control that are analyzed in the same run are outside of 2 SD in the same direction. The second way is if there are two 1_{2S} rule violations in a row over two different runs for one level of control. This rule is indicative of systematic error.

R_{4S}: A rule that is broken when the difference or range between two control values within a run is greater than 4 SD. It is indicative of a random error.

4_{1S}: The 4_{1S} rule can be violated in two ways. The first is when four values in a row of the same level of control all fall on the same side of the mean. The other way is when two levels of control are used in a run and each has had two values in a row fall on the same side of the mean. This rule is indicative of a systematic error.

10_x: The 10_x rule can be violated in two ways. The first is when 10 consecutive runs for one level of control all fall on the same side of the mean. The other way is when the results are all on the same side of the mean for both levels of control for 5 days. This rule is indicative of systematic error.

Zero-order reactions: Used in enzyme measurements. The rate of the reaction is directly proportional to the concentration of the enzyme that is being measured and independent of the substrate (or reagent) concentration. The substrate concentration is kept in excess and the rate-limiting step is the concentration of the enzyme that is being measured.

Answer Key for In-Text Revised Practice Problems

1. 0.743
2. 17.3
3. 5.69
4. 5.89
5. 5.56
6. 7.74
7. 2.32
8. 5
9. 4
10. 6
11. 2
12. 5
13. 5
14. 68.1
15. 58.5
16. −12
17. −68.1
18. −7
19. −9
20. 6
21. 9
22. 32
23. 183.73
24. 0.063
25. 25
26. −7
27. −4
28. −6
29. −33
30. −3
31. 0.94
32. 23.8
33. 82
34. 46.6
35. −15
36. −2.5
37. 2.73
38. 5
39. 7.57
40. 1.3
41. 6.2
42. 32.7
43. $^3/_4$
44. $^1/_5$
45. $^1/_2$
46. $^1/_3$
47. $^1/_{18}$
48. $^4/_7$
49. $^{39}/_{40}$
50. $^7/_8$
51. $^7/_{40}$
52. $^3/_{14}$
53. $1^1/_2$
54. $2^1/_2$

Answers to Chapter 2 Practice Problems
1. 6.8354×10^3
2. 8.14×10^2
3. 7.0000×10^3
4. 3.519×10^{-1}
5. 8.54×10^{-2}
6. 7.53×10^{-4}
7. 3.58×10^{-6}
8. 2.10×10^6. Using the rule (Rule 3) for multiplication with exponents, $[(b \times 10^a)(c \times 10^d)] = (bc)^{a+d}$, and substituting into it the numbers from the problem, the

following equation is derived:
$[(3.26)(6.44)]^{3+2} = 2.10 \times 10^6$.

9. 9.12×10^5

10. 4.89×10^{-1}. Using the rule (Rule 3) for multiplication with exponents, the following equation is derived: $[(7.91)(6.18)]^{-3+1}$, which equals 48.9×10^{-2}. 48.9×10^{-2} can be expressed as 4.89×10^{-1}. This can be verified by solving the problem without using scientific notation. $7.91 \times 10^{-3} = 0.00791$ and $6.18 \times 10^1 = 61.8$. Multiplying 0.00791×61.8 yields 0.488 or 4.89×10^{-1}.

11. 5.93×10^{-5}

12. 3.2×10^7. Using the rule (Rule 4) for multiplying a number in scientific notation by an exponent, the following equation is derived: $[(5.5)(5.5)]^{(3)(2)}$, which equals 32.5×10^6. This equation can also be expressed as 3.2×10^7.

13. 2.2×10^{19}

14. 1.1×10^{-3}. This equation initially was 10.9×10^{-4}.

15. 4.7×10^{-7}

16. 2.3×10^2. Using the division rule (Rule 5), the following equation is derived:

$$\frac{8.1 \times 10^4}{3.5 \times 10^2} = \frac{8.1 \times 10^{4-2}}{3.5} = 2.3 \times 10^2$$

17. 4.9 or 0.49×10^1

18. 3.246

19. 4.4×10^{-2}

20. 5.92×10^2

21. 3.6×10^{-2}

22. 3.5×10^3

23. -5.6×10^{-2}

24. 0.9365

25. 0.6742

26. -0.4672

27. -2.070

28. 3.7168. This is calculated by using the rules of multiplication with logarithms. Log $5.21 \times 10^3 = \log 5.21 + \log 10^3$. The log of 5.21 is 0.7168, while the log of $10^3 = 3$. Therefore log $5.21 \times 10^3 = 0.7168 + 3$, which equals 3.7168.

29. -1.3264

30. 0.1533. Using the rule (Rule 9) for division with logarithms, the following equation was derived: log $6.42 - \log 4.51 = 0.80753 - 0.6542 = 0.1533$.

31. 1.339

32. 1.5198

33. 2.3415

34. 1.8802

35. 1.3900

Answers to Chapter 3 Practice Problems

1. 55.5×10^{-6} g OR 5.55×10^{-5} g

2. 3500.0 mg

3. 5.0 deciliters

4. 5×10^5 mcL

5. 500 mcL or 5.0×10^2 mcL

6. 2.5 dL

7. 2.5×10^{-2} L

8. 2.5×10^3 mL

9. 7 cm

10. 4000 meters

11. 20 dL

12. 20×10^{-6} or 2.0×10^{-5}

13. 63.8 g

14. 1.83 meters

15. 709.8 mL

16. 7.6 L

17. 250 mg/L

18. 0.5 mg/dL

19. 1850 mg/dL

20. 1.5 g/L

21. 1.8 g/L

22. The answer is 1000 mm^2. As 1 mm is 10 times smaller than 1 cm, a square millimeter is 10×10 or 100 times smaller than a square centimeter. As there were 10 squared centimeters, 100 is multiplied by 10.

23. The SI value of a 4.0 mg/dL magnesium value is 1.7 mmol/L. By tradition we report mmol/L values to the nearest $^1/_{10}$.

24. The SI value for a 130 mg/dL glucose value is 7.2 mmol/L.

25. 177.6 mg/dL

26. 235.4 mg/dL

27. 42.8 mmol/L

28. 12.1 mmol/L

29. $53.6°F$

30. $23.0°F$

31. $96.1°C$

32. $-27.8°C$

Answers to Chapter 4 Practice Problems

1. A 20 mcL sample added to 80 mcL diluent is a $\frac{1}{5}$ dilution, or a dilution factor of 5. This is because the sample volume of 20 mcL is diluted into a total volume of 100 mL.
2. A $\frac{1}{20}$ dilution, or a dilution factor of 20.
3. A $\frac{1}{5}$ dilution, or a dilution factor of 5.
4. Also a $\frac{1}{6}$ dilution, or a dilution factor of 6.
5. A $\frac{1}{10}$ dilution, or a dilution factor of 10.
6. A $\frac{1}{20}$ dilution, or a dilution factor of 20.
7. A $\frac{1}{4}$ dilution, or a dilution factor of 4.
8. The ratio is 1:19 while the dilution is $\frac{1}{20}$.
9. The ratio is 1:6 while the dilution is $\frac{1}{7}$.
10. The ratio is 1:39 while the dilution is $\frac{1}{40}$.
11. The true value of the analyte is 600 mg/dL.
12. The true value of the analyte is 560 mg/dL.
13. The final dilution is 1/256. The dilution made was $\frac{1}{4} \times \frac{1}{4} \times \frac{1}{4} \times \frac{1}{4} = \frac{1}{256}$.
14. The final dilution factor is 256.
15. The dilution factor for tube 3 is $\frac{1}{4} \times \frac{1}{4} \times \frac{1}{4} = 64$. As the original concentration was 100, then 100 divided by 64 or 1.56 is the concentration of tube 3.
16. The dilution factor for tube 2 is 16.
17. The final dilution is $\frac{1}{3125}$.
18. The final dilution factor is 3125.
19. The concentration in tube 4 is 0.08.
20. The dilution factor for tube 3 is 125.
21. The dilution in which the last positive reaction occurred was the $\frac{1}{64}$ dilution. Therefore the patient's measles antibody titer is 64.
22. In the first well, the serum is diluted $\frac{1}{3}$, in the second well $\frac{1}{9}$, the third well $\frac{1}{27}$, the fourth well $\frac{1}{108}$, the fifth well $\frac{1}{432}$, and in the sixth well the dilution is $\frac{1}{1728}$.

Answers to Chapter 5 Practice Problems

1. The molecular weight of a molecule is the combined atomic weights of the atoms that comprise the molecule. The atomic weight of K is 39.10, O is 16.00, and H is 1.01. Therefore the molecular weight of KOH = $39.10 + 16.00 + 1.01 = 56.11$.
2. 120.4 g molecular weight

3. 96.99 g molecular weight
4. 133.3 g molecular weight
5. 99.09 g molecular weight
6. 159.61 g molecular weight
7. 74.7 g molecular weight
8. The molarity formula is M = mol/L. Using the formula XM = 3.50 mol NaCl/L, molarity = 3.50.
9. The molarity is 1.88 mol/L. The molarity formula is based on a liter quantity. When the solution quantities are different than 1 L, the quantity must be converted to liter terms. Using the molarity formula:

$$(X)M = 1.50 \text{ mol}/0.800 \text{ L}$$
$$(X)M = 1.88$$

Molarity = 1.88 mol/L

10. The molarity is 2.12 mol/L. In this problem the amount of moles must first be established. The molecular weight of NaOH is 40.00. Using the molarity formula and substituting into it the data from the problem:

$$(X)M = \frac{\left(\dfrac{85.0 \text{ g NaOH}}{40.00 \text{ gmw NaOH}} \right)}{1.00 \text{ liter of solution}}$$

Solving for X:

$$XM = \frac{2.12 \text{ moles}}{1.00 \text{ liter of solution}}$$

Molarity = 2.12 moles/L

11. 0.15 Molar (Be careful to use 0.500 L in your calculation.)
12. This problem is asking for the amount of grams of KCl needed to make the solution. The gram molecular weight of KCl is 74.55. Using the molarity formula and substituting into it the data from the problem:

$$0.750M = \frac{\left(\dfrac{X \text{ gKCl}}{74.55 \text{ g molecular weight KCl}} \right)}{0.200L}$$

Solving the equation:

$$(0.750)(0.200) = \frac{Xg}{74.55 \text{ gmw}}$$

$$0.150 = \frac{Xg}{74.55 \text{ gmw}}$$

$$(0.150)(74.55) = X \text{ gram}$$

$$11.2 \text{ gram} = X$$

Therefore 11.2 g of KCl are weighed and qs to 200 mL with solvent.

13. 1.75 g of NaCl are weighed and qs to 75.0 mL with solvent.

14. 24.07 g of $MgSO_4$ are weighed and qs to 500 mL with solvent.

15. 111.8 g of KCl are weighed and qs to 600 mL with solvent.

16. 7.292 g of HCl are weighed and qs to 500 mL with solvent.

17. 4.800 g NaOH are weighed and qs to 100 mL with solvent.

18. The gram equivalent weight is 36.46, the same as the gram molecular weight.

19. The gram equivalent weight is 40.00, the same as the gram molecular weight.

20. The gram equivalent weight is 44.44 because the gram molecular weight is divided by the valence of 3.

21. The gram equivalent weight is 33.03.

22. The gram equivalent weight is 55.49.

23. 0.133 normal

24. 0.499 normal

25. 11.30 normal

26. 0.326 normal

27. 1.37 normal

28. 5.50 N HCl

29. 5.00 N H_2SO_4

30. 5.250 N H_3PO_4

31. 1.7 N $CaCl_2$

32. 2.5 N NaOH

33. 1.5 N KOH

34. 3.50 M NaOH

35. 0.01 M $MgSO_4^{+2}$

36. 1.50 M H_2SO_4

37. 0.15 M HCL

38. 0.833 M K_3PO_4

39. The molality formula is similar to the molarity formula except that molality is based on kilogram quantity, not liter quantity. The molecular weight of NaCl is 58.44; therefore, using the molality formula:

$$X \text{ Molal} = \frac{\left(\dfrac{75.0 \text{ g NaCl}}{58.44 \text{ g molecular weight}}\right)}{1.00 \text{ kg solvent}}$$

$$(X \text{ Molal})(1.00) = \frac{75.0}{58.44}$$

$$X \text{ Molal} = 1.28$$

Therefore the solution has a molality of 1.28 mol/kg.

40. 0.469 mol/kg

41. 167.7 g KCl

42. 4.99 mEq/L. To convert mg/dL to mEq/L, convert mg/dL to g/L, then solve for normality.

$$10.0 \text{ mg/dL} = 0.100 \text{ g/L}$$

$$Eq/L = \frac{\left(\dfrac{0.100g}{\dfrac{40.08 \text{ g molecular weight}}{2(\text{valence})}}\right)}{1.00 \text{ liter of solution}}$$

$$Eq/L = \frac{\dfrac{0.10}{20.04}}{1.00 \text{ liter}}$$

$$Eq/L = 0.00499 \text{ Eq/L} = 4.99 \text{ mEq/L}$$

43. 3.29 mEq/L

44. 333 mg/dL

45. 408 mg/dL

46. 135 mmol/L

47. 4.00 mmol/L

48. The molecular weight of glucose is 180.16; 500 mg/dL is equal to 5000 mg/L. Using the molarity formula:

$$mM = \frac{\left(\dfrac{5000mg}{180.16 \text{ g molecular weight}}\right)}{1.00 \text{ liter of solution}}$$

$$mM = 27.75$$

The 500 mg/dL glucose standard is equal to 27.75 mmol/L glucose.

49. 135.1 mg/dL

50. The gram molecular weight of creatinine is 113.12. Using the formula in practice problem 48, the answer is 1.06 mmol/L.

51. 12.0 g of NaCl are present in a 12.0%$^{w/w}$ solution. If water is the solvent, then the 12.0 g of NaCl are added to 88 g of water.

52. There are 10.0 mL of HCl in 90.0 mL water to make a final 10.0%$^{v/v}$ HCl solution.

53. 15.0 g of NaOH are present in 100 mL of a 15.0%$^{w/v}$ solution of NaOH.

54. There are 20.0 g of KCl/100 mL of solution. Using ratio and proportion, the amount present in 10.0 mL is as follows:

$$\frac{20.0 \text{ g KCl}}{100 \text{ mL solution}} = \frac{X \text{ g KCl}}{10.0 \text{ mL solution}}$$

$$(20.0)(10.0) = (100)(X)$$

$$200.0 = (100)(X)$$

$$2.00 = X$$

Therefore, there are 2.00 g of KCl in 10.0 mL of a 20.0% $^{w/v}$ solution of KCl.

55. There are 35 g of HCl/100 mL of solution. Using ratio and proportion, the amount present in 50.0 mL can be determined to be 17.5 g.

56. In a 15.0%$^{w/v}$ solution, there are 15.0 g/100 mL. To determine the amount of grams per 1.00 L, use ratio and proportion:

$$\frac{15.0 \text{ g}}{100 \text{ mL}} = \frac{X \text{ g}}{1000 \text{ mL}}$$

Crossmultiplying the equation yields the following:

$$(15.0)(1000) = (100)(X)$$

$$15,000 = (100)(X)$$

$$150g = X$$

This solution contains 150 g KCl/1.00 L. Next use the molarity formula to determine the molarity of the solution:

$$X \text{ Molar} = \frac{\left(\dfrac{150 \text{ g KCl}}{74.55 \text{ g}}\right)}{1.00 \text{ liter of solution}}$$

$$X \text{ Molar} = 2.01 \text{ Molar}$$

Therefore a 15.0%$^{w/v}$ KCl solution has a molarity of 2.01.

57. 0.69 Molar

58. 2.70 Molar

59. Using the ratio and proportion formula for concentrations, the following equation is derived:

$$(75.0)(X) = (25.0)(500.0)$$

$$(75.0)(X) = 12500.0$$

$$(X) = 166.67 \text{ or } 167$$

Therefore 167 mL of stock ETOH is measured out and qs'd to 500 mL using deionized water to prepare 500 mL of a 25.0%$^{v/v}$ EtOH solution.

60. 4.500%$^{w/v}$ tris buffer solution

61. 60.00 mL of stock 25% $^{v/v}$ acetic acid is required.

Answers to Chapter 6 Practice Problems

1. Using the formula A = 2−log % T, the % T concentration can be converted into absorbance:

$$A = 2.0 - \log\%T$$

$$X = 2.0 - \log 25\%$$

$$X = 2.0 - 1.3979$$

$$X = 0.602$$

2. 0.131

3. 0.495

4. To convert from absorbance values to % T values, the same formula is used:

$$A = 2.0 - \log\%T$$

$$0.188 = 2.0 - \log\%T$$

$$-1.812 = -\log\%T$$

Removing the negative signs from both sides of the equation yields the following:

$$1.812 = \log\%T$$

$$\%T = \text{antilog } 1.812$$

$$\%T = 64.86$$

5. The % T value is calculated in the same manner as in problem 4. The absorbance of 1.625 is equal to a % T of 2.37.

6. 18.6% T

7. Using the Beer's law formula A = abc, the concentration of the substance is 2.78×10^{-5} M.

8. The LDH concentration is 125 IU/L.

9. The pH of a buffer is determined by the Henderson-Hasselbalch equation:

$$pH = pK_a + \log\left(\frac{[A^-]}{[HA]}\right)$$

$$pH = 3.6 + \log\left(\frac{0.50M}{0.80M}\right)$$

$$pH = 3.6 + [(\log 0.50) - (\log 0.80)]$$

$$pH = 3.6 + -0.204$$

$$pH = 3.39$$

10. Using the Henderson-Hasselbalch formula, the pH of blood can be determined:

$$pH = 6.1 + \log\left(\frac{\text{Bicarbonate}}{\text{Carbonic acid}}\right)$$

The majority of carbonic acid in the blood is in the form of dissolved carbon dioxide (dCO_2). Rather than measure the concentration of dCO_2, the dCO_2 can be calculated by multiplying the pCO_2 by its solubility coefficient of 0.0306 mmol/L/mm Hg. Therefore:

$$pH = 6.1 + \log\left(\frac{31.0\text{ mmol/L}}{(0.0306\text{ mmol/L/mmHg})}\right)$$

$$(45\text{mmHg})$$

$$pH = 6.1 + \log\left(\frac{31.0\text{ mmol/L}}{1.38\text{ mmol/L}}\right)$$

$$pH = 6.1 + \log 22.5$$

$$pH = 6.1 + 1.35$$

$$pH = 7.45$$

11. 25.6 mmol/L

12. Uncompensated respiratory acidosis

13. Compensated metabolic acidosis

14. Uncompensated metabolic alkalosis

15. The anion gap is calculated by subtracting the concentrations of chloride and bicarbonate from the sodium concentration. Some laboratories include the potassium concentration as part of the included cations that are measured. The anion gap for this problem is 2 mmol/L.

16. The serum osmolality is calculated by the following formula:

Calculated osmolality (mOsmol/kg H_2O)

$$= 1.86[NA^+] + \frac{[\text{glucose}]}{18} + \frac{[\text{BUN}]}{2.8}$$

Calculated osmolality (mOsmol/kg H_2O)

$$= (1.86)(147) + \frac{410}{18} + \frac{20}{2.8}$$

Calculated osmolality (mOsmol/kg H_2O)

$$= 273.4 + 22.78 + 7.1$$

Calculated osmolality (mOsmol/kg H_2O)
$$= 303$$

17. The osmolal gap is the difference between the measured osmolality and calculated osmolality. The calculated osmolality for this problem is 287 mOsm/kg and the measured osmolality is 290 mOsm/kg. Therefore the osmolal gap = 290 − 287 = 3 mOsm/kg.

18. The concentration of LDL cholesterol can be calculated with the following formula:

LDL cholesterol

$$= \text{Total cholesterol} - \left[\text{HDL chol.} + \left(\frac{\text{Trig}}{5}\right)\right]$$

LDL cholesterol

$$= 255\text{ mg/dL} - \left[30\text{ mg/dL} + \left(\frac{250}{5}\right)\right]$$

LDL cholesterol = 255 mg/dL − 80 mg/dL

LDL cholesterol = 175 mg/dL

Answers to Chapter 7 Practice Problems

1. For every g/dL of protein, the specific gravity is falsely elevated by 0.003. As there are 2 g/dL of protein in this sample, the effect is a false elevation of 0.006. Therefore the correct specific gravity is 1.014.

2. The corrected specific gravity is 1.023.
3. For every g/dL of glucose, the specific gravity is falsely elevated by 0.004. Since the urine contains 4 g/dL of glucose, the specific gravity is falsely elevated by 0.016. Therefore the correct specific gravity is 1.026.
4. The corrected specific gravity is 1.019.
5. The amount of urine in terms of mL/min is equal to 2400 mL/1440 min or 1.67 mL/min. Using the clearance formula:

$$\text{Clearance} = \frac{(180 \text{ mg/dL})(1.67 \text{ mL/min})}{1.7 \text{ mg/dL}}$$

$$\text{Clearance} = 176.5 \text{ mL/min}$$

6. The corrected clearance is calculated by accounting for the patient's body size. From Fig. 7-2, the patient's body size is 2.08 m^2. As the clearance test is based on a body surface area of 1.73 m^2, the calculated clearance is multiplied by the product of 1.73 divided by 2.08:

$$\text{Corrected clearance} = 176.5 \text{ mL/min} \times \frac{1.73 \text{ m}^2}{2.08 \text{ m}^2}$$

$$\text{Corrected clearance} = 176.5 \text{ mL/min} \times 0.832$$

$$\text{Corrected clearance} = 146.6 \text{ mL/min}$$

7. The rate of urine production of mL per minute is calculated to be 1.15 mL/min. Using the clearance formula:

$$\text{Clearance} = \frac{(150 \text{ mg/dL})(1.15 \text{ mL/min})}{2.5 \text{ mg/dL}}$$

$$\text{Clearance} = 69.0 \text{ mL/min}$$

8. The corrected clearance is calculated by adjusting for the patient's body surface area. From the nomogram in Fig. 7-2, the patient's surface area is 1.48 m^2. Therefore the corrected clearance is as follows:

$$\text{Corrected clearance} = 69 \text{ mL/min} \times \frac{1.73 \text{ m}^2}{1.48 \text{ m}^2}$$

$$\text{Corrected clearance} = 69 \times 1.17$$

$$\text{Corrected clearance} = 81 \text{ mL/min}$$

Answers to Chapter 8 Practice Problems

1. The MCV (fL) is calculated from the following formula:

$$\text{MCV (fL)} = \frac{\text{Hct} \times 10}{\text{RBC count}}$$

Substituting into the formula the data from the problem yields the following:

$$\text{MCV (fL)} = \frac{40.0 \times 10}{4.4}$$

$$\text{MCV (fL)} = 90.9 \text{ fL}$$

2. MCV = 90.4 fL
3. MCV = 89.3 fL
4. The formula for MCH is as follows:

$$\text{MCH (pg)} = \frac{\text{Hemoglobin (g/dL)} \times 10}{\text{RBC count(millions per mcL)}}$$

Substituting into the formula the data from the problem yields the following:

$$\text{MCH (pg)} = \frac{6.0 \text{ g/dL} \times 10}{4.1 \text{ (millions per mcL)}}$$

$$\text{MCH (pg)} = 14.6 \text{ pg}$$

5. MCH = 29.4 pg
6. MCH = 33.3 pg
7. The mean corpuscular hemoglobin concentration (MCHC) is calculated by the following formula:

$$\text{MCHC g / dL} = \frac{\text{Hb(g/dL)} \times 100}{\text{Hematocrit(\%)}}$$

Substituting into the formula the data from the problem yields the following:

$$\text{MCHC g/dL} = \frac{11 \text{ (g/dL)} \times 100}{33(\%)}$$

$$\text{MCHC g/dL} = 33.3 \text{ g/dL}$$

8. MCHC = 33.3 g/dL
9. MCHC = 33.3 g/dL

10. The factor method for counting WBCs uses the following formula:
Factor = 1/area × depth factor × dilution factor
Area counted = number of large squares counted
Depth factor = reciprocal of depth [1/(1/10)] = 10
Dilution factor = reciprocal of dilution = [1/(1/20)] = 20
Therefore the factor =

$$\frac{1}{4} \times 10 \times 20 = 50$$

Multiply the number of WBCs counted by the factor to determine the WBC count/mm³: 40 × 50 = 2000/mm³

11. WBC count = 7400/mm³
12. WBC count = 4500/mm³
13. Platelet count = 380,000/mm³
14. Platelet count = 63,000/mm³
15. Platelet count = 180,000/mm³
16. WBC count = 1625/mm³. This is calculated using the formula:

$$\text{No. cells / mm}^3 = \frac{\text{No. cells counted} \times \text{depth factor} \times \text{dilution factor}}{\text{area counted}}$$

In this problem, 65 cells were counted. The depth factor is 10, the dilution factor is 10, and the area counted is 4.

17. 3375 WBC/mm³
18. 46,500 platelets/mm³
19. 952 WBC/mcL and 610 RBC/mcL
20. 36,353 WBC/mcL and 16,606 RBC/mcL
21. 88 million per mL and 2.9 × 10⁸ sperm count per ejaculate
22. 134 million per mL and 3.7 × 10⁸ sperm count per ejaculate
23. The formula to calculate reticulocytes is as follows:

$$\frac{\text{Number of reticulocytes counted per 1000 erythrocytes}}{1000} \times 100$$

Using the formula and substituting into the data from the problem:

$$\frac{52}{1000} \times 100 = 5.2\% \text{ reticulocyte count}$$

24. 1.5% reticulocyte count
25. The formula to calculate the quantity of reticulocytes using the Miller disk is as follows:

$$\frac{\text{No. reticulocytes in small and large squares}}{(\text{No. RBCs in square 2})(9)} \times 100$$

Substituting into the equation the data from the problem:

$$\frac{48 \text{ reticulocytes}}{(254 \text{ RBCs})(9)} \times 100 = 2.1\% \text{ reticulocyte count}$$

26. 1.4% reticulocyte count
27. The reticulocyte index corrects the reticulocyte count by the following formula:

Corrected reticulocyte count
$$= (\text{Patient's reticulocyte count})\frac{(\text{Patient's Hct})}{45}$$

Substituting into the equation the data from the problem:

$$\text{Corrected reticulocyte count} = (5.9\%)\frac{28}{45}$$

Corrected reticulocyte count = 1.8%

28. Corrected reticulocyte percentage of 1.7%
29. To correct the reticulocyte count when there is an increased production use the following formula:

$$\text{RPI} = \frac{(\text{Reticulocyte count})(\text{Reticulocyte index})}{\text{Maturation factor (from Table 8-4)}}$$

Substituting into the equation the data from the problem:

$$\text{RPI} = \frac{(4.6\%)(25\% \div 45\%)}{\text{Maturation factor}}$$

$$\text{RPI} = \frac{2.55}{\text{Maturation factor of 2.0}}$$

RPI = 1.3%

30. Corrected reticulocyte percentage of 0.3%

Answers to Chapter 9 Practice Problems

1. The hemoglobin concentration should rise to 12 g/dL, as the hemoglobin concentration is expected to rise by 1 g/dL for each unit of packed RBCs in patients who are not actively bleeding.
2. The patient's hemoglobin should increase to 10 g/dL.
3. The patient's hemoglobin should increase to 11 g/dL.
4. The patient's hematocrit should increase to approximately 20% to 23%. Each unit of packed RBCs is expected to increase the hematocrit percentage by two to three percentage points. As the patient received three units, the hematocrit should increase between six and nine percentage points.
5. The patient's hematocrit should increase to approximately 18% to 22%.
6. The patient's hematocrit should increase to approximately 14% to 17%.
7. The clotting factor activity should increase by 38% to 50%. For every two units of fresh frozen plasma the clotting factor activity is expected to increase by 15% to 20%. Since the patient received five units, the increase is 38% to 50%.
8. The increase in clotting factor activity should be between 60% and 80%.
9. The patient's platelet count should rise approximately by 90,000 platelets/mcL. Each unit of platelet concentrate is expected to increase the platelet concentration by 10,000 platelets/mcL. Because nine units were transfused, the total platelet count should rise from 30,000/mcL to 120,000/mcL.
10. The patient's platelet count should rise by approximately 40,000 to 100,000 platelets/mcL because each pheresis pack contains an equivalent amount of platelets as 4 to 10 random platelet concentrate units.
11. Eight vials of RHIG should be given. The calculation results in a value of 6.8. The result is rounded to the nearest whole number (7), and an extra vial is given as a precaution.

12. Four vials of RHIG should be given because the calculation for the amount of vials results in a value of 2.3. This is rounded to 3, and an extra vial is given as a precaution.
13. The probability of finding a unit negative for the Jka+b+ antigen is 50%.
14. The probability of finding a unit negative for both K-k+ and Le a-b- antigen is 1.56%.

Answers to Chapter 10 Practice Problems

1. 175,000 CFUs/mL
2. 272,000 CFUs/mL
3. When the concentration of organism is less than 1000 CFUs/mL, the sample is not indicative of a urinary tract infection and may simply be due to contamination.
4. CFUs greater than 100,000/mL indicate probable infection.
5. Tube 11

Answers to Chapter 11 Practice Problems

1. 3.0×10^7 pg/mL
2. 0.12 pg or 1.2×10^{-1} pg
3. 6.2×10^7 ng
4. 2.8×10^{-3} mg
5. 10 mL of diluent is needed (30 mL of stock solution needed).
6. 71.3 mcg/mL
7. 9.1×10^{-2} pmol/mcL
8. 59.4 mcg/mL

Answers to Chapter 12 Practice Problems

1. 546
2. 544
3. 538
4. 48.8
5. 7.00
6. 1.3%
7. The mean is 328 mg/dL.
8. The median glucose value is 328.5 or the average of 328 and 329 mg/dL.
9. The modal value is 330 mg/dL. Notice that this example does not exactly follow a gaussian distribution, as the mean, median, and modal numbers are not all the same.
10. The variance is 23 mg^2/dL^2.

11. The standard deviation is 4.8 mg/dL, or the square root of 23 mg^2/dL^2. Notice that the units for the standard deviation are the same as the units for the data values.

12. The coefficient of variation is 1.5%.

13. There is approximately a 68.2% probability that a control result will fall within +/− 1 SD of the mean.

14. 47.75% probability

15. 99.7% probability

16. 4.5% probability

17. 0.3% probability

18. The plus and minus 2 standard deviation range would encompass all values including and between 65 and 85.

19. The plus or minus 3 standard deviation range for this group of data ranges from 220 to 280.

20. 170

Answers to Chapter 13 Practice Problems

1. A shift can be caused by many things. Some examples are expired reagents or a change in lot numbers of reagents without recalibrating the method.

2. A trend can be caused by changes over time, such as a refrigerator that is losing its ability to keep reagents cold, or by allowing QC material to evaporate over a number of days.

3. The main number of a Westgard rules number informs you of how many QC levels may have violated the rule. For example, using the 1_{2S} rule, the number 1 lets laboratorians know that it is only one level of QC that is affected. The subscript number describes the QC level that has been potentially exceeded, and the letter s refers to standard deviation.

4. Some causes of random error can be a bubble in the sample cup, a loose pipette tip, or an electrical surge. Random errors usually do not occur again once their cause has been discovered and rectified.

5. Some causes of a systematic error are improperly made QC, an instrument that is out of calibration, and dirty optics that interfere with Beer's law methods. The errors

impact the overall system of operation of the analyzer or method.

6. The R_{4S} rule cannot be violated across runs for one level of control.

7. The 4_{1S} rule can be violated by both levels of control if both levels of control exceed +/− 1 SD for two consecutive runs.

8. The 10_x rule can be violated if the results for one level of control consecutively fall on the same side of the mean for 10 values or if results for both levels of control fall on the same side of the mean for five consecutive values.

9. There is a 1_{2S} warning rule violation for level 1 on day 6 and again on days 9 and 10. On day 8 the 1_{3S} rule was violated, and on day 9 for level 1 there is a 2_{2S} rule violation across runs from day 8 1_{3S} warning rule violation. On day 10 there is also another 2_{2S} rule violation.

For level 2, there is a 1_{2S} warning rule violation on day 1, and again on days 3 and 5.

10. There is a 1_{2S} warning rule violation on day 5 for Level 1, and a 2_{2S} rule violation for Level 1 on day 6. For Level 2 control there is a 1_{3S} rule violation on day 4.

Answers to Chapter 14 Practice Problems

1. 99.6%
2. 97.8%
3. 99.5%
4. 99.9%
5. 91.8%
6. No, the calculated F value of 1.56 is below the critical value.
7. 1.33
8. −0.88
9. With the calculation:

$$SEE = \sqrt{\frac{\sum (y_m - y_c)^2}{n - 2}}$$

where:

y_m = the measured value of y

y_c = the calculated value of obtained from the regression formula

10. The correlation coefficient infers if the values of one method are statistically the same as the values of another method. A perfect r value would be 1.000.

Answers to Chapter 15 Practice Problems

1. To solve this problem, use the ratio and proportion formula for anhydrous and hydrated compounds. The formula is as follows:

$$\frac{\text{anhydrous chemical molecular weight}}{\text{hydrated chemical molecular weight}}$$
$$= \frac{\text{gram of anhydrous chemical}}{\text{gram of hydrated chemical}}$$

The molecular weight of NaH_2PO_4 is 119.98, while the molecular weight of $NaH_2PO_4 \cdot 3 H_2O$ is 174.04. Substituting the data into the formula yields the following:

$$\frac{119.98 \text{ gmw}}{174.04 \text{ gmw}} = \frac{15.0 \text{ g}}{\text{X g}}$$

Crossmultiplying yields the following:

$$(119.98)(X) = (174.04)(15.0)$$
$$(119.98)(X) = 2610.60$$
$$X = 21.8$$

Therefore 21.8 g of $NaH_2PO_4 \cdot 3 H_2O$ are dissolved into water and qs to 100 mL.

2. This problem asks for the amount of hydrated $CuSO_4$ needed to prepare 75.0 mL of a 20.0%$^{w/v}$ solution. First determine the amount of copper sulfate that would be present in 75.0 mL versus 100 mL by using ratio and proportion:

$$\frac{20.0 \text{ gram}}{100 \text{ mL}} = \frac{\text{X gram}}{75.0 \text{ mL}}$$
$$(20.0)(75.0) = (100)(X)$$
$$1500.0 = (100)(X)$$
$$15.0 = X$$

Therefore, in 75.0 mL of solution, 15.0 g of copper sulfate is needed. The gram molecular weight of $CuSO_4$ is 159.61. The gram molecular weight of $CuSO_4 \cdot 5 H_2O$ is 249.71 because of the five water molecules. By substituting the data given into the equation, the following equation is derived:

$$\frac{159.61 \text{ gmw } (CuSO_4)}{249.71 \text{ gmw } (CuSO_4 \cdot 5H_2O)}$$
$$= \frac{15.0 \text{ g } (CuSO_4)}{\text{X g hydrated}}$$

Crossmultiplying yields the following:

$$(159.61)(X) = (249.71)(15.0)$$
$$(159.61)(X) = 3745.65$$
$$X = 23.5 \text{ grams}$$

Therefore 23.5 g of $CuSO_4 \cdot 5 H_2O$ are dissolved into 75.0 mL of water.

3. The density of a solution defines how many grams of solvent are in 1.00 mL of solution. A solution with a density of 0.910 contains 0.910 g of ammonium hydroxide in each 1.00 mL of the solution. However, the purity of the solution is 28.0%$^{w/w}$, which means that for every 100 g of the solution, 28 of those grams are ammonium hydroxide. To determine the amount of pure NH_4OH in 1.00 mL of solution, the density of the solution is multiplied by its purity:

$$\left(\frac{0.910 \text{ g}}{1.00 \text{ mL}}\right)\left(\frac{28.0 \text{ g}}{100 \text{ g}}\right) = 0.255 \text{ g per } 1.00 \text{ mL}$$

Therefore in 1.00 mL of concentrated ammonium hydroxide solution there are 0.255 g of ammonium hydroxide.

4. To determine the molarity of a concentrated solution, first determine the amount of solute in 1.00 mL as demonstrated in problem 3:

$$\left(\frac{1.42 \text{ g}}{1.00 \text{ mL}}\right)\left(\frac{70.0 \text{ g}}{100 \text{ g}}\right) = \frac{0.994 \text{ g pure } HNO_3}{1.00 \text{ mL}}$$

Next determine the quantity of pure nitric acid in 1.00 L by ratio and proportion:

$$\frac{0.994 \text{ g}}{1.00 \text{ mL}} = \frac{X \text{ g}}{1000 \text{ mL}}$$

$$X = 994 \text{ g in } 1.00 \text{ liter}$$

Last, use the molarity formula to determine the solution's molarity:

$$X \text{ Molar} = \frac{994.0 \text{ g}}{63.02 \text{ gmw}}$$

$$X \text{ Molar} = 15.8 \text{ M}$$

5. The formula for calculating the concentration of unknowns using a single standard is as follows:

$$\text{Conc of unknown} = \frac{(\text{Abs unknown})}{(\text{Abs standard})}$$

$$\times \text{ Concentration of standard}$$

Substituting the data from the problem into the equation:

Concentration of unknown

$$= \frac{0.681}{1.250} \times 300 \text{ mg/dL}$$

Concentration of unknown $= 163 \text{ mg/dL}$

6. 269 mg/dL
7. Using ratio and proportion, the following equation is derived:

$$\frac{35 \text{ mEq}}{1000 \text{ mL}} = \frac{X \text{ mEq}}{900 \text{ mL}}$$

Crossmultiplying the equation yields the following:

$$(35)(900) = (1000)(X)$$
$$31,500 = 1000X$$
$$32 = X$$

The sodium concentration can be expressed as 32 mEq/900 mL.

8. To solve this problem, first convert the units of deciliters into milliliter units.

$$\frac{50 \text{ mg}}{100 \text{ mL}} = \frac{X \text{ mg}}{1500 \text{ mL}}$$

Crossmultiplying the equation yields the following:

$$(50)(1500) = (100)(X)$$
$$75,000 = 100X$$
$$X = 750 \text{ mg/1500mL}$$

The glucose concentration can be expressed as 750 mg/1500 mL.

9.
$$\frac{525 \text{ mg}}{100 \text{ mL}} = \frac{X \text{ mg}}{1825 \text{ mL}}$$

$$(525)(1825) = (100)(X)$$
$$958,125 = 100X$$
$$X = 9581 \text{ mg or } 9.58\text{g/1825mL}$$

10. 1000 mg/1750 mL is comparable to 1000 mg/24 hours, as the collection period time and volume are interchangeable.
11. 40 mEq/12 hours

Index

Page numbers followed by *"f"* indicate figures, *"t"* indicate tables, and *"b"* indicate boxes.